DENTAL RADIOLOGY

DENTAL RADIOLOGY

ARTHUR H. WUEHRMANN, D.M.D., A.B.

Professor of Dentistry (Retired),
University of Alabama in Birmingham School of Dentistry,
Birmingham, Alabama

LINCOLN R. MANSON-HING, D.M.D., M.S.

Chairman and Professor of Dentistry,
Department of Dental Radiology,
University of Alabama in Birmingham School of Dentistry,
Birmingham, Alabama

FOURTH EDITION

with 404 illustrations

THE C. V. MOSBY COMPANY

Saint Louis   1977

FOURTH EDITION

Copyright © 1977 by The C. V. Mosby Company

Previous editions copyrighted 1965, 1969, 1973

Printed in the United States of America

Distributed in Great Britain by Henry Kimpton, London

The C. V. Mosby Company
11830 Westline Industrial Drive, St. Louis, Missouri 63141

Library of Congress Cataloging in Publication Data

Wuehrmann, Arthur H
 Dental radiology.

 Bibliography: p.
 Includes index.
 1. Teeth—Radiology. 2. Skull—Radiology. I. Manson-Hing, Lincoln R., joint author. II. Title.
RK309.W78 1977 617.6′07′572 76-55692
ISBN 0-8016-5642-7

CB/CB/B 9 8 7 6 5 4 3 2 1

As with prior editions, this text is dedicated to those teachers and investigators whose efforts have contributed to the information compiled in this volume.

Preface

Dental radiology, or roentgenology, is composed of technical and interpretive procedures that interdependently result in useful diagnostic data. Technical procedures depend on a comprehension of morphologic and physical sciences, and interpretation must be correlated with microscopic, clinical laboratory, and clinical findings. Although technic and interpretation continue to form the core of dental radiology, they no longer constitute the entire scope of the science. X-radiation is only one form of radiant energy available to the dental practitioner, the teacher, and the investigator. The scope of dental radiology has broadened within recent years to encompass, at least potentially, many physical and biologic phenomena. With these advances has come a responsibility to protect the health of involved individuals from needless, useless, and wasteful exposure to ionizing radiation of all types. Federal regulations relating to diagnostic x-ray systems and major components are now in effect. Certification of competency for all users of ionizing radiation on human beings is in the offing. The future presents a tremendously stimulating challenge to dentistry and to the dental radiologist.

A single book no longer can cover completely all aspects of this constantly expanding field. The science crosses the lines of many diverse disciplines, and one volume cannot serve as a suitable reference for the student, the general practitioner, and the individual interested in specific, in-depth aspects of the science. It became necessary early in the development of this book to focus on and define its purpose. This book is written for the dental student and for the general practitioner; some of the chapters are applicable to the training of dental auxiliaries. Dental specialists, of course, should be thoroughly conversant with the technical aspects of this text and with the interpretive portions that apply to their specialty. This text is not designed to serve the dental specialist as an in-depth reference. Portions of the text are deliberately superficial; others are rather detailed. For example, Chapter 16 (Diseases of radiographic importance) is restricted to radiographic findings, and often only one illustration is used to depict a disease entity that can have a variety of radiographic appearances. Conversely, Chapter 5 (Intraoral radiographic technics) and Chapter 15

(Common diseases of teeth and supporting structures) are treated in a rather detailed fashion. To fully comprehend the subject of dental radiology, students will need to attend the lectures of their teachers and read the works of other authors, which will supplement most chapters by providing information on some aspects of the field not mentioned in this text.

Several departures from conventional texts will become obvious even on superficial perusal. One requires specific attention. References, except those related to specific quotations, have been deleted for the most part. However, the reader will find a list of suggested readings at the end of the book. This list is arranged in sections comprised of chapters of similar content. There is no desire to avoid giving proper credit, but much of this text is devoted to a compilation of information that through use has become general knowledge. Furthermore, it is our belief that multitudinous references in a text designed for general purposes tend to encumber rather than enhance the text's value.

This book is dedicated with the utmost sincerity to those individuals who through their past efforts have made it a reality. It is difficult, if not impossible, to acknowledge the assistance of all persons who have cooperated in this venture. Prior editions have acknowledged our debt of gratitude. The assistance of Dr. Orlen N. Johnson and his colleagues at the Bureau of Radiological Health, U.S.P.H.S. in revising portions of Chapter 4 for this edition is acknowledged with appreciation. Most important, as our dedication states, we give thanks to and acknowledge those who in the past supplied the information collated in this text. Also, we express our thanks to those unhonored and unsung contributors, our wives.

Arthur H. Wuehrmann

Lincoln R. Manson-Hing

Contents

CHAPTER 1

Fundamentals of radiography

Radiography is the production of a photographic image of an object through the use of x-rays. In dentistry it is used to provide information about underlying oral structures not visible to the eyes. The practice of radiography requires some knowledge of radiation physics and photographic chemistry, and the acquisition of a high degree of skill. Radiography is both a science and an art. In this chapter the fundamentals of radiography are discussed under the following headings: history, x-radiation, fundamental concepts of matter, x-ray machine, generation of x-rays, x-ray beam, absorption of x-rays, x-ray films, and latent image and film processing. Material presented in this chapter is closely interrelated with that in Chapters 2 and 3.

HISTORY

The foundations for the discovery of the x-ray date back as far as the seventeenth century, when the sciences of magnetism and electricity were started with the discovery of magnetism. Experiments with electricity, vacuum tubes, and cathode rays laid the groundwork for the discovery of the x-ray by Wilhelm Conrad Roentgen in November 1895.

As professor of physics at the University of Würzburg, Germany, Roentgen was experimenting with cathode rays when, quite by accident, he noticed the fluorescence of barium platinocyanide crystals that were some distance from his activated Crookes-Hittorf tube. Roentgen immediately recognized the significance of his observation and investigated it thoroughly. Finding that the phenomenon was caused by a previously unknown ray, he called it the x-ray. Roentgen established most of the properties of the x-ray and reported his findings in December 1895, in March 1896, and in May 1897. The diagnostic possibilities were recognized at once by many, and thousands of papers and books were soon published on the practical use of the new rays. Use of the x-rays in dentistry began as early as 1896, when x-ray films were made of the teeth and jaws.

1

X-RADIATION

The exact nature of radiation in general has yet to be proved. Experiments indicate that x-rays behave like waves in some instances and like particles in other instances. X-rays are thought to be made of discrete units of energy called quanta (singular, quantum) or photons that travel with a wave motion. The concept of waves can be obtained by observing the ripples or waves created when the still surface of a pool of water is disturbed. The distance between the crests or troughs of the waves is called the wavelength. The wavelengths of x-rays are so short that they are measured in Angstrom units (Å). An Angstrom unit measures $\frac{1}{100,000,000}$ cm.; x-ray wavelengths used in diagnostic radiography range from about 0.1 to 0.5 Å.

X-rays behave very much like light. This is not surprising; both of these radiations belong to the same family of electromagnetic radiations (Fig. 1-1), in contrast to corpuscular radiations, such as alpha and beta particles, which are composed of particles or bits of matter. X-rays and light affect photographic plates in a similar manner, are not affected by magnetic fields, and travel in straight lines and at the same speed (about 186,000 miles per second). X-rays and light cast shadows of objects in a like manner. The major difference in behavior between these two radiations is the ability of x-rays to penetrate some opaque objects. This property of x-rays is associated with wavelength; the shorter the wavelength, the more penetrating and the more energetic is the x-ray photon. Other interesting properties of x-rays include their ability to produce fluorescence and phosphorescence in over 1,000 substances, their ability to ionize atoms, and the fact that they are invisible.

Since the x-ray is an ionizing and penetrating radiation, it is not surprising that these rays are used in almost all scientific fields. Some uses of these rays are given in Table 1-1. The fact that x-rays are invisible gives rise to the need for special detecting and recording devices. In radiography this device is the photographic, or radiographic, film. Although the exact nature of x-radiation is unknown, much is known about its behavior and effects. This is in no way different

Table 1-1. Some uses of x-radiation

Subject	Use
Radiology	Diagnosis in dentistry and medicine
X-radiation therapy	Treatment of neoplasms
Industrial and art "radiography"	Examination of gross structures (castings, welds, old paintings, etc.)
Spectroscopy	Identification of elements—their atomic numbers and structure
Photochemistry	Ionization of chemicals producing oxidation, reduction, etc.
Radiobiology	Alteration of cells and tissues for experimental purposes
Crystallography	Analysis of molecular structure
Sterilization	Preservation of food

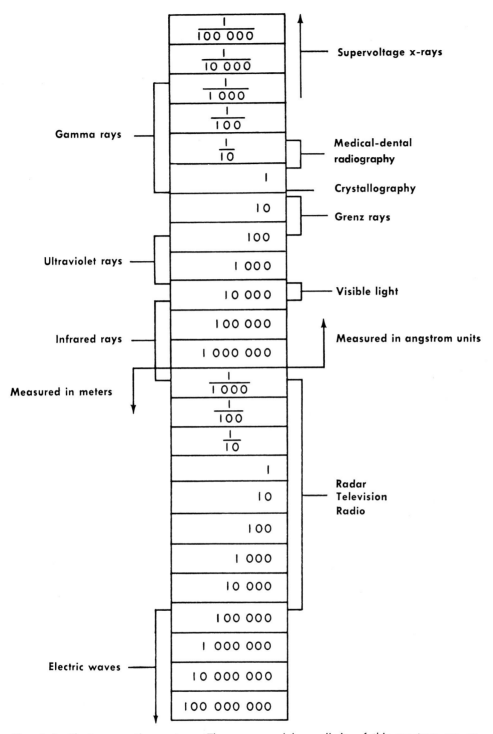

Fig. 1-1. Electromagnetic spectrum. The upper and lower limits of this spectrum are as yet undefined. The shorter waves are measured in Angstrom units, and the longer waves are measured in meters or in seconds per cycle, that is, the time in seconds that one cycle of the wave takes to pass a fixed point.

from knowledge of the other forms of energy, such as heat, light, electricity, and magnetism, wherein the exact natures of these forms of energy are also unknown.

FUNDAMENTAL CONCEPTS OF MATTER

Matter, of which all earthly things are made, is composed of atoms. Atoms in turn are made of many types of subatomic particles. X-rays are produced when some subatomic particles interact with atoms. It is necessary for the radiologist to understand the basic structure of atoms.

Atoms consist of two major parts (Fig. 1-2), a centrally located nucleus and one or more electrons orbiting around the nucleus. The nucleus consists of protons (positively charged particles), neutrons (neutrally charged particles of about the same size as protons), and many other smaller particles. The particles in the nucleus are bound together by strong nuclear forces. The number of protons in the nucleus is specific for each element and is known as the element's atomic number. The number of neutrons equals the number of protons in the lighter elements but becomes disproportionately larger in the heavier elements. An electron weighs only $\frac{1}{1.836}$ the weight of a proton. The number of electrons in an electrically neutral or stable atom equals the number of protons in the nucleus. The electrons travel around the nucleus in definite orbits. These orbits, or shells, consist of definite energy levels for each element. The innermost shell

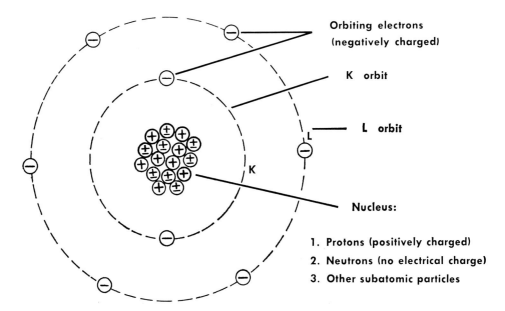

Orbiting electrons (negatively charged)

K orbit

L orbit

Nucleus:

1. Protons (positively charged)
2. Neutrons (no electrical charge)
3. Other subatomic particles

Fig. 1-2. Diagram of an oxygen atom according to present fundamental concepts of matter. The neutral atom has a number of positively charged protons in the nucleus equal to the number of negatively charged orbiting electrons.

is called the K shell; the next, the L shell; then M, N, O shells; and so forth for as many shells as the atom may possess.

X-RAY MACHINE

A prerequisite to the study of the x-ray machine is a background of basic physics. It is thus best to begin with a simple review of some basic electrical terms.

Electricity

An electric current can travel in either direction along a wire or conductor. It can be an alternating or a direct current (AC or DC). An alternating current travels first in one direction, builds up from zero to a peak potential (voltage), and drops to zero again. It then reverses its direction, builds up from zero to a peak potential, and drops to zero again. If the changes in potential are plotted on a graph, a sine wave is obtained (Fig. 1-3). The change in the direction or polarity of the current is shown by plots above and below a line representing zero potential. The term *cycle* refers to a complete curve above and below the line. The time it takes the current to complete one cycle varies with different alternating currents. These currents are commonly classified by the number of cycles they complete each second, for example, 60 cycles AC.

Voltage is the term used to describe electrical pressure or force. The volt is the unit of measurement. The kilovolt (kV) is equal to 1,000 volts. In an alternating current the voltage is constantly changing; thus the term kilovolt peak (kVp) is used. Here, the measurement is made at the greatest potential difference, or at the peak of the sine wave (Fig. 1-3).

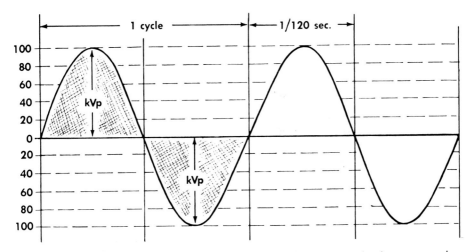

Fig. 1-3. Diagram of a sine wave of a 60-cycle electric current operating at a peak potential of 100,000 volts (100 kVp).

The *ampere* is the standard unit used in measuring the amount of an electric current that is flowing through a circuit; the milliampere (mA) is equal to $\frac{1}{1,000}$ ampere.

A *transformer* consists of two coils of electric wire insulated from each other. The magnetic field around the input coil induces an electric current in the second coil. The voltage in the second or output coil is in direct proportion to the voltage in the first or input coil as the number of turns of wire in the second coil is related to the number of turns in the first coil:

$$\frac{V \text{ (output)}}{V \text{ (input)}} = \frac{\text{number wire turns in second coil}}{\text{number wire turns in first coil}}$$

These devices can be used to raise (step up) or lower (step down) the voltage of an AC electric current by a high factor.

The *autotransformer* makes one coil do the work of two. It can be used only for making minor changes in voltage. If such a transformer has 100 loops in the coil and an AC current of 110 volts is put into the coil, then any two of the 100 loops tapped for the output circuit would have a voltage of $y/100 \times 110$ volts (where y is the number of loops between the taps of the output circuit). Two different ways in which an autotransformer is used in most modern machines are shown in Fig. 1-4.

The *rheostat* (or choke coil) is a device that increases the resistance to the passage of an electric current through a wire. It reduces or controls the amount of current that flows through a circuit and thus controls the amperage or amount of the flow of electricity.

The *ammeter* and *voltmeter* are basically the same type of instrument (galvanometer) since both are operated by the magnetic field that every electric current possesses. When placed within a circuit, these instruments measure the amount of current passing through the wire; when placed across the circuit (see milliammeter and voltmeter, Fig. 1-4), they measure the difference in potential or voltage between the two wires.

Wiring diagram

The modern dental x-ray machine is composed of many different electric and electronic parts. A dentist does not need to know all these various parts, but he should have an understanding of the basic electrical units. The simplified wiring diagram of an x-ray machine, shown in Fig. 1-4, satisfies this objective. It can be seen that the machine basically consists of a step-up and a step-down transformer, an autotransformer, an x-ray tube, a rheostat, a voltmeter, a milliammeter, and a timer.

X-ray tube and related parts

The x-ray tube (Fig. 1-5) used in dental machines is a Coolidge, or hot filament, tube. It consists of an anode and a cathode enclosed in a highly evacuated glass tube. The glass is sometimes thin where the x-rays emerge from the tube. The cathode, or negative electrode, consists of a molybdenum focusing cup (or a depression in the molybdenum cathode) in which is set a tungsten filament similar to that of an ordinary light bulb. The anode, or positive electrode, consists of a thin tungsten button set in a rod of copper, the other end of which is attached to a radiator or some other cooling device, such as an oil bath, outside of the glass tube.

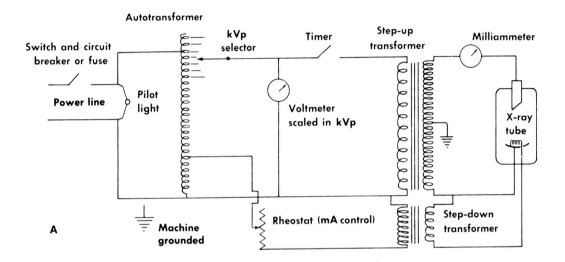

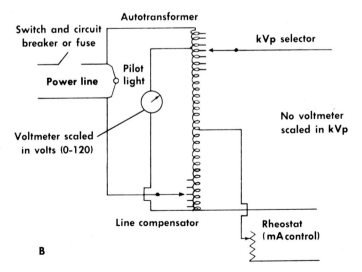

Fig. 1-4. A, Simplified wiring diagram of the basic electrical circuits and parts of an x-ray machine. **B,** Alternative voltage-regulating system.

Continued.

Fig. 1-4, cont'd. C, Dental x-ray machine. To the wall plate, *1,* is attached the tube head support, *2,* and tube head, *3.* The control panel, *4,* is enlarged in proportion to the tube head and folding support for seeability. This panel permits a choice of milliamperage and kilovoltage in addition to exposure time and can be used for up to three different tube heads. The timer cord is not shown. (**C,** Courtesy General Electric Co., Medical Systems Division, Milwaukee, Wis.)

The x-ray tube is supplied with two electrical circuits, the anode-cathode circuit and the filament circuit. Dental x-ray machines must operate at a set voltage; fluctuations in line voltage must be controlled. An autotransformer used as a line compensator or as a kilovolt peak selector combined with a suitably placed voltmeter can control the fluctuations. The filament circuit of the x-ray tube needs low voltage; thus a step-down transformer is used in this circuit. The heating of this filament by the electric current must also be controlled; a rheostat or choke coil is placed in this circuit and is operated by the milliampere-adjusting knob on the control panel of the machine.

The step-up transformer is used to produce potentials of as much as 100,000 volts between the cathode and the anode of the x-ray tube. This potential can be varied by changing the voltage to the input side of the step-up transformer. A voltage change is accomplished by connecting the input circuit to a variable number of coils in the autotransformer; the knob that operates this is the kilovolt peak selector on the control panel of the machine. The voltmeter, calibrated in kVp to register the potential across the x-ray tube, actually measures the voltage of input current of the step-up transformer. This calibration is possible since the factor by which the step-up transformer raises the voltage of the electric current does not vary. The milliammeter measures the amount of current flowing in the high-tension circuit across or through the x-ray tube. Its position in this

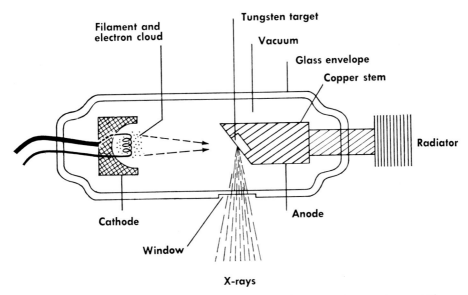

Fig. 1-5. Diagram of a dental x-ray tube, electron beam, and x-ray beam. When an electric current (50 to 100 kVp in dental radiography) is applied to the tube circuit (between the anode and the cathode), each electron is driven from the cathode to the anode in a direction perpendicular to a tangent of the curved surface of the cathode adjacent to the electron. The electrons are thus focused on the target of the anode.

circuit indicates that whenever this meter registers a flow of current, x-radiation is being produced. The step-up transformer is located in the head of the x-ray machine. Because of this arrangement, small flexible low-tension electric wires can be used between the base and the head of the x-ray machine and the maneuverability so necessary for dental x-ray equipment is enhanced.

Timer

The timer activates the high-tension current across the x-ray tube. In some machines, the filament circuit is activated and the filament is fully heated when the line current is turned on. In other machines, the filament is partially activated by the line current, but its temperature is minimal; full activation of the filament is accomplished when the timer button is pressed. In the latter instance, a slight delay between pushing of the timer button and activation of the high-tension current occurs. Many types of timers, operating on a mechanical, electrical, or electronic basis, are available. Their accuracy varies from $\frac{1}{4}$ to $\frac{1}{30}$ second in the order mentioned. Although accuracy is important, consistency is of prime concern. Exposure times that will produce satisfactory film density can be selected (see p. 76 and Fig. 4-5) for a timer that is consistent even though the time intervals may not be entirely accurate.

Timer intervals have traditionally been expressed as fractions and whole numbers of seconds. The *American National Standard for Exposure Time Designations for Timers of Dental X-ray Machines*[*] now designates the unit of exposure as an impulse and defines the impulse as $1/n$ second with n-cycle alternating current. Thus the impulse is $\frac{1}{60}$ second with 60-cycle alternating current (see p. 5 and Fig. 1-3). The standard calls for timer impulse designations of 1, 2, 3, 4, 5, 6, 8, 10, 12, 15, 19, 24, 30, 38, 48, 60, 75, 96, 120, 150, 190, 240, and 300. Any of these numbers placed over 60 (for example, $\frac{19}{60}$ or $\frac{48}{60}$) gives the exposure time in seconds. Manufacturers are asked, but are not legally obligated, to use the impulse system.

GENERATION OF X-RAYS
Electron beam

X-rays are produced or generated at the surface and within the tungsten button of the anode by the bombardment of the anode with electrons coming from the cathode. When the filament in the cathode is electrically heated, a cloud of electrons is formed in the vacuum outside of the filament wire. The temperature of the filament that determines the size of the cloud or number of electrons is controlled by the rheostat, which regulates the amount of electricity that is supplied to the filament. The size of the cloud determines the amount of electricity that can flow between the cathode and the anode since these two parts are sep-

---

[*]Copies of this standard can be obtained from the American National Standards Institute, 1430 Broadway, New York, N.Y. 10018.

arated by a vacuum. When the high voltage circuit between the cathode and anode of the x-ray tube is activated, the electrons are repelled from the cathode and attracted to the anode. Travel of these electrons is not impeded, since the gases in the tube have been removed by a high vacuum. The speed with which these electrons travel across the gap between the cathode and the anode depends on the potential difference (kV) between the two electrodes; this potential is controlled on the x-ray machine panel by the kilovolt peak selector and is registered by the voltmeter. The electrons, in traveling across this gap, are focused by the focusing cup of the cathode to impact on a rectangular area (focal spot) on the surface of the tungsten button, or target, of the anode. A diagram of this electron beam impacting on the focal spot is shown in Fig. 1-6.

Of all the kinetic energy (speed or motion) carried over by the electrons from the cathode to the anode, only about 0.2% is converted into x-radiation at 65 kVp. When higher voltages are used, the conversion percentage is slightly greater. The remaining energy goes to form heat, which is dissipated into the head of the x-ray machine with the aid of the radiator attached to the anode. Cooling of some modern x-ray tubes is accomplished by oil immersion; other

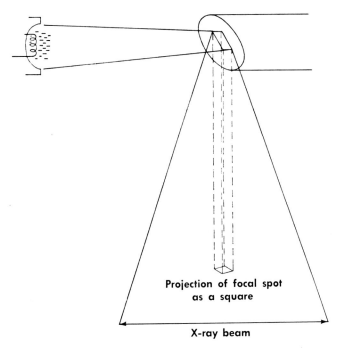

**Projection of focal spot
as a square**

X-ray beam

Fig. 1-6. Diagram of the anode, focal spot, and x-ray beam. The focal spot as seen from points within the x-ray beam appears as a square of approximately 0.8 × 0.8 mm. This square is the source of radiation or effective focal spot for the beam of radiation. The actual focal spot is rectangular and has a considerably greater area (approximately 0.8 × 1.8 mm.) than the effective spot.

tubes are cooled by the circulation of air or oil around the tube or by water circulated through a hollow anode. The heat must be transmitted to the outside of the tube case. If the heat is not removed quickly enough and the heat-storing capacity of the tube is exceeded, the tube will be severely damaged. Damage of this kind most commonly shows up as a pitted surface on the focal spot area of the tungsten target. The manufacturer's recommendations for the operating capacities of the x-ray tube must be observed.

Selection of target material

The selection of the target material on which the electrons will impact is of great importance. The ideal target material should possess the following qualities:

1. It should have a high atomic number.
2. It should have a low vapor pressure at high temperatures.
3. It should have a high melting point.
4. It should possess a high degree of thermal conductivity.

The anode should have a high melting point since most of the energy received from the electrons is converted into heat. The high anode temperatures must not cause the anode material to melt. The anode should have a low vapor pressure at high temperatures since the electron beam is directed to a very small area on the surface of the anode and some of the atoms may reach a vapor state. If a high vapor pressure is obtained, the smooth surface of the target will be disturbed and blisters may be formed. The anode should also possess a high degree of thermal conductivity since the great amount of heat formed at the focal spot must be carried to the radiator that is on the outside of the x-ray tube. The anode of a dental x-ray tube must have a high atomic number. X-rays needed to pass through dental hard tissues must possess a great power of penetration. This penetrating power is related to the radiation energy and wavelength. The shorter the x-ray wavelength, the greater will be the energy and the ability to penetrate matter. Target material must be sufficiently dense (have a sufficiently high atomic number) to stop the electron abruptly on its surface and thus to produce maximum conversion of kinetic energy into x-ray energy. The higher the atomic number, the denser is the target material and the more efficient is the production of useful x-rays.

The element tungsten (chemical symbol, W) has a high atomic number and a high melting point. It also has a low vapor pressure at high temperatures. It does not have a high degree of thermal conductivity. This defect can be overcome by embedding a thin button of tungsten in a copper stem to form the anode. The electron beam impacts on this tungsten button, or target, and the heat generated is quickly transferred to the copper, which possesses a high degree of thermal conductivity. The copper stem stores and carries the heat off to the radiator.

Focal spot

X-rays or photons are produced where the electrons impact on the target material (focal spot) (Fig. 1-6). The useful beam of x-rays emerges from this spot through a port in the tube case. The beam travels at approximately right angles to the long axis of the x-ray tube. A projection of the focal spot (effective focal spot), when viewed from any point within the x-ray beam, appears more or less like a square, the dimensions of which are equal to those of the shorter side of the rectangular focal spot. It is desirable in diagnosis radiology for the projection of the source of radiation to be as small as possible. The use of a rectangular focal spot, which is projected as a square, is called a *line focus* and is obtained by setting the surface of the target at an appropriate angle. The use of a line focus allows the x-rays to be generated over a large surface area on the target; thus less heat per unit area is produced. Therefore, greater numbers of electrons can be used, and a great number of x-ray photons result. The fact that the heat is generated over a greater area makes the target less susceptible to damage when overloading (excessive mA, kVp, or exposure time) occurs.

Energy conversion into x-radiation

The x-ray photons result from conversion of kinetic energy (carried by the electrons in the form of speed) into radiant energy; this basically is accomplished in two ways: (1) The electron can be brought to a stop through collision with the tungsten atom (the exact mechanism is unknown) and the giving up of all its energy to the formation of an x-ray photon. Glancing collisions result in the electron's giving up only part of its energy and therefore in an x-ray photon that has a longer wavelength, less energy, and less penetrating power. Most of the x-rays produced in dental machines are created in this manner. (2) The electrons can dislodge one or more orbital electrons of the atom. Fig. 1-7 is a schematic demonstration of these principles. In dental machines, only the removal of the K orbital electrons is of practical importance. To remove the K electrons of tungsten, the electrons from the cathode must possess more than 69,000 electron volts of energy; thus this phenomenon can occur only when the machine is set at 70 kVp or above. When a K electron is removed out of its orbit, an electron from an outer orbit (usually the L orbit) falls into the K orbit and in so doing releases energy in the form of an x-ray photon. The photon emitted in this manner (for example, an L electron replaces a K electron) by an atom of any one element has a definite wavelength because the energy level between the orbital electrons of the same orbits of the same element is constant. The energy level between orbits varies with different elements. X-rays so formed by different elements have wavelengths that are characteristic of the particular element that emitted them. This phenomenon is used to identify elements. These radiations are called characteristic radiations.

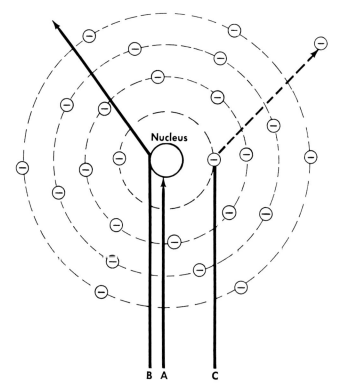

Fig. 1-7. Diagram of electrons colliding with a simulated tungsten atom (the number of electrons is insufficient for this atom to be tungsten). **A,** Giving up all of its kinetic energy. **B,** Relinquishing part of its energy. **C,** Displacing a K orbit electron.

In summary, x-rays are produced through the conversion of electric energy (potential difference between the anode and cathode) into kinetic energy (speed of the electrons in the electron beam), which is converted into x-ray energy and heat. In addition to this, when the machine is operated at or above 70 kVp, characteristic x-rays of tungsten are produced.

X-RAY BEAM
Position and shape

X-rays are created at the focal spot of the anode and travel in all directions. The x-rays used are those that travel away from the anode in a beam, the direction of which is at right angles to the electron stream between the cathode and anode and in the direction that the tungsten target faces. This intense beam of x-rays passes through the glass envelope of the x-ray tube. Some tubes have a thin area or window in the glass through which these rays emerge. This window is placed in the tube because glass absorbs x-rays and does not allow easy transmission of x-ray photons. In addition to this useful beam of x-rays, the focal spot

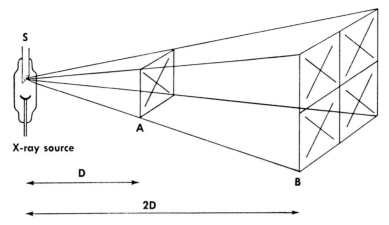

Fig. 1-8. Diagram showing the relationship of distance to the area covered by x-rays emanating from an x-ray tube. Photons emerging from the tube travel in straight lines and diverge from each other. The areas covered by the photons at any two points are proportional to each other as the square of the distances measured from the points to the source of radiation.

produces x-rays traveling in all directions. These stray x-rays are confined in the head of the x-ray machine by enclosing the x-ray tube in a leaded shield. An opening in this shield, usually covered with glass or aluminum in the form of a seal, allows the useful beam of x-rays to emerge from within the head of the x-ray machine; it is usually circular in shape. The useful x-rays, created at the focal spot, emerge from the dental x-ray machine in the form of a cone of x-radiation. Photons traveling in the very center of this cone of radiation are called the central ray. The central ray is commonly used to fix or locate the position of the x-ray beam.

Inverse square law

X-rays, like light, travel in straight lines. The inverse square law is based on this fact. This law states that the intensity of radiation is inversely proportional to the squares of the distances measured from the source of radiation to points of radiation intensity measurement. The formula for this law is

$$\frac{I_1}{I_2} = \frac{(D_2)^2}{(D_1)^2}$$

where I is intensity and D is distance. If intensity is thought of as the number of photons per unit area, one can easily see from the diagram given in Fig. 1-8 how x-ray intensity is related to distance in a beam of x-rays.

Rectification

The x-ray beam used in dentistry is not a continuous stream of radiation but comes from the tube as pulses, the frequency of which depends on the number of cycles per second (or frequency) of the alternating electric current. For example, if a 60-cycle AC current activates the tube, then 60 pulses of x-rays per second will be emitted from the tube. Each pulse of radation lasts for $\frac{1}{120}$ second. The reason that x-rays are produced in pulses is that the tube can operate only when the electric current is traveling from the cathode to the anode. When the AC current changes direction, it cannot travel across the tube, since there are no electrons at the anode to carry it across to the cathode; thus the current is blocked from traveling in that direction. This unidirection of the AC current is called rectification. Since rectification is accomplished by the x-ray tube itself without the assistance of other rectifying tubes or devices, the dental x-ray tube is said to be self-rectified.

The production of x-rays in pulses can be used to check the timing mechanism of the machine at its lower setting ($\frac{1}{30}$ to 1 second). A spinning top is used to count the number of pulses of x-rays emitted by the machine for a particular time interval. A spinning top is a disk of heavy metal with a shaft in the center on which the disk spins. A notch is placed in the edge of the disk, or a hole is drilled through the disk near its periphery. The device is spun slowly on the surface of a large film, and an x-ray exposure is made while it is in motion. The image of the hole or notch will appear at a different position on the film with each pulse of x-rays. After the film has been processed, the number and quality of the images are examined. When a 60-cycle current is used, 60 pulses of radiation occur every second the machine is in operation. Fractions of a second exposure produce a similar fraction of the 60 pulses or images. More sophisticated electronic devices ordinarily are used to verify timer accuracy.

X-ray spectrum

The x-ray beam consists of millions of individual x-rays or photons. These photons do not all have the same wavelength or energy but vary considerably in this factor. One reason is that the potential across the tube changes constantly as the AC voltage varies (Fig. 1-3). Another reason is that the electrons (when they reach the target) do not give up all of their kinetic energy in an identical fashion; they may give up energy completely through a single impact or in a series of steps through glancing collisions with the tungsten atoms. A typical graph showing the spectral distribution of the x-ray beam is shown in Fig. 1-9. The minimum photon wavelenth (maximum photon energy) obtainable at any potential between the anode and cathode can be calculated from a simple formula, as follows:

$$\frac{12.35}{kVp} = \text{minimum photon wavelength in Å}$$

Filtration

X-rays used in denistry must be able to penetrate dental tissues. The longer wavelength x-rays are of no use in diagnostic radiography and are more or less

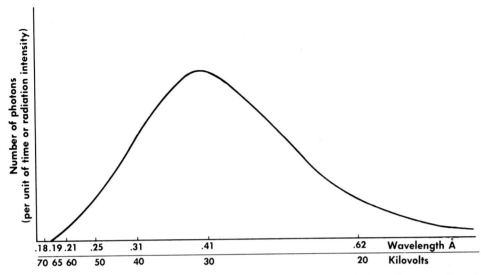

Fig. 1-9. Graph showing an x-ray beam spectrum that can result from the operation of an x-ray tube at 65 kVp.

removed from the x-ray beam by having the beam pass through aluminum disks (filters). These disks may be built into the machine by the manufacturer or may be added by the dentist. Any material that the x-ray beam passes through exerts a filtering effect on the beam. The glass of the x-ray tube, the oil surrounding the tube, and any plastic pointed cone attached to the head of the x-ray machine produces some filtering of the beam. The filtering effect of these materials is usually referred to as being equivalent to the filtering effect of specific thicknesses of aluminum. The total filtering effect of materials that the x-ray operator cannot normally remove from the machine is called the inherent or built-in filtration; the sum of all extra filters is called added filtration. Total filtration is the sum of inherent and added filtration. The overall effect of filtration on the x-ray beam is the absorption of most of the long-wave photons along with a few of the short-wave, more penetrating x-rays. After proper filtration the beam consists mainly of photons having the ability to penetrate through soft tissue, bone, and teeth to reach the film. When a beam is so filtered, it is said to be hardened or to consist mainly of the hard, more penetrating x-rays. Conversely, the beam is said to be softened and to contain more of the soft, less penetrating x-rays when filters are removed. (See also p. 42.)

Collimation

The x-ray beam is shaped or collimated to the desired size by a lead diaphragm. A diaphragm is a lead disk with a hole in its center that allows the x-rays to pass through. The lead is of a thickness (1/16 inch or more) that will absorb effectively all the x-rays in the beam except those passing through the opening. The beam can also be collimated by permitting it to enter a metal cylinder or cone and allowing only the needed portion to emerge from the other end of the cylinder. The ordinarily recommended beam size for intraoral radiography is one that has a diameter of no more than 2¾ inches at the patient's skin. Some operators prefer a rectangular-shaped column of x-rays instead of a circular column or cone of radiation. Properly used rectangular collimation reduces patient exposure beyond that accomplished with a 2¾-inch diameter round beam. The shape of the beam is controlled by the shape of the hole in the diaphragm or by the shape of the metal collimating device. (See also p. 39.)

ABSORPTION OF X-RAYS
Interreaction with matter

X-rays are absorbed by any form of matter (solids, liquids, and gases). In the main, when a photon reaches an atom, one of four things can happen: (1) It can pass through the atom without any change occurring to either the atom or the photon. (2) It can be deviated from its path by the atom without any change to the atom; the photon now becomes a photon of scattered radiation. (3) It can strike an electron of the atom and be completely absorbed (photoelectric effect). Under these conditions the electron is accelerated out of its orbit and becomes a photoelectron. This photoelectron gives up its kinetic energy by colliding with the electrons of other atoms or by interacting with the nuclei of atoms and producing electromagnetic radiation of long wavelengths. If the photoelectron originated from an inner orbit of the atom, the atom will then emit an x-ray of characteristic radiation when the inner electron is replaced by an outer electron. (4) The x-ray can hit an electron of the atom and give up only part of its energy (Compton effect). The result will be an electron that is traveling at a high rate of speed (giving up its energy like the photoelectron) and an x-ray photon that is changed in its direction and that has a longer wavelength, that is, less energy. Characteristic x-rays from the absorbing atoms may also be produced by this fourth method of x-ray absorption. Basically, then, when x-rays are absorbed by matter, positive and negative ions* are created along with secondary radiations. The energy imparted to the absorbing material by the x-rays can also result in fluorescence, phosphorescence, and heat.

Primary radiation is considered to be energy emerging from the tube head in a collimated useful beam. For purposes of this text, all other radiation is classified as secondary radiation or radiation resulting from the interaction of the primary beam of x-rays with matter. Thus, secondary radiation consists of both the scattered photons of the primary beam and the characteristic radia-

---

*Ions are electrically charged atoms or electrons. They consist of electrically positive atoms, free negatively charged electrons, or atoms that have become electrically negative through the capture of an electron. Ionization is discussed later in this chapter under x-radiation measurement and again in Chapter 4.

tions produced when inner orbital electrons are removed from atoms during the absorption of the x-ray photons. Since leakage radiation from the tube head (if present) emerges in all directions, it also can be thought of as scattered radiation. Secondary or scattered radiation travels in all directions.

The absorption of x-rays is proportional to the density of the absorbing material. The heavier the element (the more mass per unit volume), the more x-rays are absorbed. Thus it is obvious that lead is a most efficient material for absorbing x-radiation. Lead is incorporated in glass to produce an x-ray barrier material through which one can see. When rigidity is needed in a barrier material, steel and brass are sometimes used. Liquids containing heavy elements such as iodine or barium are also used in oral radiography to absorb x-rays.

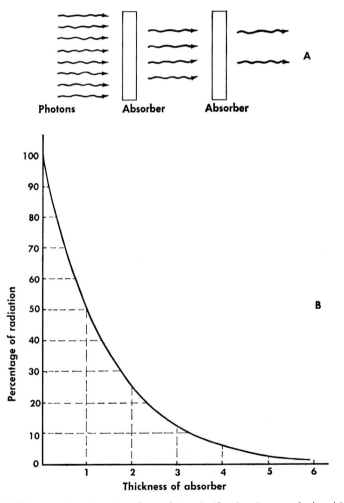

Fig. 1-10. A, Diagram showing the effect of two half-value layers of absorbing material on a monochromatic beam of x-ray photons. **B,** Graph showing the exponential curve of x-ray absorption.

Half-value layer

When an x-ray beam encounters a mass of material or a barrier, all the x-ray photons are not absorbed. If an x-ray beam consisted of photons all having the same wavelength (monochromatic radiation) and a certain thickness of the material absorbed half the photons, then doubling the thickness of the material would not result in the absorption of the remaining photons. Doubling of the material's thickness would result in the absorption of half the remaining photons. This phenomenon is shown diagrammatically in Fig. 1-10. An exponential curve results when such absorption measurements are plotted on a graph. If a certain thickness of a material reduces a monochromatic x-ray beam by 50%, the x-ray beam is said to have a half-value layer (hvl) of the thickness used, measured in terms of the absorbing material.

The quality (energy level or wavelength) of a monochromatic beam of x-rays can be identified by its absorption curve. Various metals are used as absorbers; for example, lead, copper, and aluminum. In diagnostic radiography, aluminum is the absorber of choice. The beam of x-rays from a dental machine consists of photons of many different wavelengths (heterogeneous or polychromatic radiation). The shorter wavelength photons carry more energy and are able to penetrate deeper into matter than are the longer wavelength photons. To measure the quality of a beam of heterogeneous x-rays, a method of measurement called the half-value layer of aluminum is used. This half-value layer, measured in millimeters of pure aluminum, is the thickness of aluminum that will reduce the intensity or energy of a beam of radiation by 50%. This measurement indicates the *average* quality or penetrating ability of the x-ray beam. When a heterogeneous beam of x-rays and a monochromatic beam have the same half-layer, the two beams have quite similar radiographic properties.

Monochromatic beams have photons of the same wavelength and energy. Heterogeneous beams are classified by their effective photon wavelength or kilovoltage. This effective wavelength is the same wavelength as that of a monochromatic beam that has essentially the same properties as the heterogeneous beam. The greater the half-value layer of aluminum, the more penetrating are the radiations of a heterogeneous beam; that is, the photons have greater energy and shorter wavelength. These x-rays are often called hard radiations. When the soft (long wavelength) x-rays are filtered out of a beam of x-rays, the beam is said to be hardened. In oral diagnostic radiography the half-value layer of the beam of radiation is approximately 2 mm. of aluminum.

X-radiation units of measurement

X-radiation is ordinarily measured in terms of roentgens *in air* (R).* For the purpose of this text, it is sufficient to limit the discussion to the roentgen. In addi-

---

*The symbol R instead of r has been used to comply with the recommendations of Report 10a, 1962, of the International Commission on Radiological Units and Measurements.

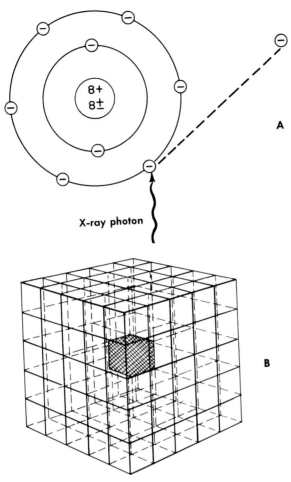

X-ray photon

Fig. 1-11. Schema of, **A,** ionization of an oxygen atom and, **B,** a 1-cm. cube of air surrounded by an infinite amount of air.

tion to the roentgen, other units of radiation measurement include the roentgen
absorbed dose (rad), roentgen equivalent man (rem), and relative biologic
effectiveness (RBE).*

A roentgen can be defined as that amount of x-radiation or gamma radiation
which will produce in 1 cc. of air (at standard temperature and pressure) ions

---

rad: A unit of absorbed energy per gram of absorbing material; *rem:* the dose of any ionizing
radiation that will produce the same biologic effect in man as that produced from the absorption of 1 R of x-radiation or gamma radiation; *RBE:* all ionizing radiations have the ability to
produce biologic effects. Certain types of radiation are more effective than others in that
smaller absorbed doses of these radiations are required to produce a particular effect. A
comparison between one type of radiation and another with respect to this ability is known
as the relative biologic effectiveness of that type of radiation. RBE is expressed in numerals,
usually from 1 to 20.

carrying one electrostatic unit of either sign. One electrostatic unit equals 2.08 $\times 10^9$ ion pairs. At the risk of oversimplification, let us envision a cube of air, 1 cm. in all dimensions. As an x-ray beam passes through it, the x-ray photons strike electrons orbiting about the nuceli of electrically stable air atoms and separate the electrons from their respective nuclei (Fig. 1-11). This action is ionization (ion pair formation); the electron is negatively charged, and the remainder of the atom becomes positively charged. In measurement of radiation, these charges are collected and measured.

X-RAY FILMS

The radiograph is basically a photographic image of an object made with the use of x-rays instead of light. The roentgen image or shadow of an object is invisible and has to be recorded before the dentist can observe it. This is done by having the x-rays expose a film (similar to that used in photography) and then processing the film to make visible the roentgen image of the object.

Intraoral film construction

The x-ray film consists of a sensitized emulsion on the surface of a transparent base. The base is made of cellulose acetate, and the emulsion consists of crystals of silver halides (mostly bromides) suspended in gelatin. Almost all intraoral x-ray films are coated with an emulsion on both sides of the base (double emulsion films). It is necessary in diagnostic radiography to know which side of the intraoral film faced the x-ray source when the film was exposed in order that the films can be properly mounted. Some means of identifying this surface

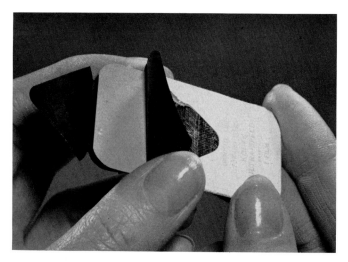

Fig. 1-12. Typical intraoral film packet as seen from the back. In the white lightproof envelope is the dental film surrounded by black paper and backed by lead foil. A herringbone pattern can be seen impressed in the foil.

must be inherent to the film. This is done ordinarily during film manufacture by indenting one side of the film; on the other side of the film this indentation appears as a bump or raised dot on the surface of the film. This latter surface is the one that faces the x-ray source when the film is correctly exposed.

Intraoral x-ray films are wrapped in an opaque material to prevent exposure to light. Light photons also activate silver halide crystals. The wrapping is sometimes stippled on the side facing the x-rays to aid in preventing the film package from slipping when it is held against the oral mucosa by the patient's finger. The wrapping is fairly waterproof to prevent the patient's saliva from reaching the film.

A thin sheet of lead foil is usually placed within the film packet behind the film. This metal foil prevents most of the secondary radiation, originating in the tissues of the patient behind the film packet, from reaching the film. The metal foil thus helps to reduce secondary radiation film fog during exposure. It also absorbs x-rays that have passed through the object and film and thus reduces exposure of the tissues behind the film. The metal foil frequently has a design stamped on it, for example, a herringbone pattern. This design or pattern will appear on the exposed film if the film packet was facing the wrong way during film exposure. A typical film packet and its contents are shown in Fig. 1-12.

Intraoral film size and speed

Intraoral film sizes have been standardized on a numerical basis, as listed in Table 1-2. (*Note:* We are opposed to the use of the 2.3 film as a periapical film, that is, without a wing.) One of us (A. H. W.) would prefer to have film sizes 1.00 and 1.0 (especially the former) deleted from the standard because these films are quite small. The diagnostic information obtained from their use in children's mouths tends to be minimal in terms of radiation absorbed.

Dental x-ray films vary considerably in speed or sensitivity to radiation. They are made to be relatively more sensitive to x-rays than to light. Much of the speed of a film depends on the size of the silver halide crystal used (grain of the film); the larger the crystal (the greater the grain size), the faster the film. The fastest available film is more than 12 times faster than the slowest film. Many films have intermediate speeds. Intraoral film speeds have been standardized on an alphabetical basis, as shown in Table 1-3. A typical box of intraoral film with size and speed clearly stated is shown in Fig. 1-13. Table 1-4 presents the film speeds of dental films manufactured in the United States.

Extraoral film

Extraoral films come in two types—nonscreen and screen film. A *nonscreen film* is one with an emulsion considerably more sensitive to x-rays than to light. These films may have a double emulsion with a thickness greater than that of intraoral films. The increased emulsion thickness makes this film fairly fast; in other words, it needs less exposure time. However, because of the increased

Table 1-2. Sizes of intraoral film*

Type-size number† (shorter dimension first)	Dimensions	
	Millimeters Tolerance ± 0.50	Inches Tolerance ± 0.20
Periapical		
1.00	20.60 × 31.80	0.811 × 1.252
1.0	22.20 × 34.90	0.874 × 1.374
1.1	23.80 × 39.70	0.937 × 1.563
1.2	31.00 × 40.90	1.220 × 1.610
Interproximal		
2.00 (Posterior)	20.60 × 31.80	0.811 × 1.252
2.0 (Posterior)	22.20 × 34.90	0.874 × 1.374
2.1 (Anterior)	23.80 × 39.70	0.937 × 1.563
2.1 (Posterior)	23.80 × 39.70	0.937 × 1.563
2.2 (Posterior)	31.00 × 40.90	1.220 × 1.610
2.3 (Posterior)‡	25.60 × 53.60	1.047 × 2.110
Occlusal	57.20 × 76.20	2.252 × 3.000
3.4		

*The American Dental Association is the proprietary sponsor of the performance standard for intraoral radiographic film (size and speed). The standard was originally developed by the American National Standards Institute (ANSI) Committee PH 6. This Committee was disbanded in 1974. An American National Standards Institute designation PH 8 was given to the American Dental Association as the proprietary sponsor of the film standard. Information about size and speed standards can be obtained from the Council on Dental Materials and Devices, American Dental Association, 211 East Chicago Avenue, Chicago, Ill. 60611. The American National Standards Institute, Inc. is located at 1430 Broadway, New York, N.Y. 10018.

†*Note:* The digit at the left of the decimal point in the type-size number indicates the use of the film (i.e., periapical, interproximal, or occlusal). The digit (or digits) at the right of the decimal point denotes the film size (i.e., size 00, 0, 1, 2, 3 or 4).

‡Films of this size may be provided without a wing.

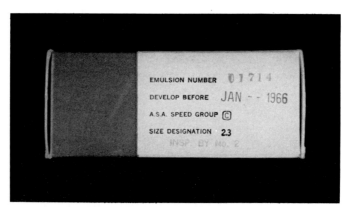

Fig. 1-13. Pertinent information concerning film size and emulsion factors is clearly marked on the outside of the film box. (Courtesy Rinn Corp., Chicago, Ill.)

Table 1-3. Speed of intraoral film*

Speed group	Speed range† (in reciprocal roentgens)‡
A	1.5- 3.0
B	3.0- 6.0
C	6.0-12.0
D	12.0-24.0
E	24.0-48.0
F	48.0-96.0

*See footnote to Table 1-2.
†The upper range limit of each speed range shall be excluded from that range.
‡A roentgen is a measurement of radiation exposure or quantity. In this table, A is the slowest (least sensitive) film and F is the fastest.

Table 1-4. Group ratings of dental radiographic film speed*
(data verified by manufacturer†)

Film brand	Manufacturer or distributor	Speed group	
		ANSI PH 6.1 1970	Reciprocal roentgens‡
Periapical film			
None		A§	1.5-3.0
None		B	3.0-6.0
Minimax Extra Fast	Minimax Co.	C	6.0-12.0
Kodak Ultra-Speed (Morelite)	Eastman Kodak Co.	D	12.0-24.0
Minimax Triple X	Minimax Co.	D	12.0-24.0
Rinn Super (Plus Light)	Rinn Corp.		
None		E	24.0-48.0
None		F	48.0-96.0
Bite-wing film			
Minimax Extra Fast	Minimax Co.	C	6.0-12.0
Kodak Ultra-Speed (Morelite)	Eastman Kodak Co.	D	12.0-24.0
Minimax Triple X	Minimax Co.	D	12.0-24.0
Rinn Super (Plus Light)	Rinn Corp.		
Occlusal film	Eastman Kodak Co.	D	12.0-24.0
Kodak Ultra-Speed (Morelite)			

*Efforts were made to obtain verification of data from the Minimax Co., but no response from the company was forthcoming. We have included data based on available advertisements by the Minimax Co.
†See footnote to Table 1-2. Table excludes films of foreign manufacture. The method of calculating film speeds is described in J.A.D.A. **59**:472, 1959.
‡The upper limit of each speed range shall be excluded from that range.
§Alphabetical sequence is from slowest (least sensitive) to fastest. Speed groups A and B were available in the past but are no longer available. Groups E and F may become available in the future. The table includes these groups for the purpose of completeness.

emulsion thickness, the processing time usually must be increased 50% more than that for the other films. Film processing is discussed later in this chapter. Nonscreen film is used in a cardboard holder or envelope. The conventional sizes employed in dentistry are 5 × 7 and 8 × 10 inches. The cardboard holder has a definite exposure side. A sheet of an x-ray–absorbing material is placed in the back of the film holder to absorb the x-rays after they have passed through the film.

A *screen film* is a film with an emulsion sensitive to visible light and more specifically to the blue light of the visible light spectrum. The most common sizes used in dentistry are 5 × 7, 8 × 10, and 10 × 12 inches. While x-radiation–sensitive emulsions are activated by x-rays, they are also sensitive to visible light but to a much lesser degree. Similarly, although screen film is most sensitive to blue light, it is also exposed by x-rays but to a much lesser degree. The screen film is used between two fluorescent screens in a rigid holder or cassette. The fluorescent screens are made of tiny calcium tungstate crystals or other phosphor crystals bound together in a uniform layer on a firm base. Upon striking these crystals, the x-rays create a blue light, which in turn exposes the screen film. The efficiency with which these screens produce blue light depends on the size of the fluorescent crystals. Screens are commonly classified as (1) slow or detail screens, (2) medium or par-speed screens, and (3) fast or high-speed screens. When screen film is used with fluorescent screens, the film must be in intimate contact with the screens since it is mainly the light from the screens that exposes the film. Any space between the film and screens will result in unsharp or blurred images in the radiograph. Intimate film-screen contact is obtained through the use of springs or clamps.

Film properties

Film properties (those inherent in the film itself) include density, contrast, and detail or definition.

The density and contrast of a film are best shown by the sensitometric or H and D curve* of the film (Fig. 1-14). This curve is obtained by plotting film density against exposure time. When a film is exposed by x-rays and subsequently processed, it becomes dark. The more the film is exposed to x-rays, the blacker it becomes when processed. When the conditions under which the film is exposed and processed are standardized, the blackness in the finished film is a function of the exposure time. This is seen in the H and D curve.

Density is the degree of blackness present in the processed film. It is measured in terms of light transmission on a percentage or logarithmic scale and

---

*A Hurter-Driffield (H and D, D $\log_{10}$ E, or sensitometric) curve is a curve that illustrates graphically the relationship of radiation exposure of the photosensitive material to the resulting density of the silver deposit in the processed film. This curve is named in honor of two early research workers in the field of photographic sensitometry.

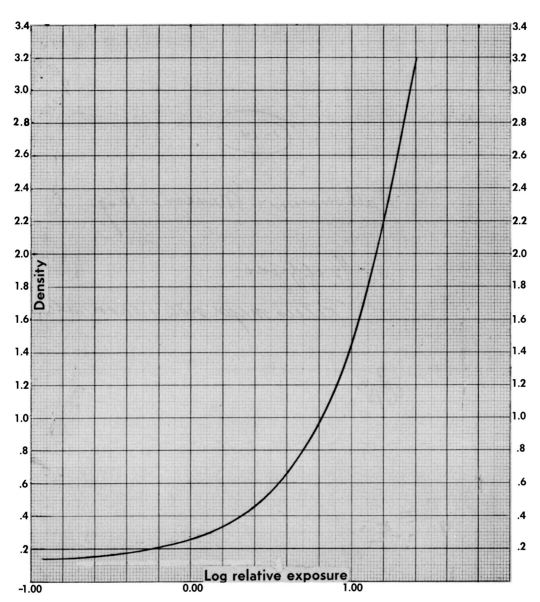

Fig. 1-14. Typical sensitometric curve for x-ray film. The slope and location of the curve vary with different films and with exposure and processing procedures. Light-sensitive films produce a different curve, particularly in the upper density ranges.

is most often expressed in the latter form. For example, if a film permits only one tenth of a beam of light to pass through it, the film is said to have a density of 1 ($\log_{10}$ of $10 = 1$). If the film is blacker and allows only a hundredth of a beam of light to pass through it, the film is said to possess a density of 2 ($\log_{10}$ of $100 = 2$).* Although film density varies between different parts of a radiographic image, the term *density* is usually applied clinically to mean the overall blackness or darkness of the entire radiograph. It should be noted that exposure time is not linear in its relationship to film density; however, there is a rather linear relationship above, and somewhat below, density 0.5. This more or less linear area is spoken of as the useful slope of the curve. Basically, diagnostic radiography uses a film density range of 0.25 to 2. Darker films can be used, but special high-intensity illuminators or view boxes must be available for one to see the rather black images in the film. Densities less than 0.25 are not practical for dental radiography.

The speed of a particular film refers to its ability to produce a radiographic image with greater or lesser amounts of radiation. With an H and D curve, film speed is determined by the position of the curve along the abscissa (horizontal axis of the graph given in Fig. 1-14). If a second film produces a similar curve but is to the right of the one seen in Fig. 1-14, the second film, though possessing similar characteristics to the first film, will have a slower film speed and will need more radiation to produce comparable densities.

Contrast† is the gradation of the differences in film density in different areas of a radiograph. If a film is exposed to x-rays and many different areas on the film receive different amounts of radiation, the processed radiograph may or may not show different blacknesses or densities between all of the areas. If many different film densities can be seen between the totally clear and totally black areas of the radiograph, the contrast gradation is said to be one of long-scale or low contrast. If, on the other hand, only a few different densities can be seen between the black and clear areas of the radiograph, the film contrast is said to be of short-scale or high contrast. On the H and D curve, the inherent contrast of a film, or the ability of the film to show contrast, is seen as the steepness of the useful slope of the curve. The contrast of a radiographic film is measured as the steepness of a line drawn from density 0.25 to density 2 on the H and D

---

*Expressed another way, if the source of light (incident light) has 5,000 light units and the light emerging through the film (transmitted light) has 500 light units, the ratio of incident to transmitted light is 5,000 to 500 or 10. The logarithm (to the base 10) of 10 is 1. If the film is darker and only 50 light units are transmitted, the ratio is 100; the logarithm of 100 is 2. Thus the density of the measured areas would be 1 and 2, respectively. If the ratio of incident light to transmitted light is less than 10 (that is, the film is quite light), the logarithm will be a decimal ranging downward from 0.99. If the ratio exceeds 100, the logarithm will be between 2.0 and infinity. Densities in excess of 2 are quite black.

†The subject of contrast is difficult to present in a concise manner. A full evaluation would require a disproportionate amount of textual material. The subject is presented in practical terms, an approach that tends to oversimplify.

curve of the film. The two densities used are essentially the densities of the very clear and very black areas of a diagnostic radiograph. The steeper the slope, the shorter will be the scale of contrast.

In a diagnostic radiograph, contrast is determined not only by the ability of the film to show contrast, but also by the range of x-ray intensities resulting from the absorption of varying amounts of x-radiation by different parts of the object. The contrast change produced by the object is sometimes called subject contrast. Contrast in the diagnostic radiograph is also affected by the voltage applied to the x-ray tube, that is, kVp. The object used to show radiographic contrast is the step wedge or penetrometer. This wedge is usually made of aluminum and is constructed so that there is a constant increase in the thickness

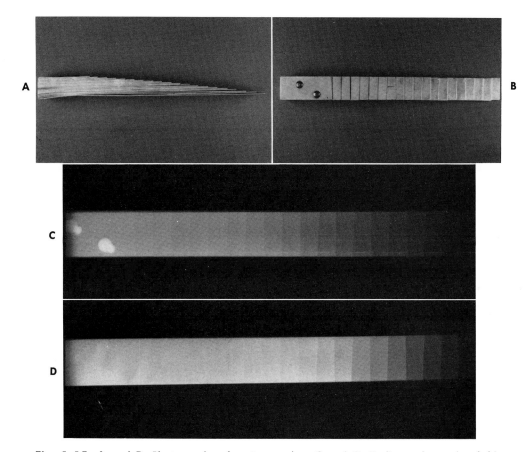

Fig. 1-15. A and **B,** Photographs of a step wedge. **C** and **D,** Radiographs made of this wedge, demonstrating a long scale of contrast (middle) and a short scale of contrast (below). The same object and type of film was used, but the kVp of the machine was changed to vary the radiographic contrast. The mA was also changed to maintain approximately a constant film density.

of aluminum between the tube and film. A long-scale or low-contrast radiograph of the wedge shows less density difference between two steps of the wedge when compared to a radiograph possessing short-scale contrast. This effect is demonstrated in Fig. 1-15. Note that the number of observable steps increases with long-scale contrast. (Contrast is further discussed in this chapter under film processing and in Chapters 2 and 3.)

When *detail* and *definition** are used to describe inherent film quality, they refer to the ability of a film to reproduce the sharp outlines of an object. A radiograph that has good detail will show the images of very small objects. The size of the silver halide crystals in the film affects detail. This is commonly called the film grain. Basically, fine-grain film has good detail but slow film speed, whereas large-grain film has poor detail but fast film speed. It should be noted that in dental radiography detail of the radiographic image is affected mainly by the conditions under which the image was projected onto the film (Chapter 2) and, in part, by film-processing conditions.

LATENT IMAGE AND FILM PROCESSING
Latent image formation

The silver halide crystals in the film emulsion are changed whenever they absorb x-ray photons. The result of x-ray absorption is precipitation or formation of a speck of silver in each affected crystal. This speck of silver consists of only a small amount of the total silver contained in the entire crystal. The remainder of the silver in the crystal remains in its original form until the film is processed. Collectively, these specks of silver are called the latent image. The halide radicals (bromide) that were combined with the precipitated silver escape through the emulsion in the form of a bromine gas. This separation of the silver and bromine within the crystal (latent image production) can also be produced by other forms of energy, such as heat, chemicals, electricity, and mechanical energy, for example, bending the film. When an x-ray beam exposes a film, very little (about 2%) of the radiation passing through the film is captured by the film. The recording of the roentgen image by a photographic process is thus not a very efficient method.

In order for the radiographic image to be seen, the film must be processed. Processing consists of developing, rinsing, fixing, washing, and drying the film. To do this, a light-free room (darkroom) suitably equipped with safelights and so forth is necessary. The darkroom is discussed in Chapter 9. The film is removed from its package and is processed under light-safe conditions. (See also p. 50.)

---

*The terms *detail, definition, sharpness,* and *resolution* are used in a variety of ways by different authors. Technically, each term has a particular meaning. For the purposes of this text they will be thought of as being synonymous.

Developing

The film is placed in a developing solution and developed according to the manufacturer's recommendations. It is developed for a specific amount of time at a certain temperature within a limited range of temperature. The action of the developing agents on an exposed silver halide crystal is to continue the process of precipitating the silver in the entire crystal until all of the silver is deposited at the site of the crystal and the bromine is released into the developing solution. The unexposed crystals, or those not containing the silver specks or latent image, are not affected by the developing solution. Film-processing technic is discussed in Chapter 9. The contents of a typical x-ray developer and the purpose of each chemical found in the solution are listed in Table 1-5.

The data given in Table 1-5 are indicative of why most manufacturers recommend a time-temperature system of developing. More than one developing agent is present in the developer solution, and one of them (hydroquinone) is sensitive to changes in temperature. This results in the relative overactivity of the Elon at temperatures that are too low and a corresponding relative overactivity of the hydroquinone at temperatures that are too high. These two developing agents affect film contrast differently; thus the temperature of the developing solution affects radiographic contrast. The higher the temperature, the shorter the time needed to develop the film. A chart listing the time-temperature relationship is usually supplied by the manufacturers of processing solutions.

Exposed films are sometimes developed by sight. The films in the developer are repeatedly observed with the safelight and are considered developed when the image of the object is clearly seen. Film in this condition appears cloudy because of the unexposed crystals in the emulsion. Developing of exposed film by sight is not recommended except in known overexposure of the film by x-rays. The time-temperature system of developing is superior to the sight or visual method because it is the only practical way that a controlled, standardized, and consistently accurate film-developing process can be achieved.

Fixing

After it is developed, the film is rinsed in water for at least 30 seconds and is then placed in the fixing solution. Rinsing is done to remove the alkaline developer on the surface of the film and film rack and to prevent its being carried over to the acid fixer, where it would deteriorate the fixing solution. The contents of a typical x-ray fixer and the action of each chemical in its solution are listed in Table 1-6.

The developed film is left in the fixer for a total of 10 to 15 minutes, but the radiograph can be used prior to total fixing. This matter is discussed more extensively in Chapter 9. The fixer solution removes all of the unexposed or undeveloped silver halide crystals and rehardens the emulsion, which has

Table 1-5. Radiographic developer

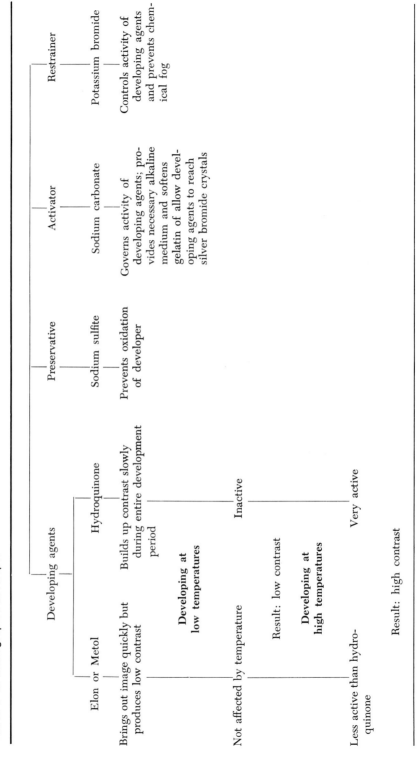

Table 1-6. Radiographic fixer

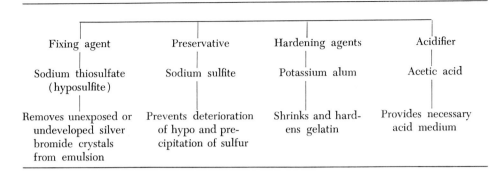

Fixing agent	Preservative	Hardening agents	Acidifier
Sodium thiosulfate (hyposulfite)	Sodium sulfite	Potassium alum	Acetic acid
Removes unexposed or undeveloped silver bromide crystals from emulsion	Prevents deterioration of hypo and precipitation of sulfur	Shrinks and hardens gelatin	Provides necessary acid medium

softened during the developing process. When a quick view of the x-ray image is necessary, the film may be read wet. The film must be placed in the fixer until it clears (the unexposed areas become transparent); it may then be removed from the fixing solution, rinsed in water, and taken into the light for viewing. Such a film, if kept wet, can be left in an average illuminated room for hours; however, it must be returned to the fixing solution to be permanently fixed. Failure to properly fix films permits any residual silver halide crystals in the emulsion to give the film a fogged appearance. In addition, sufficient time in the fixer is necessary to harden the emulsion.

After fixing, the film is washed in running water for 20 to 30 minutes. The time varies with the rate of water flow. Washing removes the chemicals of the fixing solution from the emulsion. Failure to wash a film properly will result in chemical stains producing a brown discoloration after a period of time. The film is dried in a dust-free area; circulating dry air that is warm but not hot is used. The dried films are mounted in film mounts or are stored in envelopes. Sharp corners on films should be rounded before the film is stored. Sharp corners can scratch other films when more than one film is placed in the same envelope. The value of the radiograph as a permanent record cannot be overemphasized.

CHAPTER 2

Factors relating to the production of the radiograph

A multitude of factors enter into the production of a radiograph. In the main, the quality of the radiograph and the safety of the patient and operator are the two most important aspects to be considered. Factors related to radiation hazards and protection are discussed in Chapter 4. The factors pertaining to radiographic quality that are of interest to dentists are presented in this chapter in three basic groups: (1) factors related to the radiation beam, (2) factors concerning the absorbing media or object, and (3) factors pertaining to the recording of the roentgen image of the object. The reader should be aware that subject matter in this chapter is interrelated with that in Chapters 1 and 3.

RADIATION BEAM FACTORS

Variations in the makeup of the x-ray beam greatly influence the quality of a radiograph. These factors pertain mostly to the x-ray machine. The operator has little control over the actual x-rays.

Exposure time

Exposure time is the interval during which the x-rays are being produced. A change in any one factor involved in the production of a radiograph can basically be compensated for by an adjustment in one of many other factors. The factors that can be varied or adjusted easily are usually exposure time, kilovoltage peak (kVp), and milliamperes (mA) (Table 2-1). In dental radiography, exposure time is the factor most commonly used to compensate for changes in other variables because exposure time is most easily understood and most easily changed. It is quite common to see radiographic technics standardized to the point that only the exposure time varies.

Present thinking about exposure time intervals is discussed on p. 10. Exposure time and milliamperage exert direct control over total photon production. These two factors often are multiplied to form a common factor of milliampere seconds

Table 2-1. Approximate relationship of kVp and mA to exposure time

mA°	Exposure time	kVp°	Exposure time
5	2	55	2
10	1	65	1
15	⅔	75	½
20	½	90	¼

°All other variables are constant.

(mAS). In the future, the common factor is likely to be milliampere impulses (mAI). However, although changes in exposure time do not affect other radiographic factors, changes in milliamperage do modify other variables, for example, the effective kilovoltage or wavelength of the x-ray beam. For this reason, exposure time and milliamperage are dealt with separately. Note that mAS is a measure of total photon production and not a measure of energy. To measure total energy of the beam for any exposure, one must also consider the effective wavelength or energy of the photons in the beam.

The effect of exposure time on the quality of a radiograph is seen mainly in density. The greater the exposure time, the greater are the total photon production and the resultant film density. The relationship of exposure time to film density seems to be frequently misunderstood. Film density alterations from a usable but *very* light to a *very* dark film and vice versa require exposures that vary by a factor of approximately eight times. Thus, to bring a very light film to an optimal density, the exposure time must be increased by three or four times. To reduce the density of a very dark film to the optimal level, the exposure time must be reduced to one third or one quarter of the prior time. Within this range, the operator must make a judgment concerning any required exposure time changes. Changes of 20% from a prior exposure are ordinarily not noticeable to the human eye. Density is defined and discussed in Chapters 1 and 3.

To a limited degree, contrast also is affected by exposure time. Contrast increases with increased film exposure. However, various levels of illumination must be used to observe this contrast, which can lie in very light or very dark areas of the radiograph. One can relate the effect of exposure time to contrast from another aspect. The human eye can see things only within a certain range of densities and contrast. If a film has had too much or too little exposure time, the densities of parts of the radiograph may be too dark or too light, respectively, to fall within the range of human vision. In such cases, parts of an object shown in a radiograph may not have enough contrast to be seen properly. For all practical purposes, contrast is not affected by exposure time as long as the film density is reasonable. Contrast is defined and discussed in Chapters 1 and 3.

Milliamperage

Milliamperage is measured in the high-voltage tube circuit. Milliamperage relates to the amount of electricity passing through the filament circuit of the x-ray tube. The filament current controls successively the temperature of the filament in the x-ray tube, the size of the electron cloud, the current in the high-voltage circuit, and the number of x-ray photons·produced by the tube; in other words, it controls the rate of x-ray photon production. As stated before, when coupled with exposure time (mAS), milliamperage directly affects total photon production and thus the density of the radiograph.

Kilovoltage

Kilovoltage or kilovoltage peak (kVp) refers to the potential difference between the anode and cathode of the x-ray tube. The higher the kVp, the greater is the potential difference between the anode and cathode and the greater is the energy of the photons produced. These shorter wavelength, high-energy photons result in an x-ray beam with more penetrating power. Higher kVp's are used when the object to be examined is thick or has great density. Kilovoltage also changes the number of x-ray photons produced. Thus, increased kVp produces more useful photons in terms of penetration and a greater tube efficiency on the basis of photon quantity per unit of time.

Exposure time is affected by kVp. An increased kVp increases the number of photons; and since some individual photons carry more energy when kVp is increased, fewer photons are needed to expose the film to the desired density. Proper film density is easily accomplished by reducing the exposure time, but it also can be readily accomplished by reducing the milliamperage or increasing the tube-film distance. For practical purposes, the relationship of exposure time to kVp on dental machines is such that an increase of approximately 15 kVp necessitates halving of the exposure time; conversely, a reduction of 15 kVp means that the exposure time must be doubled to maintain proper film density.

Radiographic contrast, or the contrast of an object seen in the radiograph, is affected by kilovoltage. The lower the kVp, the greater is the contrast. The higher the kVp, the longer is the scale of contrast. Increased kilovoltage also increases the amount of scattered radiation and thus further reduces the visible contrast of the radiograph through the production of film fog (see p. 44).

The effect of kilovoltage on x-ray absorption by the object is of importance. The film needs a certain amount of energy in order to be exposed. When more penetrating x-rays are used, x-ray energy reaches the film with less absorption by the object. This x-ray property can be stated as follows: the higher the kVp, the lower the skin dose and the greater the depth dose of x-rays. This property is used extensively in deep x-radiation therapy. In extraoral radiography, this property is of value in reducing the x-ray exposure of the patient. However, in intraoral radiography, in which the film is in the oral cavity, increased kVp, while reducing the x-ray exposure of the tissues between the film and the source of radiation, increases the exposure to the tissues behind the film. In terms of total energy absorbed by the patient in intraoral radiography, increased kVp probably has only a small total effect on patient dose reduction.

Tube-film distance

The distance from the x-ray tube or target (radiation source) to the film greatly affects the intensity of radiation at the film position. This relationship is stated in the inverse square law. The effect of distance on exposure time is easily calculated if the inverse square law is applied in a slightly different manner. Obviously, if the intensity of radiation is reduced, the exposure time must be increased to maintain proper film density. In other words, exposure time is inversely proportional to radiation intensity (photons per unit area). Now, by using the inverse square law, one can see that exposure time is proportional to the square of the distance measured from tube to film. For example:

$$\frac{\text{Old exposure time}}{\text{New exposure time}} = \frac{\text{old distance}^2}{\text{new distance}^2}$$

This formula can be applied whenever the tube-film distance (TFD) or exposure time needs to be changed. Other factors such as mA and kVp must be kept constant when this formula is applied.

The effect of tube-film distance on the radiation dose to the patient is of interest whenever the tube is close to the patient and the film is relatively far from the tube. For instance, envision a situation in which the tube is 1 inch from the patient's skin and the tube-film distance is 8 inches. If the tube is moved 1 additional inch away, an increase in exposure time for the film will probably not be necessary. However, the exposure at the skin per unit area is reduced by

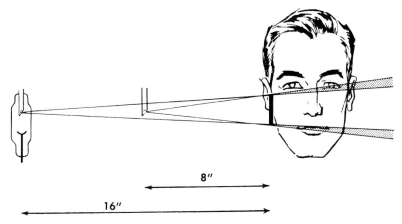

Fig. 2-1. Diagram showing the amount of tissue irradiated by the primary beam of radiation when the tube-skin distance (TSD) is 16 and 8 inches. The exposed skin area near the tube is the same for both distances. The shaded area depicts the increase in tissue being irradiated by the shorter TSD.

approximately 75%. In x-ray therapy, long tube-skin distances (TSD) are used for treatment of deep lesions and short tube-skin distances, for surface lesions. In extraoral diagnostic radiography, long tube-film distances assist in reducing patient exposure.

In intraoral radiography, an increased tube-film distance reduces the total amount of tissue within the primary beam of radiation. This is because the x-rays originate from a small source (focal spot) and diverge to form the cone of radiation. When the size of the beam of radiation at the patient's skin is kept constant by the use of different collimators (see p. 78, and also pp. 71 and 72), the closer the tube is brought to the skin, the more the primary beam diverges behind this skin area and the more tissue is irradiated (Fig. 2-1).

The interrelationship of mA with TFD is the same as the interrelationship of exposure time with TFD (as TFD changes either or both mA and exposure time must be changed). For practical purposes, changes in TFD do not affect kVp, but it is quite common to see changes in TFD related to mAS. It should be noted that when the TFD is increased, the x-ray beam covers a larger area at the film position. Control over beam size at the film position must be exercised through the use of a collimator, which is a device that limits the diameter of the x-ray beam.

The tube-film distance consists of tube-object plus object-film distances. Both of these distances play an important part in radiographic quality. The role of these distances in diagnostic radiography and radiation protection is discussed in Chapters 3 and 4.

Focal spot size

It is desirable in diagnostic radiography that the size of the focal spot or source of x-radiation be as small as possible. Dental x-ray tubes use a rectangular focal spot (line focus) to produce the x-ray photons over a large surface area. Its use prevents overheating and damage to the target of the x-ray tube. When this spot is projected (in other words, when the spot is seen from any point within the beam of radiation), it appears as a square, the sides of which measure approximately the same as the short side of the rectangular focal spot. This projected or effective spot shape and size are determined by the manufacturer. Such a design provides maximum x-ray production for a given tube while maintaining a more or less symmetrical and small focal spot for the x-ray beam (Fig. 1-6).

The size, or more specifically the effective size, of the focal spot is important in making x-ray pictures, or radiographs. The role of focal spot size in this aspect of radiography is discussed in Chapter 3. It should be noted that the operator exercises no control over the actual size of the focal spot in the dental x-ray tube. However, any movement of this spot during exposure of the x-ray film causes the source of radiation to be larger, as far as the film is concerned. The head of the x-ray machine must be stabilized in order to provide the smallest possible source of radiation.

Collimation

In diagnostic radiography, collimation refers to control of the size and shape of the x-ray beam. The opening in the shield of the head of the x-ray machine through which the beam emerges is usually circular; it could be rectangular. If the opening is circular, the radiation beam is cone shaped. A rectangular opening creates a beam having the shape of a pyramid. A basic rule of radiation hygiene calls for the use of a radiation beam that is as small as practical. The beam should cover the area or object being examined and should be larger only to the extent of allowing for small errors in the alignment of the beam, object, and film. For intraoral radiography, the diameter of a circular beam of radiation at the patient's skin need be no greater than 2¾ inches. If a rectangular beam is used, its dimensions at the skin should be approximately 1½ × 2 inches. Use of rectangular collimation necessitates rotation of the collimator to accommodate for films placed either horizontally or vertically. These dimensions allow for easy coverage of intraoral periapical film and are ordinarily satisfactory in fulfilling the purposes of occlusal film use. For extraoral radiography, the beam should be collimated to be only slightly larger than the area being examined.

One of two methods of collimation is usually employed in dental radiography: (1) diaphragms (round or rectangular) or (2) metal cylinders, cones, and rectangular tubes. Further comments about collimation in this chapter relate primarily to circular x-ray beams; rectangular collimation is discussed on pp. 17 and 71. Examples of round collimation accessories are shown in Fig. 2-2. The *diaphragm* consists of a metal plate or disk usually made of 4-pound* lead. A hole is cut in the *exact* center of the disk to allow the x-ray beam to escape. The shape of the beam is determined by the shape of the hole in the diaphragm. The diaphragm, like all collimators, is placed over or in the opening in the head of the x-ray machine through which the useful beam emerges. The placement of an additional or new diaphragm is easily accomplished. In most machines, the diaphragm can be retained by the removable cylinder or cone. *Metal cylinders* or *cones* are open at both ends and allow the x-rays to pass through. The shape of the outer opening of the cylinder or cone determines the shape of the radiation beam. The sides of the collimating cylinder or cone need not be as thick as a diaphragm, because the x-rays penetrate the material at an angle. A thin metal cone can present the same amount of material as a thicker barrier (diaphragm) placed perpendicular to the radiation beam. Metal cone collimators usually are made of steel; in addition to collimating the beam, they are very effective in absorbing the scatter radiation coming from the filter.

The required dimensions of either the end of the metal cone or the hole in the diaphragm are easily determined for any desired beam size if the position of the focal spot in the machine head is known. It is a simple matter to draw on a piece of paper the shape of the desired beam from the focal spot to the position

---

*Four pounds to the square foot, that is, approximately 1/16 inch thick.

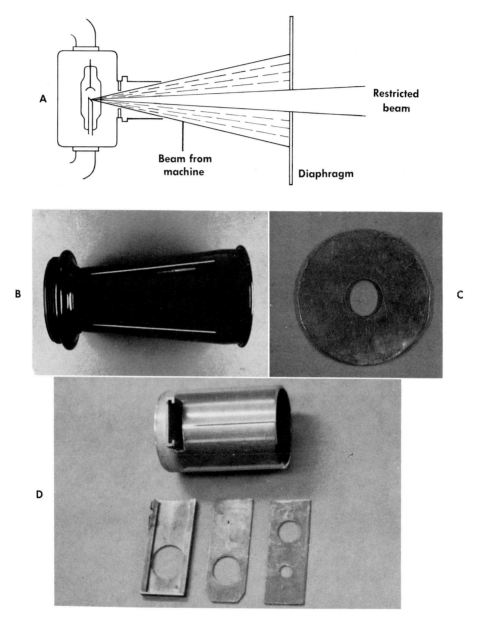

Fig. 2-2. A, Diagram illustrating beam diameter reduction. The diaphragm can be supplanted by a metal cone or cylinder of the same diameter as the hole in the diaphragm. **B,** Metal cone and, **C,** typical lead diaphragm. Another approach to x-ray beam collimation is seen in **D.** A lead-lined plastic cylinder in which a grooved receptacle has been permanently installed is shown. A sample receptacle is shown below (left). The hole in the receptacle is centered exactly in the center of the cylinder, and the lead inserts shown below (center and right) are inserted into the groove and held in a constant position. The holes in the insert must be centered exactly in the center of the receptacle opening. Illustrations in Chapter 7 show the device in use.

where the desired beam size is required. The beam drawing will give the correct measurement of the desired beam of radiation at the position of the diaphragm or outer cone opening. A new diaphragm or cone can be made to these dimensions.

To determine the position of the focal spot, a large film is exposed at any known film position. The film is processed, and the size of the beam shown on the radiogram is measured. By drawing the resultant beam size measurement and the diaphragm opening measurement at their respective positions, it is possible to draw in the beam shape and find the position of the focal spot or source of radiation (Fig. 2-3). If a large film is not available, one can substitute smaller films taped together in the shape of a cross. Different-shaped metal markers, for example, paper clips and coins, can be placed on the small films before the exposure is made. These markers permit the operator to reassemble the films in their proper positions after processing. A modification of this method using a single small film is also practical. Two straight pins are placed parallel to each other and a short distance apart on cellophane tape or paper; the tape or paper is placed over the diaphragm opening. A small film is exposed and processed. The distance between the images of the pins seen on the radiograph is measured. The focal spot position is now determined from the various known measurements: the ratio of the distance measured between the pins and between the images of the pins is the same as the ratio between the focal spot–diaphragm and focal spot–film distances (Fig. 2-3).

When the x-ray beam size is restricted to the smallest possible dimensions, the amount of tissue being irradiated can be held to a minimum. Also, the pro-

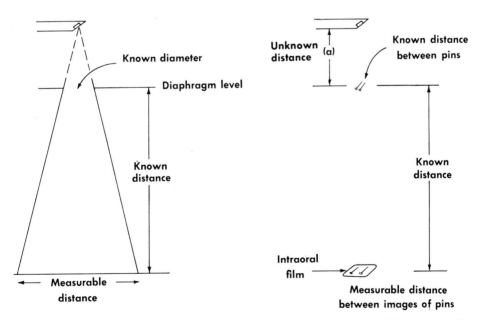

Fig. 2-3. Technics for determining the position of the focal spot in relation to the diaphragm.

duction of secondary radiation fog (see p. 44) is minimized and a radiograph with little fog density is produced.

Filtration

The x-ray beam from a dental machine consists of photons of many different wavelengths. The beam thus has a polychromatic spectrum. The shortest wavelength and most penetrating x-rays are determined by the kVp. The beam contains many long wavelength x-rays that possess little ability to penetrate calcified tissues. These long wavelength x-rays are of little value since they cannot reach the film in practical amounts and actually constitute a hazard; they contribute appreciably to the x-ray dose of the patient. X-ray beams used in dentistry should be filtered by 1.5 to 2.5 mm. of aluminum (equivalent) total filtration. A more accurate way of measuring the quality of the x-ray beam is by determining its half-value layer. Dental x-ray beams should have a half-value layer of at least 2 mm. of aluminum.

When filtration is increased, the x-ray beam is hardened. In other words, the half-value layer is increased or the effective wavelength of the beam is decreased. The effect on film quality is an increase in the scale of contrast. Density is affected because increased filtration also results in absorption of some of the useful penetrating x-rays. When filtration is increased, a slight increase in exposure time is sometimes needed. Filtration is increased by placing one or more sheets of commercially pure aluminum of the desired thickness in the path of the x-ray beam. Filters usually are placed at the base of the pointed or open-end cone. This is also the position of the diaphragm; these two parts of the machine are usually found together. When metal cone collimators are used, the filter must be placed at the inner end of this cone, a desirable procedure because the filter produces secondary x-rays when the primary x-rays pass through it. The patient is effectively protected from this secondary radiation if the filter is placed at the inner end of a collimating metal cone.

Equipment efficiency

Dental x-ray machines vary in both construction and efficiency. The quality and quantity of the x-ray beams thus vary from machine to machine, even at similar mA, kVp, and exposure times; mA and kVp meters may not register correctly, and timers may be inaccurate. It is more accurate to evaluate a machine's x-ray beam by its intensity of radiation and its half-value layer. Because of the variation in efficiency between machines, it is not unusual to find that one machine requires more or less exposure time than another machine to radiograph the same object.

OBJECT FACTORS

The object being examined is basically an x-ray–absorbing medium. As such, two factors play an important role in radiography of the object. These factors are (1) thickness and (2) density of the various parts of the object. When an x-ray beam passes through an object, an x-ray or roentgen image of the object is produced. The film is the means by which one records and observes this roentgen image. The quality of the roentgen image is reduced or masked by secondary radiation; the production of these radiations by the object is therefore of importance. Note that the radiograph is a picture of a three-dimensional object and that various structures are superimposed on each other. The amount of any one tissue through which the x-ray beam has to pass to reach the film varies with the shape of the object and the direction of the x-ray beam.

Object thickness

The film requires a certain amount of radiation to form a latent image. The thicker an object, the more radiation is needed to get through the object to the film. Usually radiation is increased by increasing the mA and/or exposure time. This assumes that the x-rays have the ability to penetrate the object or, in other words, that the percentage of x-ray absorption by the object is not unduly great. Such is the case when 60 kVp or more are used in the examination of teeth and jaws. When the object thickness is greatly increased, it is often advisable to use the higher kVp's. Higher kVp's reduce the exposure time and minimize image blurring because of movement. A reduction in exposure time also can be accomplished by increased mA and/or film speed. Note that the operator has no control over the thickness of the object with the exception that, in some instances, the x-ray beam can be directed at the object from a more favorable direction. Secondary radiation produced while the object is being exposed increases with increased object thickness.

Object density

Object density refers to the weight per unit volume of the object. In dental radiography, object density is a very interesting factor. The diagnostic intraoral radiograph is used to show changes in the enamel. Enamel has the highest density of all body tissues, and the x-rays have to penetrate, in posterior teeth, approximately 8 mm. of this material. The same intraoral radiograph is expected to show small changes in the thin bony lamina dura surrounding the tooth. Lesions in the enamel and the lamina dura produce changes in the amount of x-ray absorption by these structures. These changes must be of a sufficient magnitude if the film is to record them. As a result, intraoral film density is usually a compromise between a less exposed film that will show periodontal lesions optimally and a more exposed film that will show carious lesions more clearly.

X-rays are absorbed proportionately to the total mass through which they pass. This total mass is calculated by multiplying the effects of the thickness and density factors of the object. Thus a small amount of enamel may absorb the same amount of x-rays as a great amount of soft tissue. In such a case, these two objects would produce the same film density on a radiograph. In intraoral radiography, the calcified tissues are usually shown and the soft tissues are not seen. However, when there is enough soft tissue to absorb sufficient x-rays to create an image, these tissues begin to appear on the radiograph. Such is the case when the shadows of the nose and lips appear on intraoral radiographs.

The density of the tissues being examined plays an important part in the creation of film fog due to secondary radiation. With dense objects, the secondary radiation produced is greatly absorbed in the object itself. The result is that soft tissues tend to produce more secondary radiation fog on a film than do hard tissues. This effect is easily seen if one compares a radiograph made of a patient's head with one made of a dry skull.

Object density affects the total mass that the x-rays have to penetrate. Like thickness of the object, increased object density also necessitates an increase in the mA, kVp, or exposure time factors.

Soft tissues vary little in density. They all approximate the density of water. Thus, changes in soft tissues are not observed on the usual dental radiographs. However, when much less x-ray exposure is used and/or there are gross soft tissue changes, these changes may appear in a dental radiograph. Thickness of and secondary radiation from soft tissues are the important factors to be considered when soft tissues are present in the field under examination.

IMAGE-RECORDING FACTORS

When an x-ray beam passes through an object, an x-ray, or roentgen, image of the object is produced. This image is recorded in the form of a latent image by the film. The latent image becomes a visible image when the film is processed. The basic factors that affect the recording of the roentgen image are the following: (1) reduction of secondary radiation, (2) films and film storage, (3) intensifying screens, and (4) film processing.

Reduction of secondary radiation

The presence in the roentgen image of any secondary radiation (including scattered, stray, leakage, or any other radiation not belonging to the primary beam) is undesirable. This secondary radiation reaches all parts of the film and produces film fog in the radiograph. When the radiograph is viewed on an illuminator or view box, film fog appears to the diagnostician as though a masking mist or thin veil were present between his eyes and the image on the film. Since the major portion of secondary radiation originates in the object itself, most protective devices are aimed at reducing the secondary radiation coming from this source.

In intraoral radiography, the production of secondary radiation is minimized through the use of as small a beam of x-rays as possible. Proper collimation of the x-ray beam is mandatory in dental radiography. The film packet, whether it is intraoral, a cardboard film holder, or a metal cassette, has a sheet of x-ray–absorbing material behind the film. After the x-rays pass through the film or film-screen combination, they are of no further use in radiography. These unwanted rays are absorbed partially or totally by the metal backing behind the film. Not only is living tissue behind the film protected from being unnecessarily irradiated, but also secondary radiation production behind the film is reduced. In addition to this, much of any secondary radiation produced in areas behind the

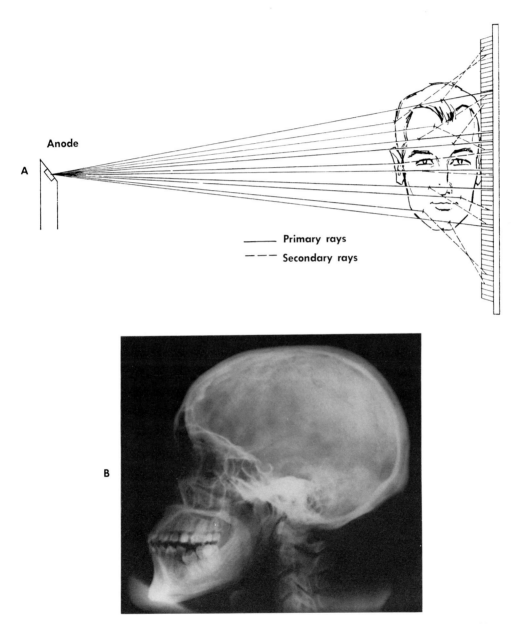

Fig. 2-4. A, Diagram illustrating the use of a grid in reducing secondary radiation reaching the film. **B,** Radiograph produced without use of a grid.

Continued.

film because of the primary beam being larger than the film is prevented from reaching the recording medium.

In extraoral radiography, the same methods used for reducing secondary radiation in intraoral radiography are also utilized. However, two additional methods are also of practical importance. These methods involve the use of a stationary or moving grid. A grid is a sheet of radiolucent material in which is

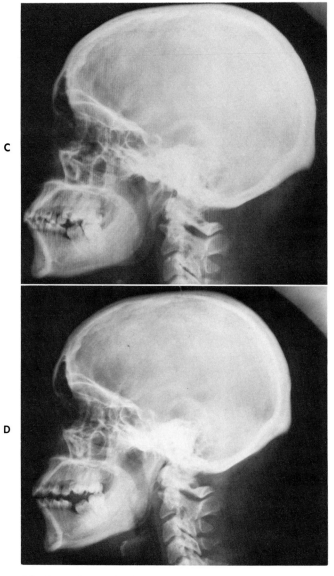

Fig. 2-4, cont'd. C, Radiograph showing typical grid lines. **D,** Radiograph produced using a Potter-Bucky diaphragm.

embedded strips of lead (Fig. 2-4). The strips of lead all slant toward a point some distance away. This point is where the anode of the x-ray machine must be placed. Grids are designed to operate at a particular tube-grid distance. The grid is placed between the object and the film. When used correctly, the grid allows most of the x-rays originating from the anode and passing through the object without a change in direction to reach the film. However, most of the secondary radiation originating in the object and traveling in all directions is absorbed by the lead strips. One objection to the stationary grid is the production of white lines, representing the lead strips, on the finished radiograph. When a grid is used and much of the secondary radiation reaching the film is removed, the exposure time has to be increased, in many cases as much as three times.

In order to obtain a radiograph with the use of a grid but without the grid lines, the grid can be moved in front of the film during film exposure. Such a moving grid is called a Potter-Bucky diaphragm. The grid is moved at a constant speed beginning just before film exposure and ending after the exposure. Since the lead strips are positioned over different areas of the film at different times, they will not appear on the finished radiograph; however, because of the grid shift, the exposure time is almost double the time of a stationary grid.

The effectiveness of a grid in reducing secondary radiation is dependent on the ratio of the distances measured on the radiolucent material between the lead strips. The ratio of the depth of this material to the distances measured between

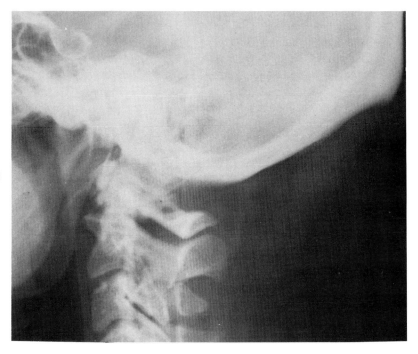

Fig. 2-4, cont'd. E, Enlarged section of **C.** Note grid lines.

the lead strip, for example, 8:1, determines the ability of the grid to reduce secondary radiation. The greater the grid ratio, the more effective is the grid; however, the greater the ratio, the more accurate the operator must be in getting the anode or source of radiation in the correct position.

Films and film storage

Radiographic films consist of a transparent base coated with a sensitized emulsion of uniform thickness. The sensitive element of the emulsion consists mainly of silver bromide crystals. These crystals are sensitive to white light; thus x-ray films are kept in lighttight packets or containers. X-ray films can be divided into two types: those very sensitive to x-rays, such as the intraoral and nonscreen films, and those very sensitive to the visible light given off by screens, that is, screen films.

The number and thickness of the various emulsions are of importance. Films coated with an emulsion on both sides of the base require only one half the x-ray exposure needed by a single emulsion film to produce the same film density. Similarly, if thicker emulsions are used, as is the case with nonscreen films, more x-ray–sensitive material is present and less exposure time is needed to give a useful film density. Remember that thicker emulsion films need increased processing time.

Radiographic films vary in speed and contrast. Of these two factors, speed is more important because film contrast varies little between the several films available to the dental profession. Such is not the case with film speeds. A multitude of dental films varying greatly in speed are available to the dentist (see Chapter 1). The faster the film, the less is the amount of x-radiation needed to expose it and to produce a radiograph of useful density. The use of less radiation reduces the radiation hazard to patient and operator; the use of fast films in this respect is of considerable importance.

In the main, the faster the film, the greater is the size of the silver grain in the finished radiograph and the less is the sharpness of the radiographic image. However, the increase in grain size ordinarily is imperceptible to the viewer's eyes. When fast films are used, it is extremely important that proper processing procedures be carried out. Fast films are affected more easily by errors in darkroom technic.

When very fast dental films are used, radiographs can be made with exposure times as short as $\frac{1}{30}$ second. Many x-ray timers are not accurate for such short exposures. However, these films can still be used, and the benefit of radiation dose reduction can be obtained by adjusting other factors. One easy method is to use less mA; another is to increase the tube-film distance.

Film storage is very important if films are to be kept unfogged for any length of time in the dental office. The chief dangers to stored film are excessive temperature, excessive humidity, and exposure to chemicals and stray radiation. Films should be stored in a cool place. Since the darkroom should be cool, it is quite convenient to store films in the darkroom. Films should not be stored where stray radiation from x-ray machines or radioactive materials can reach them. Films can be protected from these radiations by being stored in a steel- or lead-lined box. In the x-ray room it is important that unexposed and exposed films be stored in metal dispensers and containers. Several makes of these x-ray accessories are available commercially.

The expiration dates of stored films should be noted, and films should be used before these dates. It is good practice to use the oldest of the stored films first and not to store more films than is necessary. Film storage in the darkroom is discussed in Chapter 9.

Intensifying screens

Intensifying screens consist of tiny calcium tungstate crystals bonded in a uniform layer on a firm base. These screens generally are used in pairs with a double emulsion screen film between. The screens contact the film; this contact is maintained by the use of metal boxes or cassettes that have a spring arrangement to ensure screen-film contact. The screens are permanently fixed inside of the cassette. Firm contact is important because unsharp radiographs are produced when screen-film contact is poor. The calcium tungstate crystals fluoresce when struck by x-rays and emit a blue light. The screen film is very sensitive to this blue light and is exposed rapidly by it. This method of recording the roentgen image of an object requires much less radiation as compared to when the x-ray film alone is used.

Screen film in screen cassettes is used when x-ray film alone would require an excessively long exposure time and result in an appreciable amount of patient irradiation, as when thick body parts such as the skull are to be examined. The image seen in screen films is slightly less sharp than that seen in nonscreen films. However, the shorter exposure time results in much less patient movement; thus, movement unsharpness is greatly reduced.

Screens vary in speed. In other words, they vary in ability to produce blue light because of variations in the thickness of the layer of crystals and in the size of the crystals. The thicker the layer of crystals and the larger the crystals used, the faster is the speed of the screen. Thin crystal layers are used in the screen that is between the film and the object. This allows the x-rays to get through to the film and to the screen behind the film. Thick crystal layers are used on screens placed behind the film in order to capture as much as possible the roentgen image of the object. Large crystals are more efficient than small crystals. However, large crystals expose larger areas of the film with their light, and a reduction of radiographic image sharpness results. The operator must select the proper screens for a particular projection, and the choice is a compromise between the need for image sharpness and the need for reduced exposure time.

In selecting screens, it is necessary to know the relationship of the speeds of the screens. The medium or par-speed screen is most commonly used. Both films and screens are energy dependent. Within the kilovoltage range commonly used in dentistry, Patterson screens, in comparison with light-sensitive x-ray film used without screens, have an approximate intensification factor as follows: detail screens, ×10; par-speed screens, ×30; and high-speed screens, ×50. The speed factor depends on the screen and film being compared. Radiographic density is not the only quality affected by the use of screens; contrast is also affected. Contrast is greater when screens are used. In other words, the scale of contrast is reduced or shortened and can be compensated for by an increase in kVp. Care and cleaning of screens are discussed in Chapter 9.

Film processing

Film processing is very important in the production of a radiograph. All the care and time taken in exposing a film can be lost by poor processing technic. Proper film processing makes visible all of the latent image without producing artifacts; high-quality radiographs cannot be produced without satisfactory dark-room equipment and a good processing technic. Proper developing is accomplished over a time-temperature range. The optimum time and temperature for developing films is usually 4½ minutes at 68° F. When films are developed at higher temperatures, the contrast of the radiograph is increased; conversely, when developed at lower temperatures, radiographs show lowered or a longer scale of contrast. If films are not developed for the full length of time required by a specific temperature, the radiograph lacks density. Should density be correct under such conditions, the operator is overexposing and underdeveloping the films. Properly exposed films do not visibly increase in density when the developing time is increased as much as 50%. However, excessive developing time results in increased fog.

When a radiograph is properly rinsed, fixed, and washed, the unexposed areas appear clear and transparent. When any of these processing steps are done with insufficient time, the film may contain unexposed silver bromide crystals or other chemicals, and the film will be discolored either immediately or with the passage of time. Film left in the fixer solution over long periods of time loses some of the silver forming the radiographic image. The result is a radiograph that has lost density.

Many errors can occur during film processing. Many different artifacts can be produced by faulty film processing; some of these are shown along with other types of artifacts in Chapter 3. The fundamentals of film processing are discussed in Chapter 1; film-processing technic is described in Chapter 9 with other procedures and considerations pertaining to the darkroom.

The radiograph

The diagnostic radiograph is the end product of the proper use of dental x-ray equipment. When satisfactory x-ray machine, film, and darkroom equipment are available and are properly used, radiographic quality depends mainly on the ability of the clinician to expose the film properly. The understanding of film exposure technic is based on a knowledge of the ideal radiographic projection. In this chapter the ideal radiographic projection is discussed, the factors affecting radiographic quality are summarized, and some common artifacts seen in radiographs are demonstrated.

IDEAL RADIOGRAPHIC PROJECTION

The objective of radiography in dentistry is to cast shadows of dental structures in such a way that these shadows will be most informative. The ideal radiograph thus demonstrates certain image qualities. These qualities are (1) an image that is sharp, (2) an image that is shaped like the object, and (3) an image that is of the same size as the object.

In order to achieve the best possible results, five principles pertaining to projection geometry should be observed during film exposure. These principles are as follows:

1. Source of radiation should be as small as possible.
2. Tube-object distance should be as great as possible.
3. Object-film distance should be as small as possible.
4. Film should be parallel to an easily identifiable plane of the object.
5. Central ray of the beam of radiation should be perpendicular to the film.

The first three principles deal with the production of image sharpness. The other two require the alignment of the x-ray beam, object, and film in such a manner that the radiographic image of the object can be easily identified and easily evaluated. Desirable machine, object, and film relationships are shown in Fig. 3-1.

In projection geometry, the sharpness of a shadow is determined by three factors. These factors deal with the size of the *penumbra or partial shadow*. It must be remembered that this initial unsharpness is increased in the finished

51

radiograph by such items as grain size of the film, use of screens, and movement of the patient. Only factors pertaining to penumbra formation are discussed in this chapter.

The penumbra is that part of a shadow of an object that is larger than a point and yet represents a single point on the object. The penumbra is thus the amount of unsharpness of the image. When visible light projects a shadow of an opaque object, only the edges of the object show unsharpness because the light does not penetrate the object. That part of the shadow where all of the light is absorbed is called the *umbra*. The umbra is thus the area of total shadow and the pe-

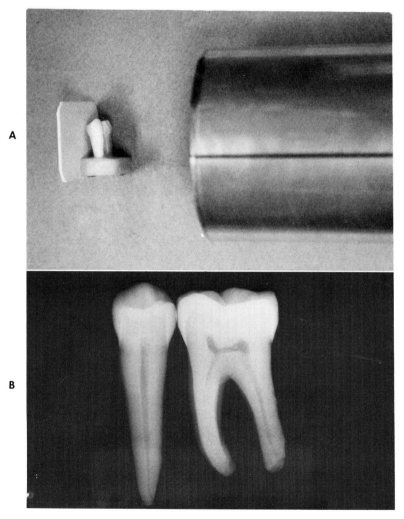

Fig. 3-1. A, Ideal machine, object, and film relationship for radiography of teeth. **B,** Radiograph of two teeth showing the radiopaque enamel and radiolucent pulp chamber.

numbra, the area of partial shadow. In radiography, umbras exist only where the object or parts of the object essentially absorb all of the x-rays.

The penumbra is created by the size of the source of radiation and is affected by the tube-object and object-film distances. This principle is shown in Fig. 3-2. Since x-rays travel in straight lines, a source of radiation that is infinitely small would cast no penumbra. However, a point source is not possible with x-ray tubes; as a result, penumbra formation will inevitably result. The larger the source of radiation, the greater is the unsharpness of the image. Note that when the head of the x-ray machine shakes during the exposure of the film, the effect is an increase in the size of the source of radiation. The closer the source of radiation is to the object, the greater the size of the penumbra at the film position. The opposite is true for the relationship of the film and object. Here, when the object is brought closer to the film, the size of the penumbra is reduced.

In intraoral radiography, the film should be positioned parallel to the long axes of the teeth, a relatively easy vertical plane to identify when the patient is sitting in a chair. Concurrently the film should be positioned parallel to the buccal surfaces of the teeth being examined. This horizontal plane is also easily

Text continued on p. 62.

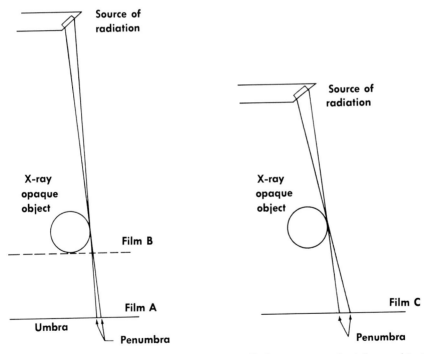

Fig. 3-2. Penumbra formation. Maximum object–radiation source and minimum object–film distances reduce the size of the penumbra, as does a small source of radiation. Alterations in object–radiation source distances are shown.

Table 3-1. Basic effects of radiographic factors

Factor	Density	Contrast* (scale of)	Sharpness	Distortion
kVp	Increases with kVp	Increases with kVp		
mA	Increases with mA			
Exposure time	Increases with exposure time			
Films	Increases with increased film speed	Varies with make of film	Decreases with larger grain size	
Screens	Increases	Decreases	Decreases with larger grain size and thicker film	
Screen-film contact			Decreases with poor contact	
Processing	Increases or decreases	Decreases with increase in temperature		
Fog	Increase with increase in fog production	Decreases with increase in fog production		
Grids and collimation	Decreases	Increases (by fog reduction)		
Filters	Decreases with increased filtration	Increases with increased filtration		
Object	Decreases with thickness and density	Decreases with thickness; varies with density	Decreases with thickness	
Target-object distance	Decreases with greater distance		Increases with greater distance	Magnification decreases with increased distance
Object-film distance	Decreases with greater distance		Decreases with greater distance	Magnification increases with greater distance
Focal spot size			Decreases with increased size	
Movement (tube, film, or object)			Decreases	
Alignment (tube, film, and object)				Decreases with proper alignment

*Contrast ranges from black to white (clear). The scale of contrast within the range can be short or long. High or short-scale contrast is seen in a film that is predominantly black and white. Low or long-scale contrast is seen in a film that shows many intermediate gray tones between black and white. *In this table, an increase in contrast means a lengthening of the gray scale;* an increase in contrast means a low contrast, *not* a tendency toward a black and white or high-contrast film.

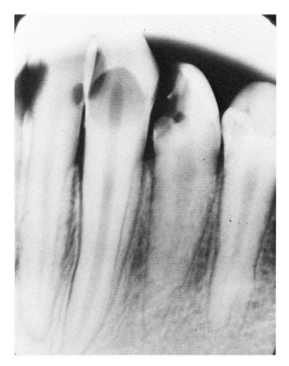

Fig. 3-3. Cone cut. The clear, unexposed area resulted because the beam of radiation did not completely cover the film (in addition, this film was not placed sufficiently deep in the floor of the mouth to receive the shadow of the cuspid apex).

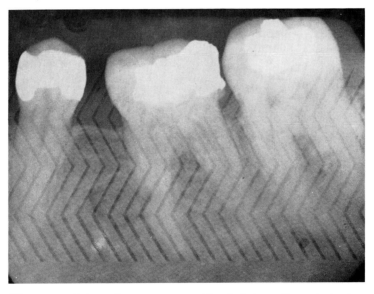

Fig. 3-4. Film exposed through nonexposure side. A light radiograph having a herring-bone or some other characteristic pattern results when the film is placed with the non-exposure side toward the teeth.

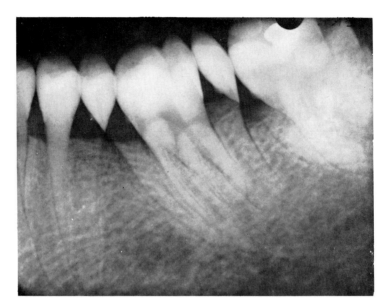

Fig. 3-5. Double exposure. Excessive density and two images result when a film is exposed twice.

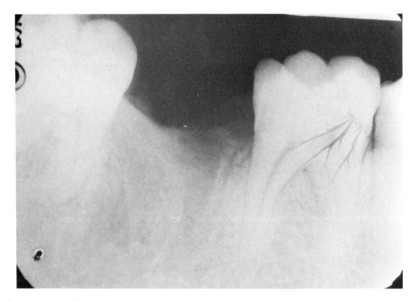

Fig. 3-6. Static electricity. Multiple black linear streaks can result if static electricity is produced when films are forcefully unwrapped or if the film is flexed to make it less stiff.

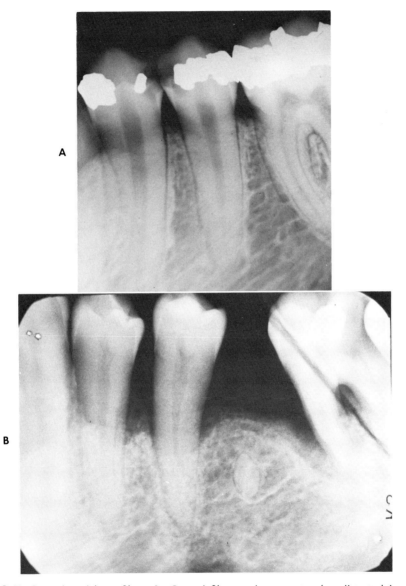

Fig. 3-7. Curved and bent films. **A,** Curved film produces a streaky, distorted image. **B,** A black line occurs where the film is bent.

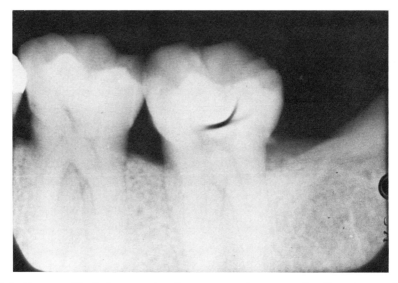

Fig. 3-8. Pressure. Black lines result when pressure is put on the film. Fingernails often cause such pressure marks (this film was also not placed sufficiently deep in the mouth to receive the tooth shadow completely).

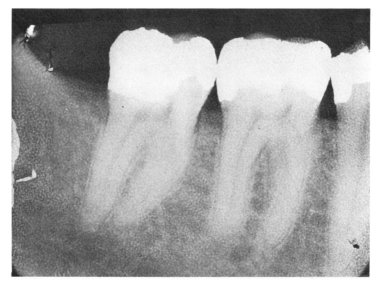

Fig. 3-9. Reticulation. The film emulsion often cracks when subjected to great changes in temperature between the different processing solutions. The temperature variation must go from warm to cold.

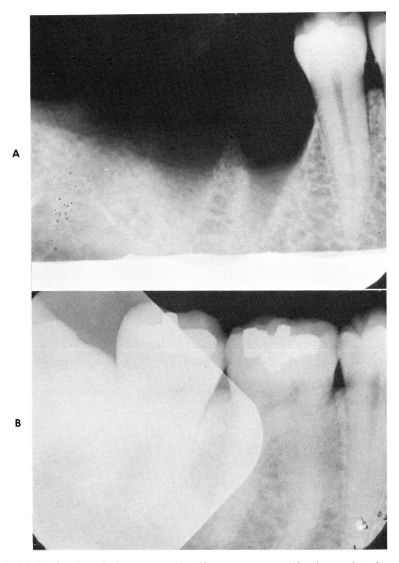

Fig. 3-10. Undeveloped clear areas. **A,** Clear area caused by incomplete immersion of film in the developer. **B,** Clear area caused by films sticking to each other while in the developer. A similar appearance can occur if the film sticks to the side of the tank.

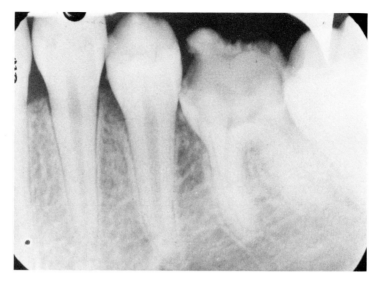

Fig. 3-11. Unexposed areas. Bits of heavy metal between the tube and film, for example, metal chips in the pointed cone, prevent film exposure. This radiograph shows a clear area because of the presence of a piece of lead foil backing in front of the film in the film packet.

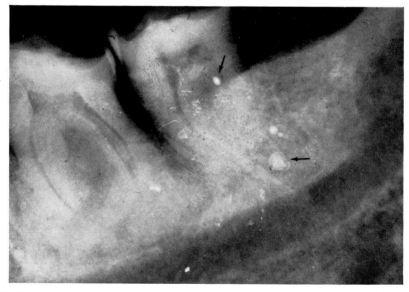

Fig. 3-12. Undeveloped areas. Accumulation of dust, air bubbles, or drops of fixer on the film surface can prevent proper development. White dots or marks result.

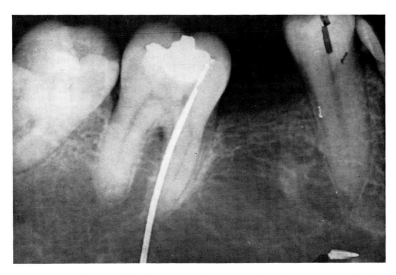

Fig. 3-13. Scratched films. White lines result if the emulsion is scratched off the film base. Careful examination of the surface of the film will differentiate these lines from other white or clear lines.

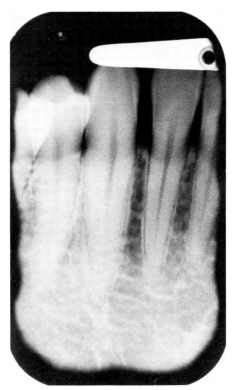

Fig. 3-14. Wet and leaking packets. Black, exposed borders are due to light entering a poorly sealed film wrapper. White smudges, when present, can be due to wet paper in the packet sticking to the emulsion during developing.

identified. The central ray of the beam of radiation should be directed perpendicular to the film in both horizontal and vertical planes so that a shadow of the teeth is shaped like the teeth; in other words, the image of the object is not distorted. These shadows are easily identified and evaluated.

RADIOGRAPHIC QUALITY

Radiographic quality or the diagnostic quality of the image seen in a radiograph is affected by the density, contrast, sharpness, and amount of distortion of the radiographic image. In radiography, the term *density* refers to the overall blackening of the film. *Contrast* or gradation is the difference in density between the areas of the radiograph that have different densities. *Sharpness* or resolution is the ability of the radiograph to define the images of objects clearly. The terms *detail* and *definition* are often used synonymously with sharpness and resolution. However, *detail* is sometimes used to denote image unsharpness caused only by film factors, whereas *definition* is sometimes used to denote image unsharpness caused by projective geometry. *Distortion* is the change in the shape of the image as compared to the object. *Magnification* of the image is sometimes spoken of as false distortion. All x-ray images are magnified and suffer from some distortion because of unequal magnification of the various parts of the object. Those factors of practical importance that affect radiographic density, contrast, sharpness, and distortion are given in Table 3-1. The above qualities are discussed in Chapters 1 and 2. Table 3-1 summarizes prior comments.

ARTIFACTS

In any evaluation of a radiograph, film faults and artifacts must be considered. A multitude of errors can be made during the production of a radiograph; however, some occur more often than others. Some of the more common film faults and artifacts are shown in Figs. 3-3 to 3-14. Other quite common ones, not shown, are (1) distorted images from improper alignment at the tube, object, or film; (2) finger marks from improper handling of the film, especially when the emulsion is softened during processing; (3) chemical stains from an unclean darkroom, chemicals on the operator's hands, or insufficient washing of the film; (4) blurred images from movement of the object, film, or tube during film exposure or from poor screen-film contact; (5) dark or light films from errors in any one of the factors controlling density; (6) unexposed areas from blemishes on intensifying screens; and (7) completely clear films because of a malfunctioning machine or because of placing films in the fixer first instead of in the developing solution.

The question of whether an area on a radiograph represents an artifact is answered easily in most cases. The simple procedure of making another radiograph of the same area usually resolves the problem.

CHAPTER 4

Hazards and protection

Complete coverage of the hazardous effects of ionizing radiation on vital tissue would require more pages than can be devoted to the subject in this text. The purpose of the discussions that follow is to provide (1) a basic understanding of phenomena related to radiation hazards and (2) a knowledge of radiation protection methods applicable to people associated with the dental office. In addition, the need for and the scope and advisability of legally established regulatory measures governing the use of ionizing radiation in dental offices are discussed.

By way of introduction and for purposes of emphasis, it is important to criticize the casual attitudes of those practitioners who have not observed fundamental precautionary measures. These practitioners apparently have not suffered untoward effects and are complacent. Actually, they have no way of detecting minor physical alterations. Furthermore, they can make no estimate of the shortening of the life-span and of genetic changes as these factors concern themselves and their progeny. A callous attitude of some practitioners can breed casualness in other practitioners. Hopefully, the discussion in this chapter will encourage concern and care for all persons who are subjected to x-radiation in dentistry.

National and international position statements about radiation effects and levels of radiation that are tolerable for man (risk estimates) vary. Although all agree that exposure to ionizing radiation should be minimized, methods of quantifying radiation effects and differences in philosophy among groups of scientists lead to variations in published documents. These controversies are discussed in the 1975 National Council on Radiation Protection and Measurements (NCRP)* Report No. 43, entitled *Review of the Current State of Radiation Protection Philosophy.* The NCRP is among the groups having differing concepts.

From a practical standpoint, dentistry need only take the position that all necessary steps will be taken to limit patient and office personnel exposure to x-radiation. Such steps include the use of modern x-ray equipment (or the modernization of older equipment when necessary), the production of high-quality

---

*7910 Woodmont Avenue, Washington, D.C. 20014.

63

radiographs (excellence of chairside and darkroom technic) using the most sensitive film emulsions available, and a certainty that radiographic interpretive competency is optimum. No exposure to x-radiation should be permitted without expectation of a commensurate benefit. Aspects of x-radiation use delegated to auxiliary personnel are the responsibility of the dentist. He must lead his office staff in being certain that the risk-versus-benefit equation is weighted heavily toward excellence of health service. This text is designed to help the profession accomplish this objective.

RADIATION—ITS EFFECT ON LIVING TISSUE

The effects of radiation on vital tissues vary over an extremely broad range because of many diverse physical and biologic circumstances. Two generalizations can be made:

1. Ionization is the underlying phenomenon by which changes occur.
2. All ionizing radiation is hazardous, but the degree of hazard varies materially.

This section is designed to provide an understanding of basic concepts that relate directly to advocated protection procedures for the dental office. We hope that this knowledge will assist the practitioner in negating the concern about radiation exposure expressed by many intelligent patients. The following factors are emphasized: ionization, direct and indirect effects of ionizing radiation, tissue variability, whole-body radiation as compared to specific-area radiation, individual variability, latent period, radiation of genetic tissues, and effects on somatic tissues.

Ionization

Ionizing radiation, of which x-radiation is only one type, affects living tissue through a process that causes electrically stable atoms and molecules to become electrically unbalanced. Briefly, all living substances are composed of atoms arranged together in a particular fashion known as molecules. Each atom, and hence each molecule, has an electrical stability or balance; the number of positive charges equals the number of negative charges. When a quantum of ionizing radiation strikes an electron in a molecule of living tissue, it may displace this particle and leave that specific molecule with an electrical imbalance. The molecule or, if one prefers, the atom making up a part of the molecule has now been ionized. The bulk of the molecule has one more positive charge than negative charges, and one electron from the molecule or a fractionated segment of the molecule exists as a separate entity. A strong tendency exists for atoms to seek electrical stability. The atom or molecule may accept a negative charge from somewhere else and in so doing may form a new chemical. Under such circumstances, the cell of which the molecule is a part can be altered. Or, as shown in Fig. 4-1, substances not compatible with body tissue may be produced. The basic effect of ionization is molecular alteration and creation of new chemicals.

The human body is composed of an infinite number of molecules, each made up of a complex system of atoms. Each atom is composed of a nucleus and orbiting electrons. Living tissue is largely a void through which a quantum of radiation energy can pass without touching anything. Should a quantum strike a subatomic particle, it probably would not destroy the cell of which that specific particle is a part. The degree of cell alteration probably depends on the essentiality of the irradiated cellular substance. In any event, there are many more similar cells; the destruction of a single cell would not have an observable deleterious effect. Subjective symptoms occur only when the amount of radiation is sufficient to damage a relatively large number of cells that either are irreplace-

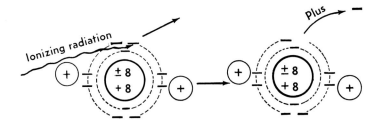

Ionizing radiation disrupts the electrical balance of water by displacing one electron and creating an ion and a free electron (water less one electron and a free electron).

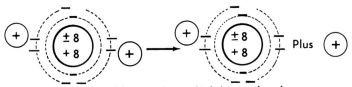

The electrically unstable water ion which has a plus charge makes itself electrically stable by liberating a positive ion (in this case the nucleus of the hydrogen atom).

Free radicals (i. e., elements with neutral charges and with unpaired orbital electrons) will go to any extent to pair their electrons.

The two free radicals shown below combine by pairing their unpaired electrons to form H_2O_2.

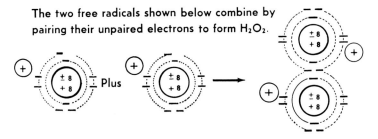

Fig. 4-1. Bombardment of water by ionizing radiation can result in many breakdown products. A typical reaction, the production of H_2O_2 from H_2O, is illustrated.

able or have been damaged in such numbers that the remaining cells cannot take over the functions of the destroyed units in an adequate fashion.

Direct and indirect effects of ionizing radiation

The effect of ionizing radiation on tissues may be (1) direct or (2) indirect. Direct effects are those caused in a specific area by radiation. Exposed cells or various-size segments of tissue are altered *directly* by ionization. If the cell is to die from radiation effects, it usually does so at the time of mitotic division.

Indirect effects may exhibit themselves in several ways. It is entirely possible for substances that are incompatible with body tissues to be produced through the exposure of tissue to ionizing radiation. An example of this is the conversion of water to hydrogen peroxide (Fig. 4-1). The hydrogen peroxide, rather than the radiation, causes cellular dysfunction. A second example of an indirect effect is the chemical alteration of certain important body secretions. Radiation can alter the chemical composition of enzymes, inhibitors, hormones, and so forth, and make them partially or perhaps totally ineffective. The indirect effect is related to the amount of radiation exposure.

Tissue variability

Certain tissues are more susceptible to ionizing radiation than are others. The degree of susceptibility in most instances appears to be related to cellular differentiation and to the rapidity of cellular reproduction. The following tissues and organs are listed in the order of their susceptibility.
1. Blood-forming tissues and reproductive cells
2. Young bone, glandular tissue, and epithelium of the alimentary canal
3. Skin and muscle
4. Nerve tissue and adult bone

Although not as sensitive as some tissues to radiation, certain specialized body areas cannot reproduce themselves. Thus the amount of ionizing radiation received by such cells must be limited. Discussions with both professional and lay people about the effects of ionizing radiation must be preceded by a clear understanding of the amount and type of tissue to be irradiated.

Whole-body radiation

Whole-body radiation, as the term implies, is radiation that exposes the entire body. A rad of whole-body radiation means that each gram of tissue in the entire body receives 1 rad of irradiation. Under normal clinical circumstances, even in instances in which large portions of the body are being radiated for therapeutic purposes, it is not conceivable that the entire body would be exposed. It is obvious that the effects of ionizing radiation directed simultaneously at all the cells of the body would have a more profound general effect than would radiation limited to a smaller area. Considerations relative to whole-body radiation are of no practical importance to the dentist except that they serve to delineate whole-body from specific-area radiation.

Specific-area radiation

The use of x-radiation in dentistry is directed to a small segment of the body. Only a limited number of the total body cells are exposed to ionizing radiation. In medicine, larger body areas are often involved. Even in therapy, the exposure is directed toward a predetermined part of the living organism and is limited in coverage to a degree consistent with the necessary treatment. The effect on an *individual cell* is basically the same whether the whole body or a specific area is irradiated, but the effect on the entire organism increases with the number of exposed cells. A rad of specific-area radiation means that *each* gram of tissue *in the irradiated area* receives 1 rad of irradiation.

Individual variability

Some people are more susceptible to disease processes than are others. The ability of individuals to respond defensively against bacteria and viruses varies. In a similar manner, animals of the same species show different abilities to cope with ionizing radiation. This can be illustrated by an experiment in which 100 mice are simultaneously exposed to sufficient whole-body radiation so that 50% of them die in a specified period. This dose is known as the median lethal dose (LD 50). Of these 100 mice, a certain percentage will die if given only one half or one fourth of the LD 50 dose. Others will live in spite of having been given this dose. For some reason not entirely known at present, certain of the mice are more able to resist effects of ionizing radiation. It is important for users of ionizing radiation to recognize that individual variability does exist and that rules governing the use of ionizing radiation must be oriented toward those people whose ability to resist is minimum.

Latent period

It also is important for the practitioner to understand the term *latent period*. The latent period is that period of time interposed between exposure and clinical symptoms. The latent period, for example, of excessive exposure to sunlight is measured in terms of hours. The skin does not redden as soon as it is exposed to sunlight. Erythema and discomfort from sunburn become evident only hours after exposure. The latent period for x-radiation varies with the dose. The more severe the dose, the shorter is the latent period. The latent period for some minimum exposures to x-radiation is as long as 25 years. The existence of this latent period is another reason for caution when ionizing radiation is used.

Radiation of genetic tissues

Except for a limited number of tissues, all cells reproduce themselves. However, relatively few cells are responsible for the reproduction of the race. Those cells that control progeny must be considered separately from somatic cells because of their reproductive role. The human race has evolved over many generations. Mutations, most of them unfavorable, have occurred as a result of probably three basic factors: heat, chemical change, and effects of natural or background radiation emanating from the earth and the cosmos. The law of "survival of the fittest" has caused the unfavorable mutations to be lost and has supported the continuance of beneficial alterations. The relative degree to which alterations from heat, chemical reaction, and radiation have had a role in human evolution is not presently well understood. Whatever the effect of ionizing radiation, it is now clear that such effects probably will be increased with the increased use of ionizing radiation.

Prior to the discovery of x-radiation and radioactive materials, the human population was subjected to only natural radiation. During the last half century, gonadal radiation has increased gradually for all human beings, particularly those having high standards of living. This increase has resulted from an expanded use of x-radiation for both diagnostic and therapeutic purposes, plus an increased use of radioactive materials for therapeutic, industrial, and military needs. Such activities are beneficial; they have actually prolonged human life. But, concurrently, they are adding to the role of radiation in evolution. If the evolutionary effects of radiation are minimal, then this increase is probably of little importance. On the other hand, if radiation has had an important role in creating evolutionary changes, any increase of gonadal radiation is probably of considerable importance. Although research is being directed toward this problem, it is likely that definitive information may become known only through observation of progeny. We in this generation have a responsibility to our progeny. Superimposed on this type of thinking is the fact that the law of "survival of the fittest" no longer is as dominant as in earlier times. We protect those members of the human race who are mentally or physically deficient and assist them in reproducing themselves.

At the moment, geneticists are concerned about the effects of ionizing radiation on the genes of the reproductive cells. The number of gene alterations in one generation, which are passed on to the next generation, can be increased by further exposure to ionizing radiation. For the most part, altered genes appear to be recessive in character. When the male and female reproductive cells unite, the dominant genes determine the characteristics of the new organism. However, recessive traits can appear in future generations through the pairing of recessive genes. Observable results of gonadal exposure from ionizing radiation can lie hidden for a number of generations. The geneticist's concern does not center about the reproductive results of persons living today unless they have been subjected to relatively massive doses of ionizing radiation. Concern is for future generations.

Effect of radiation on somatic tissues

Somatic tissues include all cells of the body other than the reproductive cells. Under normal circumstances, such cells reproduce themselves. Changes in these cells are unrelated to progeny. The effect of ionizing radiation on somatic tissues is that of alteration or destruction of particular cells. Should a large number of somatic cells be irradiated, the individual might die because of the inability of certain tissues to function properly. Ordinarily, however, the degree of cellular alteration is such that, to a greater or lesser degree, other cells can compensate for the radiation-affected units; this is particularly true for diagnostic radiography. Repair of the altered cells will be approximately inversely proportional to the degree of exposure. It is entirely possible that a threshold dose may exist, below which there will be no detectable effect from ionizing radiation. In the upper ranges of radiation exposure, it is likely that the effect and the degree of repair will be related to the amount of exposure until lethal levels are reached. Tissues that have been substantially exposed are more susceptible to subsequent radiation insult than similar tissues exposed for the first time.

PROTECTION FROM X-RADIATION HAZARDS

The increased use of x-radiation during the past several decades and the anticipated further use of ionizing radiation for health, military, and economic purposes suggest the importance of using all possible means to protect individuals from the deleterious effects of man-made ionizing radiation. This must be done concurrently with the use of ionizing radiation in man's behalf. Until recently, the responsibility for protection of the public lay in the hands of those persons who used the radiation—in the health sciences, the physician and the dentist. Now, because of the increased use of ionizing radiation for other than health science purposes, it has become the responsibility of public health authorities to regulate for the protection of those who cannot protect themselves. The health science professions have not been subjected to any regulatory measures other than those relating to physical facilities. Rather, they have been encouraged to become knowledgeable about protection methods and to exercise the prerogative of regulating their own actions without interference. It is expected that, if the professions respond properly, there will be no need for the enforcement of public health regulations insofar as health science professions are concerned; if they do not, regulatory legislation probably will develop. Protective measures must be instituted for the patient, the operator of x-ray equipment, and any associated personnel, including individuals in adjacent offices and occupants of the doctor's reception room.

Protection of the patient

Patient exposure to x-radiation through routine dental office procedures can be minimal. When the deleterious effect from exposure is balanced against the available diagnostic information obtained from the radiographic film, there is no question about the fact that the patient gains through the judicious use of x-radiation. In reality, the dentist probably malpractices when he fails to use x-radiation as needed. Concurrently, the dentist has the responsibility of minimizing patient exposure. It should be noted that many patient protection procedures also will improve film quality and reduce the total exposure received by the operator and other associated personnel.

Patient irradiation is reduced through use of high-speed films, adequate collimation, suitable filtration, use of proper exposure and developing technics, care in film placement and angulation, use of extended-cone and high-kilovoltage technics; and the use of protective aprons. Inadequate interpretation renders x-radiation use unjustifiable.

Film speed. As noted in Chapter 1, dental intraoral films currently available vary in speed by a substantial factor. Still faster films may be manufactured. Available films are quite similar in quality and appear to meet the diagnostic needs of the dental profession.

Extraoral films are generally of two types—screen and nonscreen. Screen film is designed to be used with intensifying screens, whereas the no-screen or non-screen film is planned for use in a suitable cardboard film holder. To a limited extent, film speeds vary among manufacturers within each of these two categories. The dentist or physician has little choice as to the type of extraoral film he will use other than that of deciding whether he prefers screen or nonscreen film. Nonscreen film exposes the patient to a greater amount of radiation, but this increase is justified (1) if diagnostic results are superior and/or (2) if technical aspects are simplied. Films produced with intensifying screens are of a higher contrast than those produced with nonscreen film.

The American National Standards Institute, in cooperation with film users, retailers, manufacturers, The American Academy of Dental Radiology, and the American Dental Association, has developed an American National Standard Speed Classification for Intraoral Dental Radiographic Film. Various speeds of intraoral films are listed under alphabetical groupings from A through F in Table 1-3 (p. 25). Table 1-4 (p. 25) lists dental film by speed. It is in the best interest of the patient to use the fastest possible film. The use of high-speed film requires greater care on the part of the operator since these films are more sensitive to all factors that contribute to film fog and artifacts. Extreme care must be taken in film exposure and processing. Precautions must be taken to store high-speed films at the retailers and in the dental office in strict accordance with the manufacturer's directions. Films must be processed in a clean darkroom in which the safelighting is not excessive, and they must be processed in clean, strong solutions according to the manufacturer's directions.

X-ray machine modifications. The use of high-speed films may not be compatible with the usual short-cone technics unless some modifications are made in the dental x-ray machine. This is caused by the inability of the x-ray timers, particularly the mechanical, spring-wound timers, to produce sufficiently short exposure time intervals. Several low-cost alterations can be made to older x-ray machines so that highly sensitive film can be used.

One simple method is to use an extended cone. As mentioned earlier, doubling of the target-film distance requires that the exposure time be quadrupled. A film that is four times as fast as a previously used film requires the same exposure as the former film if the distance is doubled. Methods for determining proper exposure procedures are discussed later in this chapter.

An alternative to the extended distance is to reduce the milliamperage. Dental x-ray machines are commonly operated at 10 mA. If the dental machine does not have a variable milliamperage control on the panel board, it is possible for servicemen to reduce the milliamperage by making suitable modifications inside the machine.

Another method is to add aluminum filtration in addition to the usually recommended 2.25 mm. of aluminum equivalent total filtration in order to necessitate increased exposure time. Increased filtration reduces the amount of radiation in the usable beam per unit of time. Thus, increased exposure time does not increase patient x-radiation exposure. Sufficient filtration can be added so that older timers become practical for use with fast film.

An alternative to these suggestions is the purchase of an electronic or synchronous timer that permits exposures as low as $\frac{1}{20}$ or $\frac{1}{30}$ second.

Collimation. Collimation of the x-ray beam is accomplished through the use of metallic cones or lead washers suitably placed in the path of the primary x-ray beam. This procedure is discussed in Chapters 1 and 2. Collimating devices do not materially reduce the amount of radiation received by the exposed tissues, but they do reduce radiation to those tissues that surround the area being examined by preventing unnecessary beam divergence. It is recommended that the diameter of the radiation beam used for intraoral dental film be no more than $2\frac{3}{4}$ inches at the skin surface. A beam of this diameter is more than $\frac{3}{8}$ inch wider than the greatest dimension of any periapical film. Some individuals advocate the use of rectangular diaphragms. Although this minimizes exposure of surrounding tissues, it necessitates very accurate beam positioning and rotation of the diaphragm to accommodate vertically and horizontally placed film as well as changes in head positioning. Rectangular collimation can also be obtained through the use of film holders to which is attached a facial shield (Fig. 4-2). The rectangular aperture in the shield limits the beam size. In addition, the steel film backing further limits radiation exposure behind the film. Rectangular tubes able to rotate on a turret can be used rather than circular lined cylinders to accomplish the same purpose (Fig. 4-3). Surveys of dental x-ray equipment show that the diameter of the exposure area at the skin in a few dental machines is as great as 8 to 10 inches. Many unmodified older machines have beam diameters of 4 to 5 inches.

As a result of collimating the x-ray beam, the operator may find that films appear to be cone cut (Fig. 3-3). If this is true, the operator is not justified in removing the diaphragm but is responsible for improving his technical proficiency. Cone cutting suggests that the operator is not directing the x-ray beam properly or that the diaphragm or x-ray tube has shifted in position in such a way that the x-ray beam is not centered over the diaphragm aperture. If the former is true, the operator must improve his technical proficiency. A malaligned diaphragm can be repositioned by the operator. Sometimes it may be necessary to construct a new diaphragm. A trained serviceman is required to reposition the x-ray tube.

A test for determining tube position is simple. A lead diaphragm having an aperture of no more than ¾ inch is used, and the center of the cone is placed on a marked spot in the center of an extraoral film (a cross of intraoral films can be substituted, as suggested in the discussion of collimation in Chapter 2 and Fig. 2-3). When the center of the cone is in position, an exposure is made and the film is developed. A circular exposure area that was centered on the previously marked spot should be observed after processing. If the circle is off center, either the hole in the diaphragm, the diaphragm itself, or the x-ray tube was not properly located. To retest, remove the diaphragm. Place the cone in the center of another film. The circle of exposure can now be determined by the aperture in the tube head itself. The tube should be centered over this aperture, and the exposd circle should be in the exact center of the film.

It may be necessary to change the collimation procedure for certain extraoral technics. It is obvious that the radiation beam must cover the area being examined. In general, it is important that the amount of tissue exposed to radiation be minimized without reducing tissue coverage to a size that precludes obtaining

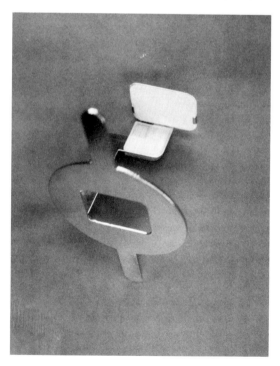

Fig. 4-2. Film holder and facial shield that produces a rectangular x-ray beam configuration prior to tissue exposure. (Courtesy Precision X-ray Instrument Co., Nashville, Tenn., and Dr. Fred Medwedeff.)

necessary diagnostic information. Collimating cones and diaphragms can be purchased from dental supply houses or can be fabricated by the dentist. A technic for fabricating the lead diaphragm is given in Chapter 2 in the discussion of collimation.

Filtration. Radiation that cannot reach the film has no diagnostic value. Such radiation has undesirable tissue effects because it is attenuated in tissue somewhere between the skin surface and the film. It becomes important to filter out of the primary x-ray beam those x-ray photons that have little or no chance of reaching the x-ray film because of their absorption by soft tissue.

This type of unusable radiation is easily eliminated by the use of aluminum filters. In medical therapeutic installations and industrial work, filters made of

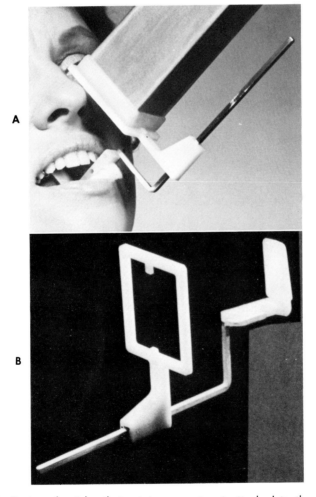

Fig. 4-3, A, Rectangular tube that rotates on a turret attached to the x-ray tube head. **B,** Film-holder beam-localizing device used with the collimator. (Courtesy Rinn Corp., Elgin, Ill.)

materials having greater densities, such as copper, are employed. In dental machines, commercially pure aluminum disks measuring approximately 0.5 mm. in thickness are interposed in the x-ray beam until the total filtration is 2 to 2.5 mm. of aluminum equivalent. Filtration is discussed in Chapters 1 and 2.

The filter should be recessed as far as possible behind the diaphragm opening. The area and thickness of the filter affect the amount of scatter radiation reaching the gonads of the patient. The smaller the filter area (for example, the long-cone diaphragm has a smaller filter area than does the short-cone diaphragm), the less scatter radiation will reach the gonads of the patient.

The dentist has two methods for determining when he has reached the proper amount of aluminum filtration. The first method is to determine the amount of inherent filtration in the machine (Table 4-1) and then add external filtration to bring the total filtration to the level suggested. It is pertinent that most machines produced since approximately 1960 are equipped with adequate filtration. In our opinion, the second method for determining the amount of needed added filtration is preferable. Aluminum measuring approximately 0.5 mm. in thickness* is cut so that it can be superimposed over the aperture in the

---

*Aluminum in sheet form such as that used for cooking purposes is satisfactory as long as it is smooth and labeled pure or commercially pure aluminum.

Table 4-1. Inherent filtration data*

Name of x-ray machine	Equivalent inherent filtration (mm. Al)
General Electric	
CDX Models E, 70 and 90	1.50
Ritter	
Models B and Dual-X	0.50
Model E (Century)	2.00–2.25
Universal	0.5 –0.75
Weber	
Raydex	0.50
Westinghouse	0.70
X.R.M.	
Models 2 and 3 (before 1956)	0.75
Models 2 and 3 (since 1956)	2.00
Model 90	2.00
Fisher (open and closed tube)	0.50?†
Philips Oralix	1.00
Prof-Ex-Ray	0.50?†
Ritter Models A, C, and D	0.50
Victor	0.75
Weber (to Model 11)	0.50
Weber Model 12	0.50?†

*From Wuehrmann, A. H.: Radiation protection and dentistry, St. Louis, 1960, The C. V. Mosby Co. First part of table from Richards, A. G., and others: X-ray protection in the dental office, J.A.D.A. 56:514-521, 1958; second part of table from Barr, J. H., and Brockman, M. K.: Radiation dosage in dental offices, Oral Surg. 13:696, 1960.
†Author apparently unable to confirm these findings.

lead diaphragm. Exposures are made of a particular area of the mouth, using increasing thicknesses of aluminum at constant mAS and kVp values. Although it is preferable to use an x-ray phantom, it is reasonable to make four or five exposures of the same area in the mouth of a patient over the age of reproduction. The films made with the successively added thicknesses of aluminum are processed together and are examined. Films showing a noticeable decrease in density indicate that the filtration used to produce them was excessive; that is, the filtration materially reduced the amount of radiation reaching the film. Filter thicknesses should be added until they cause a noticeable reduction in film blackness. The effect just described is illustrated in Fig. 4-4. Most states legally

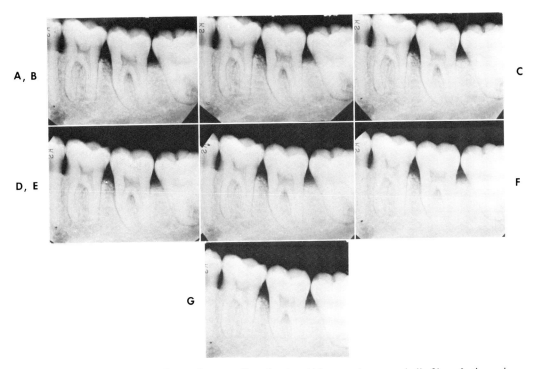

A, B   **C**

D, E   **F**

G

Fig. 4-4. Filtration and its effect on film density. Using a phantom skull, films **A** through **G** were exposed as follows: **A,** no filter and no pointed plastic cone; **B,** no filter but pointed plastic cone in place; **C,** 0.5-mm. aluminum filter added, plus pointed cone; **D,** 1-mm. aluminum filter added plus pointed cone; **E,** 1.5-mm. aluminum filter added plus pointed cone; **F,** 2-mm. aluminum filter added plus pointed cone; **G,** 2.5-mm. aluminum filter added plus pointed cone. Other constant exposure factors included 65 kVp, 10 mA, 3/4-second exposure, 0.5 mm. aluminum inherent filtration, Kodak Ultra-Speed film, a target-film distance of 22 inches, and an ionization chamber–target distance of 20 inches. The ionization chamber readings made on the surface of the simulated skin during exposure were as follows: **A,** 0.5 R; **B,** 0.38 R; **C,** 0.30 R; **D,** 0.25 R; **E,** 0.20 R; **F,** 0.17 R; **G,** 0.15 R. Total filtration to 2 mm. aluminum equivalent **(E)** does not produce any visually observable reduction in film density.

require a definite minimum amount of filtration. The dentist must be certain that he conforms with the laws in his state.

There is another concept of filtration about which the reader should be aware; this concept is not yet in vogue but may have merit. The ratio of skin exposure to film exposure (the amount of radiation necessary to produce a radiograph of suitable density) should be of concern to the user of x-radiation. When low kilovoltages and small thicknesses of filtration are used, this ratio escalates in comparison with low kilovoltages used with relatively large thicknesses of filtration. This is true even though it becomes necessary to use long exposure times to compensate for radiation loss caused by the increased filtration. Conversely, the ratio of skin exposure to film exposure does not vary nearly as widely when high kilovoltages are used with different thicknesses of filtration. Thus some knowledgeable individuals have suggested that filtration should be increased with decreasing kilovoltage and, conversely, could be decreased with increasing kilovoltage. This concept is directly in opposition to current policy.

Exposure and developing technics. Excessively long exposure times have sometimes been used in an effort to reduce development time. Even though this procedure results in films of inferior diagnostic quality, there previously was little reason to criticize as long as the operator obtained the necessary information. However, in view of efforts being made to minimize patient exposure, procedures of this type are now inexcusable. Developing technics are discussed in Chapter 9. The instructions of the manufacturer should be followed, and a time-temperature method for developing dental films should be employed.

The amount of exposure time necessary to produce films of maximum diagnostic quality varies with machines and with the kilovoltage and milliamperage employed. It is important to determine proper exposure times accurately for the x-ray equipment under one's supervision. After such factors as kilovoltage, milliamperage, distance, film speed, and so forth have been determined, a series of exposures are made. The mandibular molar area ordinarily is used because of the ease of film placement and because the exposure for this area is approximately average for all areas in the mouth. This series of exposures commences with an exposure time that definitely will result in a light film. The second exposure of the same area uses a 50% increase in exposure time. The third exposure uses a 50% increase of the exposure used to produce the second film. The 50% increase in exposure time over the prior film is continued until the resultant film definitely is overexposed.

These determinations preferably should be made on a phantom skull, but in the absence of a phantom, it is reasonable to use a dental patient who is past the age of reproduction. The accomplishment of this film series should require no more than five or six exposures. The exposed films are kept in order, are mounted together on a suitable rack, and are developed in new solution under time-temperature conditions recommended by the manufacturer. They are then rinsed, fixed, washed, and dried. The operator then observes the films and selects the film density most pleasing to him. The exposure used in producing this density is considered to be the proper exposure for the mandibular molar area. A series of films just described is demonstrated in Fig. 4-5, and the percentage changes necessary for proper exposure of other intraoral films, with the mandibular molar exposure as a baseline, are stated in Table 4-2. If high-kilovoltage technics are employed, it is possible to use a constant exposure time for the entire dentition. Exposure values for children and elderly persons may have to be decreased as

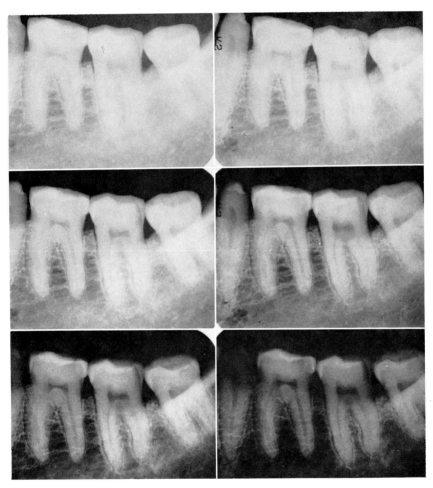

Fig. 4-5. Selection of optimum exposure times. Films ranging from minimum to maximum film density were exposed using a 16-inch target-film distance, 2.25 mm. aluminum total equivalent filtration, a diaphragm to limit the beam diameter at skin to 2.75 inches, 10 mA, 65 kVp, Kodak Ultra-Speed film, and the following exposure times: $\frac{1}{4}$, $\frac{3}{8}$, $\frac{1}{2}$, $\frac{3}{4}$, $1\frac{1}{4}$, and $1\frac{3}{4}$ seconds. All films were processed for $4\frac{1}{2}$ minutes at 68° F. on the same rack using fresh solution. A film density of choice can be selected from this group. It may be desirable to select an exposure time between any two of these intervals.

Table 4-2. Exposure variations based on correct exposure value for mandibular molar area*

Area	Increase or decrease from mandibular molar area exposure time (%)
Maxillary molars	+33
Maxillary bicuspids	0
Maxillary cuspids	0
Maxillary centrals	-15
Mandibular molars	0
Mandibular bicuspids	-15
Mandibular cuspids	-33
Mandibular centrals	-50
Posterior bite-wing film	0 to +15

*See Fig. 4-5.

much as 50%; exposure times for heavily boned or extremely obese people may in some cases have to be doubled.

Film placement and angulating procedures. One important radiation protection measure often overlooked is the degree of care used by the operator in placing films and in angulating the x-ray beam. Films should provide a maximum amount of diagnostic information without routine retakes. To have exposed the patient in producing inferior films is inexcusable in the light of present-day knowledge of x-radiation hazards. The technics for producing intraoral and extraoral films are discussed in Chapters 5, 6, and 7; darkroom processing is considered in Chapter 9. The need for meticulous adherence to acceptable technics is emphasized.

Distance and kilovoltage. It has been known for some time that the greater the radiation source–skin (hence film) distance and the higher the kilovoltage, the less radiation absorbed at or near the skin surface. Coincidental with a reduction in surface absorption is an increased radiation absorption in the deeper tissues. This knowledge is used constantly when radiation therapy is administered.

There is another important consideration related to distance (Fig. 2-1). With a constant exposure area at the skin (2.75-inch diameter for intraoral radiography), the shorter the radiation source–skin distance, the greater the volume of tissue exposed. For intraoral radiography, the tissue volume exposed for 16-, 8-, and 4-inch radiation source–skin distances varies by an approximate ratio of 1 to 1.5 to 2.5. This suggests greater patient exposure when shorter radiation source–skin distances are used, but data relating to situations of this type and to the role of kilovoltage in the integral (total) absorbed dose have not been available until recently. Recent research should be repeated and its scope expanded. Information to follow is based on presently available data, which, in addition to considering the role of distance and kilovoltage, also provide information on the use of the pointed plastic cone versus the open-end cylinder.

Any discussion of the effects of radiation source–film (or skin) distance and/or of variations in kilovoltage must assume, as a prerequisite, the production of radiographs of consistent density at a specific location in the mouth. Under controlled experimental conditions, it was found that the use of the pointed plastic cone, regardless of distance or kilovoltage, resulted in greater doses delivered to a phantom skull than did the use of the open-end cylinder. Radiation source–skin distances did influence the dose; the longer distances resulted in a lesser total dose. A kilovoltage of 90, as compared to that of 65, did not produce substantial differences in the total dose, but the use of 50 kVp with a 4.5-inch radiation source–skin distance and a pointed plastic cone resulted in a dramatic increase in the entrance (skin) dose and in the total dose. It is important to mention that the dose at the film surface (the amount of radiation necessary to produce a consistent film density) for the 50-kVp equipment was substantially greater than for equipment using either 65 or 90 kVp. Thus, film emulsion sensitivity may have influenced results. There is evidence that intraoral films are more sensitive to x-ray beams generated at 65 kVp, less sensitive at 90 kVp, and least sensitive at 50 kVp.

Lined cylinders. Unless fully justified by improved radiographic film quality, use of the traditional, pointed plastic cone is contraindicated. The plastic directly in the primary x-ray beam scatters radiation unnecessarily. An open-end plastic cylinder is preferable to the pointed cone as a position-indicating device, but it, too, will scatter any radiation that strikes it. Scattered radiation to the patient can be almost entirely eliminated by lining the inside of the cylinder with lead foil.

Non–lead impregnated plastic cylinders can be lined in the following manner: Lead foil 0.2 to 0.3 mm. (0.008 to 0.012 inch) thick is used. The foil usually can be purchased from a medical x-ray supply depot if it is not available through dental suppliers. A piece of lead foil is cut to a width of 9 inches (this assumes a cylinder having an inside diameter of 2.75 inches) and to the same length as the cylinder. The lead is rolled and smoothed onto the outside of the cylinder. It is then compressed slightly and inserted into the cylinder. The lead sleeve at the open end of the cylinder is made to contact the inside of the cylinder firmly. The overlapped lead lining is held firmly in position with a short piece of 1-inch masking tape. The entire lead sleeve is then removed, and the end with the masking tape is inserted into the cylinder; that is, the position of the lead sleeve is reversed. This permits contacting the other end of the lead foil against the sides of the open end of the cylinder. The overlapped lead lining is held in position with another small piece of 1-inch masking tape. The entire surface of the lead sleeve is then smoothed against the inner wall of the cylinder, so that the lead firmly contacts the inner surface of the cylinder. After this step is accomplished, a sufficiently long piece of masking tape is inserted so that the entire free margin of the lead on the inside of the sleeve is held firmly in place. It is essential that the masking tape adhere firmly. A woman's hand is ordinarily small enough to insert into the open end of the cylinder and can effectively make the tape adhere securely. If the lead is not held securely by the masking tape, the lead sleeve will collapse from its own weight. The free edge of the lead should come to and be burnished against the end of the plastic cylinder, thus prohibiting x-radiation from striking the plastic. Masking tape can be used to secure the open end of the sleeve to the plastic cone; alternatively, the sleeve can be fixed permanently to the cylinder with a suitable adhesive.

Protective aprons. Aprons having a lead equivalency of not less than 0.25 mm. should be used to cover the gonads and preferably the chest and gonads of all patients, especially children and adults who have not passed the age of reproduction. Care must be used in handling such aprons; when not in use they should be draped over a device similar to a towel rack. Aprons have a tendency to deteriorate and/or tear easily.

Occasionally one hears that the use of a protective apron causes the patient to become alarmed and thus encourages questions and conversations. Many patients realize that radiation has some potential for harm and will appreciate the dentist's concern. Those who question must have their fears answered. Not to use protective measures because of possible inconveniences would be unwarranted.

Radiation protection for the operator

Radiation protection standards permit users of radiation to receive approximately ten times as much radiation as the average person in the population. This larger amount absorbed by a small fraction of the total population is not considered genetically harmful, nor is it likely to cause somatic effects. In general, radiation workers may receive an *accumulated* dose to the critical organs of $(N - 18) \times 5$ rem (roentgen equivalent man).* In this formula, N is the age in years. People 18 years and younger are not expected to work with ionizing radiation. After 18 years of age, an individual should not receive more than 5 rem of whole-body radiation each year; and the dose in any 13 consecutive weeks must not exceed 3 rem. These guidelines coincide rather closely with a previous standard, which stated that users of radiation should not receive more than 100 milliroentgens (mR) of radiation per week (100 mR/week $\times$ 50 weeks = 5,000 mR or 5 R). It must be emphasized that, although these guides suggest a tolerable level of radiation, doses exceeding 25 mR/week of whole-body radiation are looked upon questioningly, and every attempt should be made to minimize the weekly dose. In some cases the above are referred to as maximum permissible doses (MPD). Note the remarks that introduce this chapter. It seems likely that the above guidelines will be reduced in the relatively near future.

---

*For our purposes, a rem can be considered identical with the roentgen, the unit of radiation defined in Chapter 1 and which, until recently, served as the basic unit for x-radiation measurement.

It is essential to reemphasize that under usual circumstances any patient radiation reduction will have a direct effect on the amount of radiation received by the operator. The term *operator* includes the dentist and all auxiliaries who expose film. The operator receives radiation in the form of secondary radiation when the primary x-ray beam strikes the patient or objects in the operatory. The operator also receives radiation exposure if he foolishly stands in the path of the primary beam. There are three important things that the operator and his assistant can do to reduce radiation exposure further. These include standing at a safe position and distance, and the use of barriers.

Position. The safest position for the operator and/or his assistant to stand during x-ray exposure is between 90° and 135° to the x-ray beam; when possible, it is best to stand behind the patient. The proper positions are shown in Fig. 4-6. When the anterior teeth are exposed, it is immaterial whether the operator stands on the right or left side of the patient. When the molar and bicuspid areas of either the right or the left side are exposed, it is preferable for the operator to stand behind rather than in front of the patient. Under the latter circumstances, the patient's head absorbs most of the x-ray scatter. It is essential to reemphasize that the operator must not stand in the path of the primary x-radiation beam.

Distance. The strength of x-radiation varies inversely as the square of the distance that an individual stands from the source of the x-radiation. The inverse square law is discussed in Chapters 1 and 2. For example, if the operator has been in the habit of standing 2 feet from the source of radiation and then moves away to a distance of 4 feet, the radiation he will receive at 4 feet will be reduced to one fourth of the previous amount (Fig. 4-7). This illustrates how important it is for the operator to stand as far from the radiation source as possible. It is recommended that the operator stand a minimum of 6 feet away from the patient

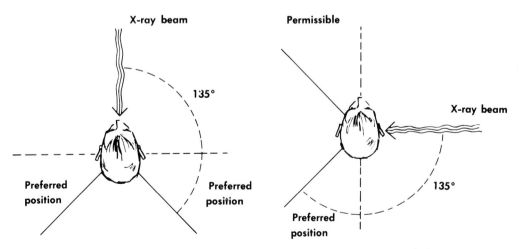

Fig. 4-6. Positions of greatest safety for dental x-ray machine operators during exposure.

and from the source of radiation. The diagram given in Fig. 4-7 illustrates the degree to which distance can contribute in reducing operator irradiation.

Barriers. The use of a barrier material interposed between the operator and the source of radiation is a most effective method of providing safety for the operator, provided that the barrier is suitably constructed. Common usage has resulted in lead ordinarily being recommended for the construction of barriers. However, other materials are equally suitable when properly used. Steel, concrete, solid brick, barium plaster, ceramic tile, and so forth, offer various degrees of resistance to radiation. If used as a barrier, their thicknesses must be greater than that of lead. The ability of these materials to absorb radiation is usually expressed in terms of lead equivalent. Decisions to use barriers depend on many factors, which are discussed under Radiation protection barriers.

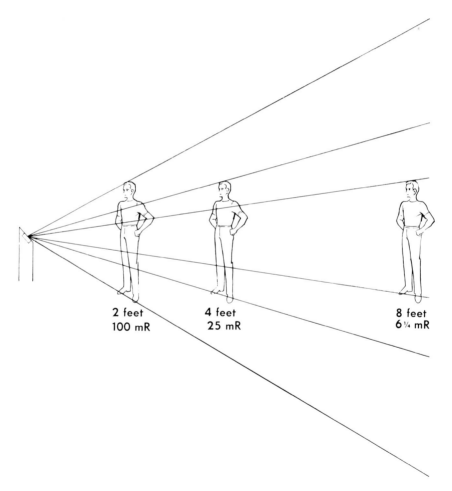

2 feet
100 mR

4 feet
25 mR

8 feet
6 ¼ mR

Fig. 4-7. Relationship of x-ray beam coverage to the distance from the radiation source. As the x-ray beam diverges, it covers an increasingly larger area. An object of constant size occupies proportionately less of this area the farther it is from the source of radiation.

Radiation protection for associated personnel

Office personnel not ordinarily responsible for radiographic procedures, individuals who may be disassociated with the dental office but whose working area may be contiguous with the dental office, and patients as they sit in another operatory or in the waiting area are included in the designation *associated personnel*. In contrast to users of radiation, the average person in the lay population is not expected to receive more than 10 rem of whole-body radiation during the first 30 years of life and not more than 5 rem (not more than 0.5 rem in any 1 year) during the following 10-year periods.

Ordinarily, the amount of radiation produced in the dental office that reaches other office personnel, people in other offices, and patients in the reception room is extremely limited. In isolated instances, however, the physical arrangement of the dental office may be such that the radiation escaping through the walls is of such magnitude as to potentially jeopardize the health of associated individuals. Each dentist must examine his office critically and, if necessary, engage the services of a radiation physicist to certify the safety of all concerned. Suitable barrier material must be installed when necessary.

Radiation protection barriers

X-radiation barrier requirements for the protection of humans are based on several factors: notably, workload, use factor, occupancy factor, maximum kilovoltage, and distance from the radiation source. *Workload* is the use of an x-ray machine expressed in milliampere seconds per week. The *Use factor* relates to the barrier itself and is defined as the fraction of the workload during which the x-ray beam will be directed at the barrier under consideration. A different use factor exists for primary and secondary radiation barriers. The *occupancy factor* is concerned with the constancy with which humans will occupy the area beyond the barrier. It is the factor (1 or less than 1) by which the workload should be multiplied to correct for the degree of occupancy of the area in question while the radiation source is "on." With a constant workload, greater barrier thickness is required with high *kilovoltages*. Calculations must be based on the assumption that the highest available kilovoltage will be used continually. The greater the *distance* between the barrier and the radiation source, the less barrier thickness required.

Barriers must be considered from the standpoint of both primary and secondary radiation. Primary radiation is that "which passes through the window, aperture, cone, and/or other collimating device of the tube housing."[*] Secondary or scattered radiation is that which is "deviated in direction during passage through matter. It may also have been modified by a decrease in energy."[*] Often, the requirements for secondary scatter are greater than for the primary beam because the use factor in conventional dental radiography for the primary beam

---

[*]National Council on Radiation Protection and Measurements Report No. 35, Dental x-ray protection.

is $\frac{1}{16}$, whereas that for the secondary beam is always 1. When differences exist, the greater barrier thickness must be used.

The NCRP Report No. 35 can be very helpful in the design of suitable barriers. Barriers are often thought of solely in terms of lead. However, other building materials can be used provided their thickness has an equivalency to the required thickness of lead. Such other building materials include steel, concrete, solid brick, barium plaster, and ceramic tile. Various thicknesses of lead-equivalent glass are available for viewing windows.

The most common form of lead used for barriers in dental installations is a sheet approximately $\frac{1}{16}$ inch thick (4 pounds per square foot). Although lesser thicknesses are available, the $\frac{1}{16}$-inch thick lead sheets are most easily obtained and generally are the most economical to use. Regardless of thickness, it must be realized that sheet lead has a great tendency to sag if not well supported. Sheets should be made to firmly adhere to a supporting structure, such as plywood, before installation. Also, if a choice exists, it is important to have the absorbing medium placed toward the operatory rather than away from it. This concept can be disregarded if the barrier is constructed of a single material, such as concrete.

REGULATORY MEASURES

It is only within the last 20 years that problems of ionizing radiation as they relate to the general public have become a public health problem. Prior to this time, the man-made radiation received by the general population was largely produced in the offices of health science personnel, and the amount of exposure was a matter of individual concern to the doctor and his patient. With the development of atomic energy and the broadening use of various types of radioactivity for military, industrial, and therapeutic purposes, the problem became important to all individuals and was recognized to require control by some central body. Originally, the control, as well as the development and promotion of various types of ionizing radiation, was the responsibility of the Atomic Energy Commission, now called the Nuclear Regulatory Commission. Today, the U.S. Public Health Service and the Environmental Protection Agency have the responsibility for safeguarding the general population from excessive exposure to ionizing radiation.

The majority of states now have regulations governing the use of ionizing radiation. At present, there are no regulatory measures that attempt to control the judgment of the physician or dentist. For example, the number of films that one may take for a specific individual is not regulated, nor is the frequency of reexamination controlled. On the other hand, many health departments, either state, country, or city, have or are developing regulatory measures that will protect the public through control of such physical factors as filtration, collimation, beam hardness, and tube head leakage.

It is in the best interest of the dental profession for each dentist to cooperate wholeheartedly with these efforts. Regulatory measures should be anticipated, and protective measures should be used voluntarily in each dental office prior to legislative action.

It is unlikely that the health professions will be told what film speed to use, since this is largely a matter of judgment. However, the fastest possible film should be used, provided that the resulting radiograph is diagnostically adequate. It is possible that regulatory measures will prohibit the manufacture of intraoral films less sensitive than speed D (see Table 1-3). The x-ray beam used for intraoral films should be collimated so that the beam diameter at the skin is no more than 2.75 inches. An amount of filtration should be added to each dental machine so that unusable long wavelength photons are eliminated from the beam. Exposure technics should be related to the proper use of the darkroom. Care must be used in film placement and in angulating to avoid the necessity of additional exposures. As additional information becomes available, the dentist should alter his procedures to best protect his patient while concurrently rendering a satisfactory diagnostic service.

Protective measures as they relate to the operator and associated personnel (see pp. 80 and 83) also should be observed. The dentist is responsible for the use of ionizing radiation in the dental office, even though other individuals operate the equipment.

Diagnostic x-ray equipment standards

Two x-ray equipment standards have been developed in recent years, one by the American Dental Association Council on Dental Materials and Devices, acting as administrative sponsor for the American National Standards Institute Committee MD 156 for Dental Materials and Devices, and the other by the federal government, specifically, the Food and Drug Administration and its Bureau of Radiological Health.

The American Dental Association document, published in the August 1974 issue of the Journal of the American Dental Association, relates to conventional dental x-ray machines and excludes cephalometric, panoramic, curved field tomographic and laminographic, and internal x-ray source equipment. The specifications are useful even though some items are quite permissive. For example, kilovoltage can vary 5 kVp from the indicated kilovoltage setting on the machine's console. Plus or minus 5 kVp means an acceptable variation range of 1 to 10 kVp between machines. A 10-kVp difference between machines is significant; it would have to be compensated for by almost doubling or halving the exposure time. In spite of such deficiencies, manufacturers are now counseled more effectively than before regarding the needs of the profession. There are no legal ramifications to the American Dental Association's specifications. The strength of the document lies in the fact that a manufacturer cannot advertise in the Journal of the American Dental Association or display a product at the association's meetings unless the product meets the association's specifications.

The federal regulations became effective August 1, 1974. They do not control medical or dental practice. They relate to diagnostic x-ray systems and major components of all types manufactured after August 1, 1974, and to the assembly of these components into new or existing x-ray systems. The regulations require manufacturers to certify equipment manufactured after August 1, 1974, as complying with the Federal Performance Standard,* and assemblers of these certified components must certify that the system has been assembled in accordance with the manufacturer's instructions. After August 1, 1979, the regulations will apply to the assembly of all x-ray equipment, new or used, if the ownership of the used equipment is transferred. In some instances, the regulations are quite specific; in others, they stipulate only the requirement of a statement by the manufacturer. For example, the kilovoltage variation situation discussed in the preceding paragraph is treated under the heading of *accuracy;* the manufacturer is required to give "a statement of the maximum deviation from the indication given by labeled control settings and/or meters during any exposure when the equipment is connected to a power supply. . . ." The Federal Performance Standard describes the power supply applicable to the regulation. At this time, the regulations do not apply to servicing or repairing of x-ray systems. The regulations, however, do establish certain criteria concerning the addition or replacement of components in an x-ray system. It is likely that amendments to the regulations will relate to servicing and repairing. Federal regulations supersede state regulations unless state requirements are identical to the federal regulations.

Neither the American Dental Association specifications nor the federal regulations directly affect the practicing dentist. They relate to the manufacturer and, in the case of the federal regulations, to the manufacturer and the assembler of x-ray equipment. Both are designed to protect the public and the profession from health hazards and from inadequacies in manufacture. It is almost certain that both will be amended as experience is gained and need for change is recognized.

Monitoring procedures

Monitoring of a dental office—the physical measuring of radiation—is best done by a competent radiation-oriented person. Equipment used in measuring the quality and quantity of radiation is expensive. However, a few procedures can be done by the dentist. He can determine the collimation and position of his x-ray beam by exposing an extraoral film or a cross of intraoral films and can make necessary corrections. The dentist can investigate and correct filtration conditions. Tube head leakage can be determined, but cannot be measured, by taping periapical films to the surface of the tube housing, particularly over joints and openings.

---

*Federal Performance Standards are available in Title 21 of the Code of Federal Regulations. Copies of the regulation may be obtained from the Bureau of Radiological Health, Food and Drug Administration, 5600 Fishers Lane, Rockville, Md., 20852.

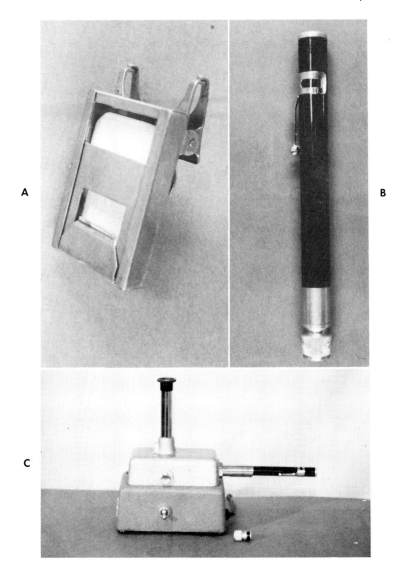

Fig. 4-8. Dose-measuring instruments. **A,** Film badge. **B,** Pocket dosimeter. **C,** Instrument in which the pocket dosimeter is charged and later read in terms of radiation exposure (charger-reader).

Dose measurements can be made by contracting for a continuing film badge service with a radiation-monitoring laboratory. In establishments with a high work load, the dentist may wish to purchase thimble ionization chambers complete with a charger-reader. The thimble ionization chamber is a device for direct reading of radiation exposure. A film badge and an ionization chamber with its charger-reader are shown in Fig. 4-8.

CHAPTER 5

Intraoral radiographic technics

Intraoral films, singly or aggregated into a complete mouth survey, must meet certain basic standards of quality. These standards are discussed to a large extent in Chapters 2 and 3. This chapter is devoted to technical procedures. As a preliminary to this topic, it is well to emphasize certain quantitative and qualitative factors essential to adequate radiographic interpretation.

The complete mouth survey is composed of a number of single films. Any survey should be designed to examine completely the teeth and teeth-bearing areas. The number of films included in a complete mouth survey must be decided by the practitioner. Some dentists take as many as 28 or 30 films per complete adult mouth series; others expose as few as 10 films for the same purpose. In our opinion, a minimum of 14 and a maximum of 17 periapical films, accompanied by a minimum of 2 and a maximum of 4 bite-wing films, are necessary for adequate interpretation of oral conditions in people with a full or nearly complete complement of teeth. The use of bite-wing films in the anterior segments of the mouth is ordinarily not necessary. We favor the 17-film periapical series for adult patients because we believe that an adequate complete mouth survey cannot be made with fewer films. Although we are opposed to the taking of additional films on a routine basis, we agree that supplemental films taken after the original series has been observed may be necessary. Although every effort should be made to minimize the amount of ionizing radiation received by the patient, it is unwise to compromise cost and the small additional amount of patient exposure with incomplete diagnostic information. Bite-wing films are of no value in edentulous areas; 14 periapical films ordinarily suffice for totally edentulous mouths. Bite-wing films are important for children; the number and size of periapical and bite-wing films vary with a child's age. Intraoral technics for children are similar to those used for adults. The psychological approach used with children differs in some cases from that used with adults. A complete mouth survey for adults is shown in Fig. 5-1.

This chapter is devoted largely to film placement and to comparison of the two major intraoral technics; exposure procedures are mentioned briefly. Quality assessment for intraoral radiographic surveys, much of which is applicable to

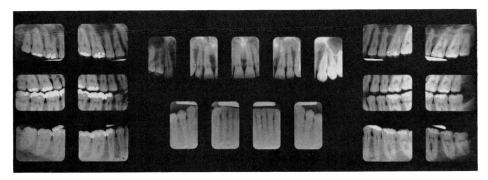

Fig. 5-1. Complete mouth periapical survey for an adult patient.

single radiographs, is stressed before technics are discussed. Specific radiographic surveys for adults, children, and patients with edentulous mouths are discussed in Chapter 10.

QUALITY ASSESSMENT

Before quality assessment is discussed, it seems appropriate to put the subject into perspective by quoting from the introductory paragraph of a paper related to the quality of dental radiographs submitted by dentists to a third party payment organization:

> From September 1973 to May 1974, an initial subjective review was conducted on over 2,000 preauthorization dental radiographs submitted to Pennsylvania Blue Shield. It was estimated (data unpublished) that at least 50% of these films were of such substandard quality that the efficacy of the proposed treatment could not be determined. This figure is startling, especially in view of the recent and probable future increase in third party payment plans. As dental care programs increase, we believe there will be a greater potential for population exposure to radiation with little apparent diagnostic benefit. No data were found on the technical quality of radiographs submitted as part of dental treatment plans, yet the ADA's *Policies on Dental Care Programs* state that "radiographs should be of such quality that they are properly diagnostic for clinical evaluation of the case involved." It became clear that a study was needed to gain reliable baseline information about the quality of radiographs submitted to third party programs.°

We believe that a similar study is needed to evaluate the quality of radiographic services for private practice patients.

The paralleling procedure for intraoral radiography is favored over the bisecting technic. This preference is based on a conviction that better quality radiographs generally can be obtained with the paralleling procedure. However, as long as quality standards are met, the technic used is irrelevant.

°From Beideman, R. W., Johnson, O. N., and Alcox, R. W.: A study to develop a rating system and evaluate dental radiographs submitted to a third party carrier, J.A.D.A. **93**:1010, 1976. Copyright by the American Dental Association. Reprinted by permission.

An article published in the Journal of the American Dental Association*
discusses in detail what is considered *acceptable* quality for a complete mouth
intraoral survey. A complete mouth survey must meet certain criteria; or, if it is
not possible to obtain desirable results using conventional methods, the survey
must be supplemented by other radiographs that, together with the intraoral
films, fulfill the criteria.†

All films must be of reasonable density. The exposed edge of the film associated with occlusal or incisal tooth surfaces (thus the portion of the film not
demonstrating calcified structures) should have a density of from 2 to 3 (see p.
26). Very little view box light should be able to penetrate this area. If there is
a choice to be made between slightly light and slightly dark films, the choice, as
far as diagnostic usefulness is concerned, should be toward the darker films. This
is because an intense viewing light can penetrate darker films and make them
useful, but there is no way to increase the density of light radiographs. Radiologic
health principles, however, negate the desirability of slightly dark films.

All interproximal spaces between adjacent teeth must be observed at least
once without tooth overlap and without extension of the buccal cusp beyond the
lingual or palatal cusp (except to the extent that the buccal cusp is anatomically
longer than the lingual or palatal cusp). Optimally, and in the interest of having
maximum quality radiographs, each interproximal space should be observed more
than once; but the quality of the survey is *acceptable* if each space is seen
once.

Each apex of each tooth must be seen at least once with no less than 1 to 2
mm. of bone surrounding it. Optimally, each apex should be seen more than
once. If the tooth apex shows actual or suspected disease, the full extent of the
area must be seen. Demonstration of the entire area may be difficult or impossible using traditional intraoral technics. In such instances, other intraoral or
extraoral technics must be used.

Finally, the distal border of the maxillary tuberosity and the upward
curvature of the mandibular ramus must be seen. Restated, all possible tooth-
bearing areas of the maxilla and mandible must be observable to be sure pathology is absent in these areas.

Even if the above criteria are met, some areas of the maxilla and mandible
are not seen on the best intraoral survey. Properly angulated extraoral lateral
oblique projections or panoramic views of the maxilla and mandible can be
helpful. However, the *routine* use of these technics is not recommended, because

---

*Wuehrmann, A. H.: Evaluation criteria for intraoral radiographic film quality, J.A.D.A. **89:**
345, August 1974.
†The California Dental Association has published (1976) a "Rating System and Quality
Evaluation Criteria for Radiographs" as part of the publication *Quality Evaluation for Dental
Care*. The rating system and criteria have been field tested. To the best of our knowledge, this
is the only professional organization that has taken this forward step.

the frequency of locating unsuspected disease in areas not directly associated with the teeth is low; the expenditure of additional radiation is not justified. Lateral oblique projections and panoramic radiography are discussed later in the text.

Panoramic-type films should not be sustituted for intraoral surveys unless, because of special circumstances not encountered in the average patient, panoramic radiographs provide diagnostic information that cannot be obtained using intraoral technics. In most cases, the substitution of panoramic views for acceptable intraoral surveys gives incomplete diagnostic information. This is true even if bite-wing radiographs accompany the panoramic radiograph.

BISECTING AND PARALLELING TECHNICS

The two commonly used intraoral technics are known by various terms but are most commonly referred to as (1) the bisecting technic and (2) the paralleling technic.* The bisecting technic is the older of the two procedures. It is used by most present-day practitioners and is taught in many dental schools. It is generally considered the easier of the two procedures. The paralleling technic was originally developed by McCormack. It was improved and popularized by Fitzgerald and is now taught in approximately half of the dental schools in the United States. We believe the results of the paralleling technic are superior to those of the bisecting technic and that it is not difficult to learn, particularly when it is taught to unindoctrinated dental students.

Basic principles of shadow casting

In order to understand the theory as well as the advantages and disadvantages of the two procedures, it is advisable to review basic principles of shadow casting. The radiographic image is a kind of shadow. The x-ray source for the shadow is the focal spot in the x-ray tube; the film records the shadows.

The fundamental rules for shadow casting, whether by light or x-rays, include the following:
1. The source of radiation should be as small as possible.
2. The distance from the radiation source to the object should be as long as possible.
3. The distance from the object to the recording surface on which the shadow is cast should be as short as possible.
4. The object and the recording surface should be parallel.
5. The radiation should strike both the object and the recording surface at right angles.

---

*The bisecting technic is also known as the procedure that follows the rules of isometric triangulation, as that which follows Ciezinsky's laws, as the short-cone technic, as the bisecting-the-angle-technic, etc. The paralleling technic is sometimes called the McCormack technic, the Fitzgerald technic, the extended-cone procedure, the long-cone technic, etc.

Theory of the paralleling technic

The paralleling technic requires a target-object distance that is as long as possible and practical. The technic also requires that the x-rays strike the object and recording surface at right angles and that the intraoral x-ray film be placed in a position parallel with a plane passing through the long axis of all teeth being examined. The latter ordinarily necessitates fairly wide separation of the tooth and the film. The only exception occurs in the mandibular molar region, where the lack of high muscle attachments and a relatively flat lingual surface permit the film to be placed vertically in the mouth, parallel with and close to the molar teeth. This lack of contact between object and recording surface would produce considerable distortion if a short target-object distance were employed. However, the use of the extended cylinder increases the target-object distance and compensates for the distortion and unsharpness that result from increasing the object-film distance. In Fig. 5-2 (solid lines) is shown the magnification created as a result of using a short target-object distance when the object and film are separated even though they are parallel. Should the object and the film not be parallel, the amount of magnification is even greater, as demonstrated in Fig. 5-3. Also illustrated in Fig. 5-2 (dotted lines) is the reduction in magnification when an extended distance is used even though the object and film are not in close approximation.

It is of value to examine the effect of a lack of parallelism between the object and the film. The x-rays (1) can strike the object at right angles, (2) can strike the film at right angles, or (3) can strike neither at right angles. The effect of proper technic coupled with the results that occur when each of the three

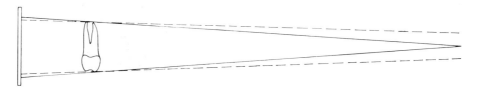

Fig. 5-2. Scale diagram of a tooth whose shadow is cast on a recording surface using an 8-inch TOD (solid line) and a 16-inch TOD (dotted line). The tooth is magnified less when the radiation source–object distance is increased.

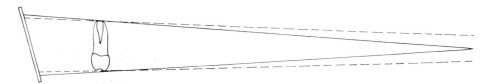

Fig. 5-3. Same situation as shown in Fig. 5-2 except that an object-film parallelism is lacking, resulting in increased magnification and disproportion (change in shape) between crown and root.

alternatives mentioned is used is shown in Fig. 5-4. Distortion in the form of magnification and/or true distortion (changes in object *shape*) occurs. The possibilities are as numerous as are the various film, object, and ray relationships. Unsharpness is not considered in Figs. 5-2 to 5-4, because the radiation source is depicted as a point.

Theory of the bisecting technic

The rules governing the bisecting technic require that the operator envision an imaginary bisector of the angle formed by the long axis of the tooth and the x-ray film; the angle is formed where the film contacts the tooth crown. With this image in mind, the operator is required to direct the middle or central ray of the radiation beam through the apex of the tooth in such a manner that it strikes the bisector at right angles.* Such angulation, if properly employed, results in a tooth image that is exactly the length of the object. The geometry of this principle is illustrated in Fig. 5-5. However, all sections of the tooth

---

*In modern practice, a small beam of radiation (2.75 inches at skin) is used; this necessitates directing the central ray through the middle of the tooth, producing slight tooth elongation.

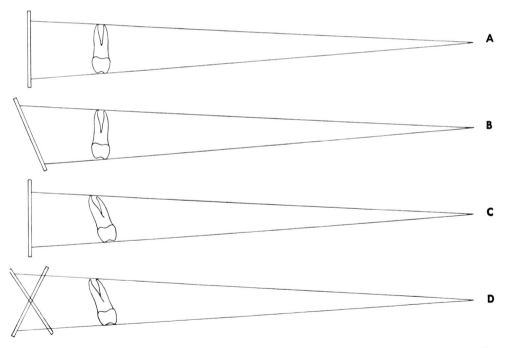

Fig. 5-4. Inaccurate shadow casting because of the following: **A,** proper parallelism of object and film and near perpendicularity of rays to both (minimum inaccuracy); **B,** faulty parallelism of object and film (central ray is perpendicular to object); **C,** faulty parallelism of object and film (central ray is perpendicular to film); **D,** lack of parallelism of object and film combined with a lack of perpendicularity of rays to either.

coronal to the apex are exposed by rays that are striking the bisector at some angle other than at right angles. As a result of the lack of parallelism between the tooth and the film, and the lack of a right-angle relationship between the rays and the tooth and film, all areas below the apex of the tooth (as well as above) are distorted. The degree of distortion can be reduced by the use of a long cylinder (16 to 20 inches TFD). The longer the distance between the radiation source and the object, the more parallel will be the rays. This principle is illustrated in Fig. 5-6.

Paralleling and bisecting technics compared

The paralleling and bisecting technics will be compared from the standpoint of the basic principles for shadow casting mentioned earlier in the chapter. In a given office, both procedures would utilize the same source of radiation. Hence, factors affecting rule 1 would be the same in both technics. The paral-

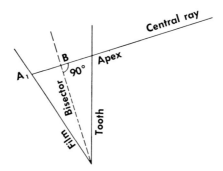

Fig. 5-5. Geometry of the bisecting technic.

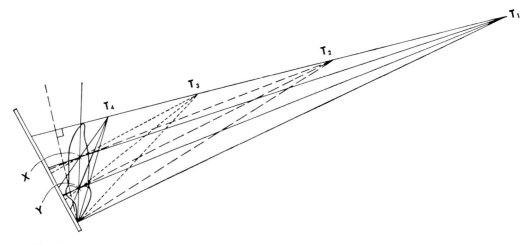

Fig. 5-6. Distortion resulting from the bisecting technic. Distortion is minimized when the target-tooth (T_4 to T_1) distances are increased. Points X and Y represent any two points on the tooth. Note that their positions change with a change in the target-tooth distance, whereas the tooth length remains constant.

leling technic ordinarily utilizes a long or extended cylinder, which increases the target-object distance of the short-cone or cylinder bisecting technic at least twofold. Thus the paralleling technic more adequately fulfills rule 2 for shadow casting. The employment of the paralleling technic using a short cone or cylinder is contraindicated because the short target-object distance produces a high degree of image unsharpness. The bisecting technic can be used advantageously with either the short or extended distance.

As will be noted when each technic is discussed individually, the tooth-film distance is somewhat greater in the paralleling technic, particularly in the coronal area of the tooth. This separation of tooth and film is due to anatomic limitations such as palatal curvature and muscle attachments. Thus the bisecting technic more closely satisfies rule 3 of shadow casting. However, this inadequacy of the paralleling technic is compensated for by the increased target-object distance.

The paralleling technic again excels in fulfilling rules 4 and 5. The paralleling technic is so named because the tooth and film are parallel. In the bisecting procedure, the film contacts the tooth at the occlusal or incisal surface and then diverges away from the long axis of the tooth. If the tooth and film are not parallel, it is impossible for the rays to strike both object and recording surface at right angles. When the bisecting technic is used, it is impossible to superimpose labial or buccal anatomic entities on their palatal or lingual counterparts; invariably when viewed on the radiograph, the labial or buccal counterpart of a similar point on the palatal or lingual surface will lie closer to the occlusal or incisal edge. This situation is not necessarily bad, but the interpreter must view the resultant films with this particular phenomenon in mind. Perhaps the disadvantages of the bisecting procedure can be summated by stating that the interpreter must read his films while applying his knowledge of the procedure's inadequacies. Conversely, the paralleling technic is more likely to portray an accurate anatomic representation of what actually exists.

Positioning of patients

When either the paralleling or the bisecting technic is used, the patient should be seated in the dental chair in a comfortable position. Ordinarily, it is helpful to have the occlusal plane of the jaw being examined parallel with the floor. This procedure is not essential unless rigid, predetermined film placement and angulation technics are used. Perfectly satisfactory films can be made with the patient in almost any position. Some operators feel that the procedure of tipping the patient backward in the chair gives them greater opportunities to observe film placement in relation to the long axis of the teeth. Probably, the greatest consideration should be for patient comfort. Chair height usually varies for exposure of maxillary and mandibular films; the chair must be higher when the lower arch is being examined.

In recent years, many dentists have equipped their dental operatories with contour chairs and have learned to do most operations with the patient in a supine position. Although intraoral technic is discussed and illustrated in this chapter with the patient in an upright position, high-quality intraoral radiographs can be produced with the patient in a supine position; this is especially true if the paralleling technic is used. McCormack, the originator of the paralleling technic, was a medical x-ray technologist. He developed the technic using medical x-ray equipment and a horizontal medical examining table; the patient could only be placed in a horizontal position. If a dental x-ray machine is to be used with the patient supine, care must be taken to install the x-ray machine so that it will function in the desired patient position.

FILM PLACEMENT AND ANGULATION PROCEDURES USING THE PARALLELING TECHNIC

In this section detailed instructions about the manner of film placement are given. The instructions commence with the placement of maxillary anterior films, proceed to the placement of maxillary posterior films, and continue to the mandibular anterior and then the mandibular posterior areas. In each instance the film placement instructions will be followed by a description of the angulation technics. The comments concern the placement and angulation of periapical films only. Technics related to the use of bite-wing films are considered separately.

Horizontal and vertical angulation

The terms *horizontal* and *vertical angulation* are used throughout this chapter. Horizontal angulation refers to the x-ray beam's direction in a horizontal plane. The x-ray tube head is held on both sides by the ends of the yoke (a typical x-ray machine is shown in Fig. 1-4). The x-ray tube head and yoke swivel on a center point in the yoke to alter the horizontal angle.

Vertical angulation is the angle of the x-ray beam in a vertical plane. The tube head turns on the yoke ends to change the vertical angle. Vertical angulation is described as being plus (positive) or minus (negative). With the horizontal plane representing zero, plus angulation means that the beam is tipped toward the floor; minus angulation indicates that it is tipped upward. The stated angulation is the amount away from zero.

The description just given is applicable when the patient is positioned so that the occlusal plane of the jaw being examined is parallel to the floor. When the patient is tipped backward in the dental chair for the convenience of the operator, the vertical and horizontal angles must be oriented toward the long axis and occlusal plane of the teeth rather than to a horizontal plane such as the floor.

Maxillary central area

Five maxillary anterior films are used to cover the area from right to left cuspids. Number 1.1 film* measuring $^{15}\!/_{16}$ by $1^{9}\!/_{16}$ inches is employed and is

---

*American National Standards Institute (ANSI) numbers for periapical, bite-wing, and occlusal film are used throughout this text. See Table 1-2.

used in a vertical position. This narrow film of approximately the same length as the standard intraoral film (1.2) is employed because of increased ease of film placement. The maxillary central film is designed to demonstrate the right and left central incisors. The film is placed so that its narrow superior edge contacts the palate approximately 1 inch distal to the location of the root apices. It is placed parallel with the long axis of the maxillary central incisors. In order to accomplish this film placement, the film may be supported by the use of cotton rolls, by strapping the film to an ordinary throat stick with tape, or by the use of a plastic film holder such as those demonstrated in Fig. 5-7. These film holders (which we developed) are not sold commercially, but they can be molded in baseplate wax and processed in acrylic by any prosthetic laboratory. It will be observed that the film holder is in the form of an arm similar to a throat stick but is bent in an offset fashion that permits the film to be set back into the mouth, away from and parallel to the maxillary anterior teeth. A slot arrangement is designed to accept film of the dimensions just mentioned. When the film is placed, with the mouth open, as illustrated in Fig. 5-8, the upper portion of the film contacts the palate while the incisal edges of the mandibular anterior teeth engage the handle of the holder and assist in immobilizing it.

The extended x-ray cylinder is directed to the anterior portion of the face so that the rays go directly through the interproximal space between the two cen-

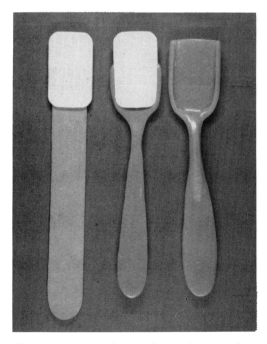

Fig. 5-7. Intraoral film taped to a throat stick or inserted into a plastic film holder (designed by us). This method is used for film placement in maxillary anterior areas.

tral incisors. If the x-ray film has been placed properly, the rays can be directed at right angles to both the teeth and the film. If the film has not been placed sufficiently far palatally, the lower edge of the film will protrude excessively below the level of the incisal edge. Obviously, the beam of radiation must completely encompass the film, or cone cutting will result.

It will be helpful when first learning this procedure to place a throat stick or some other relatively thin material on the incisal edges of the teeth and at a point approximately $\frac{1}{8}$ inch or less above the lower border of the film. This is done as a guide prior to exposure but after angulation. If the film has been properly placed, the lower border of the extended cylinder will be parallel with the line of the throat stick. If the film is not sufficiently high in the mouth, the guide plane will have a greater vertical angle than will the lower border of the cylinder. Because of the cylinder length, the x-rays, even though they do diverge slightly, can be considered parallel with each other and with the surfaces of the extended cone.

It is fortunate that the incisor teeth have a 15° to 20° inclination away from a true vertical. Thus, with the head positioned in the chair headrest so that the occlusal plane of the maxillary teeth is horizontal, the expected angulation of the x-ray tube head will be at approximately plus 15° to 20°. This is true of all maxillary teeth. Were it not for this inclination, the paralleling technic would not be feasible; the film could not be placed sufficiently high to record the apical

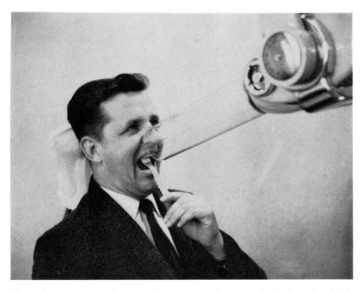

Fig. 5-8. Film placement in the maxillary central area. Cylinder should be lined with metal, preferably lead foil. Liner has been omitted in all illustrations for better visibility. Although not shown in any of the technic illustrations, the radiation protective apron, which should be used routinely, was omitted because black-and-white illustrations depicting technic are better visualized without the light-colored apron in position.

portion of the object. The separation of x-ray film from the teeth permits the x-rays to fall or to descend to a position on the film where they can be recorded. In Fig. 5-9 is illustrated diagrammatically the need for placing the film well away from the tooth and how the x-rays project the image of the tooth downward onto the properly placed film. A similar illustration is shown in the discussion of the maxillary posterior teeth because this particular point is essential to the paralleling technic.

Maxillary central lateral area

The central lateral film is placed in the same manner as the central film except that the former is turned slightly in order that the rays, as they pass through the interproximal surface of the central and lateral tooth, can strike the film at right angles. The degree of rotation varies with the arch form and the necessity for the x-rays to pass directly through the interproximal space.* In general, the narrower the mouth, the greater the amount of rotation.

Maxillary cuspid area

The procedure used for the maxillary central area and for the central and lateral areas is again employed for the cuspid tooth. The interproximal surface

---

*Whether one is using the paralleling technic or the bisecting technic, or is exposing bite-wing films, it will be of assistance, when one is learning, to insert a short piece of amalgam matrix band material interproximally between any two teeth being examined. The line that this straight piece of metal makes will act as a guide in determining proper horizontal angulation. The insertion of this metal is not done routinely; it must be removed before the film is exposed.

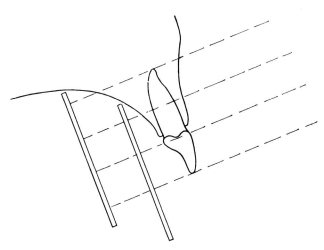

Fig. 5-9. Sagittal view of the maxillary central incisor showing proper film placement. The film must be parallel with the tooth and sufficiently far away from the tooth that the shadow can be cast on it. The film closest to the tooth is improperly placed; the shadow of the tooth apex cannot be recorded on the film.

between the cuspid and the lateral tooth is ordinarily shown without overlapping in the central lateral film. The distal surface of the cuspid will be shown on the bicuspid film. Thus it is not essential to be concerned about the interproximal surfaces when angulating for the cuspid film. The film in its plastic film holder is turned in such a manner that the flat surface of the film is at right angles to the x-ray beam as it goes directly through the cuspid tooth; this usually necessitates considerable rotation.

The film is placed as high as possible in the palate and well away from the tooth being examined. Proper film positioning and a diagram illustrating the horizontal relationship of the beam to the tooth and film are shown in Fig. 5-10. It should be noted that no fixed angulations in terms of actual degrees are suggested. Mouths vary, and angulation procedures should depend on circumstances rather than on predetermined approximate angulations. Here again, in learning proper film placement and angulation in the cuspid area, one will find it helpful to sight from the incisal edge of the cuspid to a point approximately ⅛ inch from the lower border of the x-ray film. This line, made visual rather than imaginary by a throat stick, should be parallel with the x-rays as they emerge from the cylinder.

Maxillary bicuspid area

Film positioning in both the maxillary bicuspid and molar regions requires the use of a hemostat, a rubber bite block through which is inserted the beak of

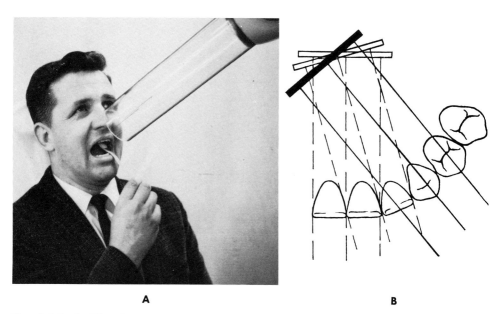

A   **B**

Fig. 5-10. A, Film placement in the maxillary cuspid area. **B,** Diagram illustrates proper horizontal angulation for the cuspid (heavy black), central and lateral, and central areas.

the hemostat, and a metal backing. The metal backing is preferably of stainless steel and is slightly smaller in dimension than the 1.2 intraoral film, measuring $1\frac{1}{4} \times 1\frac{5}{8}$ inches. An ordinary surgical hemostat may be used, but a specially designed instrument with serrations running parallel rather than at right angles with the beak is preferable. The metal backing is placed behind the film, and both are grasped by the hemostat. It is often helpful to tape the free end of the film to the metal backing in order to prevent separation. In the bicuspid view, the anterior border of the film and backing are ordinarily in contact with the rubber bite block. The arrangement of the film and instrument are shown in Fig. 5-11.

Prior to placing the film, the operator must observe the buccal inclination of the bicuspid teeth. Ordinarily, these teeth incline buccally at approximately 15° from the true vertical. Occasionally, the bicuspid teeth are quite vertically placed and almost appear to incline palatally. Having observed the buccal inclination of the bicuspid teeth, the operator rotates the hemostat in the rubber bite block so that when the planes of the bite block are parallel with the occlusal plane of the maxillary arch, the film and metal backing are parallel with the long axis of the teeth. The film is now ready to be inserted into the mouth.

Before the film is inserted, it is well to observe the plane of the buccal surfaces of the bicuspid teeth in order that (1) the plane of the film may be parallel with the plane of the buccal surfaces and (2) the x-rays may be directed through the interproximal spaces. In the average dentition, the interproximal spaces between the bicuspid teeth and between the bicuspid and first molar teeth run in a slightly anteroposterior direction. The anatomic arrangement of these teeth is shown in Fig. 5-12. A horizontal angulation that allows the beam to go directly

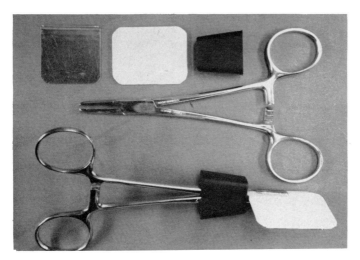

Fig. 5-11. Assembled and disassembled hemostat, rubber bite block, film, and steel backing.

through the interproximal spaces of the bicuspid teeth will ordinarily demonstrate the interproximal area between the distal surface of the cuspid and the mesial surface of the first bicuspid without overlapping.

A pen grasp is used, and the hemostat and film are inserted into the mouth with the film in a horizontal position. They should not touch the tongue or palate. When the film is sufficiently far into the mouth, its upper border is brought in contact with the palate in such a way that the distal portion of the film contacts the palate at or near the midline while the anterior portion of the film contacts the palate slightly to the *far side* of the midline. The hemostat is now rotated so that the lower border of the film swings downward and the film plane becomes parallel with the long axis of the teeth. This positioning should result in the film plane being parallel with the plane of the buccal (or palatal) surfaces. With the film held firmly in this position, the patient is asked to close on the bite block, and the operator's hand is replaced by the patient's hand. The patient is asked to exert a slight downward pressure on the hemostat handle in order to keep the film in contact with the palate. In Fig. 5-12 the horizontal positioning of the film in the mouth is illustrated diagrammatically, and the hemostat held by the patient is shown in Fig. 5-13.

The side of the extended cylinder is used as a guide, and the x-ray beam is now directed through the interproximal spaces of the bicuspid teeth in such a manner that it strikes the film at right angles. Since the hemostat handles are at

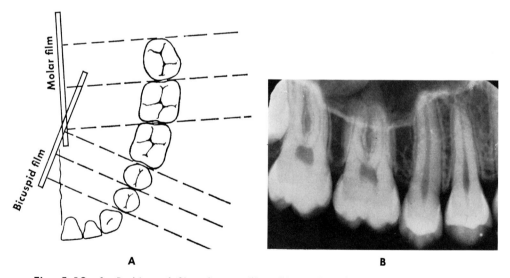

A   **B**

Fig. 5-12. A, Position of films for maxillary bicuspid and molar projections. The films must be parallel with the long axis of the teeth. The bicuspid film crosses the midline of the palate. The molar film is almost parallel with the midline. In all cases, the film must be parallel with the buccal surfaces of the teeth being examined and at or on the other side of the palatal midline. **B,** Radiograph of the maxillary bicuspid area.

right angles to the plane of the film, it is often helpful to observe the plane of the handles in relation to the upper or lower border of the cylinder. The plane of the handles and the sides of the cylinder should be parallel. Again, it will be of assistance to the beginner if he will place a tongue blade or some other suitable device on the upper border of the hemostat beak and on the cusps of the bicuspid teeth. If the film has been properly placed and if the rays have been suitably angulated, the plane of this tongue blade should be parallel with the plane of the upper or lower border of the cylinder.

It is *essential* that the film be placed at or beyond the midline of the palate rather than at some point between the teeth being x-rayed and the midline. The reason for this statement is illustrated in Fig. 5-14. Some degree of compromise is necessary if the teeth do not incline buccally, unless the patient has an exceptionally high palate. The fact that the teeth ordinarily incline buccally permits the x-ray beam to fall. The downward inclination of the x-ray beam is useful only if the film is placed sufficiently far from the teeth.

Maxillary molar area

Film placement for the maxillary molar area is almost identical with that of the bicuspid area. There are two principal exceptions: (1) The film must be placed somewhat farther distally than when the bicuspid area is examined. This necessitates that the film and metal backing not contact the rubber bite block. They should be separated by approximately ½ to ¾ inch. This distance varies and depends on the size of the maxillary arch. (2) The interproximal surfaces

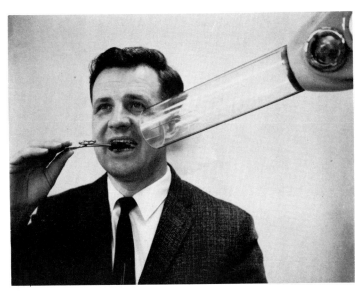

Fig. 5-13. Film and hemostat positioning for the maxillary bicuspid area. Note that the patient exerts a slight downward pressure on the hemostat handle and thus keeps the film in firm contact with the palate.

of the molar teeth, excluding the mesial surface of the first molar, are approximately at right angles to the midline of the palate. Thus, in order for the film to be perpendicular to the rays as they pass directly through the interproximal spaces, it must be placed in the mouth so that the anterior border of the film and metal backing touch the midline of the palate while the distal portion of the film and backing is located *on* or slightly to the *far side* of the midline. The film placement in the horizontal plane is shown diagrammatically in Fig. 5-12.

One view of the maxillary molar teeth, planned to show the interproximal surfaces between the first and second molars and between the second and third molars, is sufficient for a routine complete mouth survey. Supplemental films are occasionally needed but should not be made until the dentist has had an opportunity to examine initial results. There is, however, one slight modification of the technic just described, which may be helpful, particularly in examination of the third molar area or for patients who cannot tolerate a film placed distally on the palate. The principles described for the molar film placement are used except that the film is permitted to touch the rubber bite block. As the film is placed in the mouth, the distal border of the film is rotated well beyond the midline of the palate (away from the teeth being examined), while the anterior border of the film contacts the palate in the midline. Under such circumstances, the rays are projected from a somewhat more distal direction. The image of the third molar tooth is cast forward onto the film. Although improved clarity of the third molar apices often results, overlapping of the mesial surface of the third molar

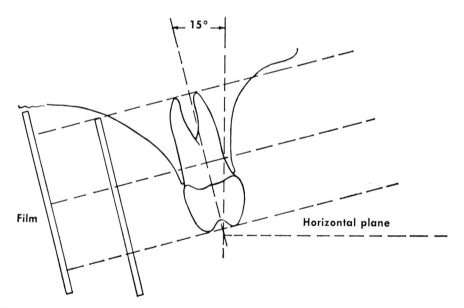

Fig. 5-14. Diagram of the maxilla in the bicuspid region, showing proper film placement. It is essential that the film be placed at or beyond the midline of the palate. The film nearest the tooth is improperly placed.

onto the distal surface of the second molar is common. Such a view is not ordinarily used as part of a routine survey.

Mandibular central lateral area

The mesiodistal width of the mandibular anterior teeth is sufficiently narrow that adequate visualization can be obtained with four anterior films. Number 1.1 film is used. The film is grasped in the hemostat beak in such a manner that when the exposure side of the film is placed in the mouth toward the teeth, the hemostat handle will protrude out of the corner of the mouth on the opposite side of the face from the teeth being examined. No metal backing is used because films of this size ordinarily are constructed with satisfactory rigidity.

A pen grasp is used to place the film in the mouth so that the lower border of the film rests under the tongue (the tongue must be relaxed in order not to traumatize the frenum) and the upper portion of the film momentarily contacts the incisal edges of the mandibular central and lateral teeth on the side being examined. The hemostat handle is now rotated; the lower border of the film pivots, and the upper portion of the film is rotated away from the incisal edges of the teeth until the film plane becomes parallel with the long axis of the central and lateral teeth. The patient is then asked to close on the bite block and to apply slight upward hand pressure on the underside of the hemostat handle so that the film is gently forced downward into the floor of the mouth.

With the film held in this position, the x-ray cylinder is angulated in such a manner that the rays go directly through the interproximal space between the

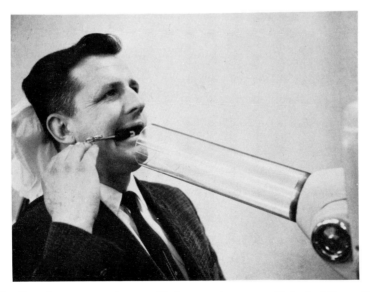

Fig. 5-15. Film placement in the mandibular anterior areas. Note that the patient gently pushes the hemostat handles upward and thus stabilizes the film in the floor of the mouth.

central and the lateral teeth and strike the film at right angles. Again, the beginner may wish to use a tongue blade to assist in estimating proper angulation. The tongue blade is placed on the incisal edges of the teeth in question and under the beak of the hemostat. The upper and lower borders of the cylinder should be parallel with the tongue blade. If the rays are not both parallel with the tongue blade and at right angles to the long axis of the teeth, the relationship between the rays, teeth, and film is unsatisfactory. In Fig. 5-15 is shown a patient holding a film for the exposure of the mandibular central and lateral teeth. The x-ray beam should be more parallel with the plane of the handle.

Mandibular cuspid area

The technic of film placement and angulation for the mandibular cuspid tooth is identical with that used for the central and lateral teeth with one basic difference. The plane of the film is rotated in such a manner that the rays passing directly through the cuspid tooth will strike the surface of the film at right angles. It is sometimes helpful to position the film to receive an image of both the cuspid and first bicuspid teeth.

Mandibular bicuspid area

A 1.2 film is used for both the mandibular bicuspid and molar areas. The muscle attachments on the lingual surface of the mandible ordinarily make it impossible to parallel the bicuspid film with the bicuspid teeth unless the film is separated from the teeth. Occasionally, the muscle attachments are sufficiently low to permit the placement of a film against the lingual tissues. A hemostat, rubber bite block, and metal backing are used. The film and the backing ordinarily contact the bite block. Again, as in the maxillary arch, the operator should observe the inclination of the mandibular bicuspid teeth and turn the hemostat handle in the bite block so that when the planes of the bite block are parallel with the occlusal plane of the mandibular arch, the film plane will be parallel with the long axis of the bicuspid teeth.

Using a pen grasp, the operator inserts the film between the tongue and the teeth. Often, it will be helpful for him to use his free hand to retract the cheek; this is done to improve visibility. With sufficient force to displace the tongue (the patient's cooperation in relaxing the tongue muscle is important), the film is placed downward into the floor of the mouth and simultaneously the anterior border is moved toward the midline of the mouth. This often takes considerable pressure on the part of the operator. Care must be used to align the film so that, in addition to being parallel with the long axis of the teeth, it is parallel with the plane of the buccal surfaces. This film should be placed sufficiently far forward to show the distal aspect of the cuspid tooth. When the film is in the correct position, the patient is asked to close on the bite block and to exert a slight upward hand pressure on the hemostat handle. As in the maxillary area, it is important that the film be placed as far as possible toward the midline. The cylinder is angulated so that the x-rays will go through the interproximal spaces and strike the teeth and the film at right angles.

There is a rather strong tendency in the mandibular bicuspid area to produce films that do not show tooth apices. In some instances, the operator will prefer to use the film with the broader dimension in a vertical position. This permits the film to be placed somewhat deeper into the floor of the mouth. Use of the hemostat in the bicuspid area is demonstrated in Fig. 5-16, and the film position for the bicuspid and molar areas is shown diagrammatically in Fig. 5-17.

Mandibular molar area

The lingual muscle attachments in the mandibular molar area are ordinarily sufficiently low to provide a rather considerable space for the placement of the mandibular films. It is almost possible to parallel teeth and film by placing the film against the lingual tissues and holding the film with the index finger of the hand on the opposite side from that being examined. This position is illustrated in Fig. 5-18. However, many operators prefer the continued use of the hemostat.

The mechanics of actually placing the film vary with different patients and with different technics. In some instances, it is completely possible to merely insert the film in its proper position; in others, it is necessary to displace the tongue manually in order to create a sufficiently wide space for the film to be inserted. If the hemostat is used, the procedure is similar to that employed in the bicuspid area. The film is placed more distally than in the examination of the bicuspid area. Thus, the film and metal backing are separated from the bite block

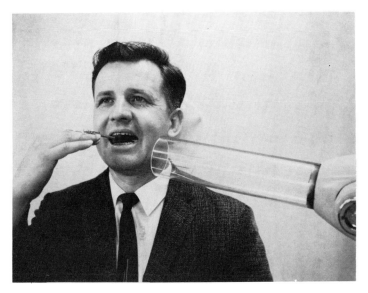

Fig. 5-16. Film placement in the mandibular bicuspid area, using the hemostat. Note that the patient exerts slight upward pressure on the hemostat handles.

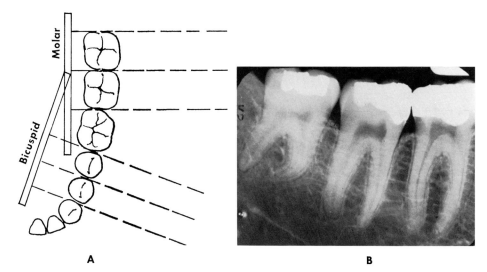

A   **B**

Fig. 5-17. A, Film position for mandibular bicuspid and molar areas. The molar film may contact the teeth, but the bicuspid film must displace the tongue and must be placed as near to the midline as possible. **B,** Radiograph of the mandibular molar area.

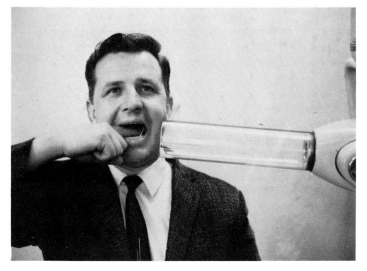

Fig. 5-18. Technic for film holding in the mandibular molar area. This is an alternate technic of the one using the hemostat, bite block, and steel backing.

by about ¾ inch. Unlike the bicuspid area, it is unnecessary to position the anterior border of the film toward the midline. As with all other periapical films, approximately ⅛ inch of the molar film should extend beyond the occlusal surface of the molar teeth. The distal border of the molar film should extend somewhat posteriorly to the distal surface of the mandibular third molar. Even if the third molar is not observable, it is essential that the film demonstrate the third molar area.

As in the case of the maxillary third molar tooth, it is sometimes advantageous, especially for exodontic purposes, to examine the third molar using a distal oblique projection. Under these circumstances, a hemostat, rubber bite block, and metal backing must be utilized. The film is placed in the floor of the mouth in such a manner that the distal portion of the film and metal backing is positioned toward the midline, thus partially displacing the tongue. The rays are angulated so that they enter the mandible considerably more distally than is customary and pass forward through the third molar area to strike the film at right angles.

Regardless of whether the distal oblique view or the customary projection is used, the operator should observe the inclination of the molar teeth prior to placing the film and should direct the rays at right angles to the tooth and to the film, which parallels the long axis of the teeth. In some instances, particularly when the first or second molar tooth has been removed, considerable lingual inclination of the mandibular molar teeth will be observed. Under these circumstances, zero or positive vertical angulation rather than negative angulation is used, and the film must be placed deeply in the floor of the mouth.

FILM PLACEMENT AND ANGULATION PROCEDURES USING THE BISECTING TECHNIC

The theory of the bisecting technic was discussed earlier in this chapter. It was noted that this is the more conventional procedure and is used by the majority of dentists. Fourteen 1.2 films are ordinarily employed in the complete mouth survey, excluding bite-wing films. Three maxillary and three mandibular films are generally taken in the anterior region with the narrowest dimension of the film in the horizontal position, and two posterior films are generally used in each of the four quadrants with the broadest dimension of the film in the horizontal position.

Anything less than 14 films ordinarily will not adequately cover the adult mandible and maxilla regardless of whether or not the mouth is edentulous. Although 14 films may suffice, it is preferable to use the same number of films advocated earlier in the discussion of the paralleling procedure, that is, 17 intraoral films: five maxillary anterior and four mandibular anterior 1.1 films, plus two 1.2 films of the posterior region of each quadrant.

In addition to the 14 or 17 periapical films, it is *essential* to use posterior bitewing films when anything other than an edentulous mouth is examined unless the proximal surfaces of all teeth can be examined clinically. Bite-wing technics are discussed later in this chapter, but it is important to emphasize at this time that the use of two 1.2 films employed with bite-wing tabs or two 2.2 bite-wing films* on each side of the mouth is preferred to the use of a single narrower and longer 2.3 bite-wing film. The preferred films demonstrate interproximal bone structure more effectively. In addition, the operator can utilize two different horizontal angulations in examining the interproximal surfaces of the posterior teeth for caries. It is often unnecessary to take two bite-wing films on each side of a child's mouth. This is particularly true until the age of 12 to 14 years, when the second molar erupts.

The short, pointed cone is often used with the bisecting technic; the open-end, metal-lined short cylinder should be used. It is important for the dentist to understand that use of an extended cylinder is not contraindicated. Any increase in the target-object distance will improve image sharpness and will contribute to diagnostic quality in the resultant film.

Maxillary central area

The periapical film, preferably the narrower type of film (1.1), is grasped by the narrow border with the operator's thumb and forefinger. The thumb is placed on the exposure side of the film; it should cover no more than ⅛ inch. The operator may stand in front of the patient or at his side. The film is placed

---

*The 2.2 bite-wing film has the same dimensions as the 1.2 periapical film. However, it is made with a bite tab.

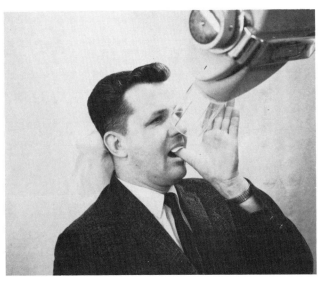

Fig. 5-19. Proper manner of holding an intraoral film in the maxillary anterior region when the bisecting technic is used.

in the palate so that the thumb and film contact the incisal edges of the anterior teeth. In this manner, approximately ¼ inch of the lower border of the film protrudes below the incisal edges of the teeth. The film should be centered in the midline with its upper border contacting the palate. The sides of the film should be parallel with the long axis of the teeth; that is, in the finished film, the image of the teeth should not cross the film diagonally.

The patient's thumb is used to hold the film in the selected position. The remaining fingers are rotated as far out of the field as possible to provide maximum visibility for the operator. When film for the central area is held, either thumb may be used. The thumb also retains the film in other areas of the maxilla. It is customary to use the thumb of the hand on the opposite side from the side being examined. It is preferable that the thumb contact the film and the palate at the upper border of the film; every effort should be made not to bend the film. The proper manner of holding the film is demonstrated in Fig. 5-19. Under no circumstances should films be held by the operator or his assistant during film exposure. Having placed the film in this position, the operator must observe the line of the film and the long axis of the central teeth (generally speaking, the anterior teeth protrude buccally at an angle of approximately 15° from vertical). These two lines form an angle. The operator now must envision an imaginary line bisecting this angle. Using the cone of his choice, that is, either the short, pointed cone or

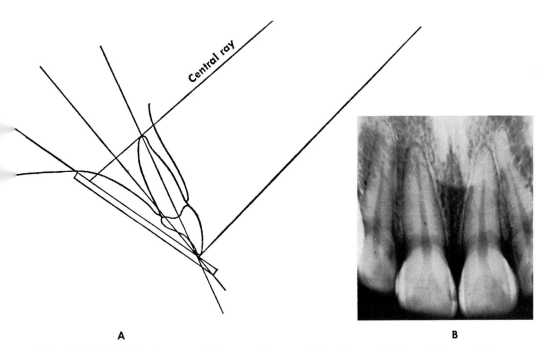

A   **B**

Fig. 5-20. A, Scale diagram of the x-ray beam relationship to the film and the maxillary central incisor in the bisecting technic. **B,** Radiograph of the maxillary central area.

an open-end lined cylinder* of any reasonable length, the operator directs the central or middle ray through the middle of the tooth† perpendicular to the imaginary bisecting line. Care must be taken to envision imaginary lines accurately if optimum results are to be obtained. Actually, this is not difficult if the operator has a reasonable capacity for object visualization. With the ray directed in this relationship to the tooth and film, an exposure is made. Proper vertical angulation is shown diagrammatically in Fig. 5-20. Horizontal angulation concepts are identical to those of the paralleling technic.

Note that no specific angulation has been given. The shape of dental arches and the positioning of teeth in these arches vary greatly. The use of predetermined angles is contraindicated if superior results are to be obtained. The operator must observe the circumstances that exist in the mouth being examined and must modify angulation procedures in accordance with needs.

Maxillary central lateral area

The technic for examining the maxillary central and lateral teeth is identical with that used for examining the midline area except that the film is positioned so that the interproximal surface between the central and lateral teeth is centered on the film.

Maxillary cuspid area

As in the case of the central lateral area, the technic employed for the cuspid area is similar to that used for the maxillary central teeth. The film is positioned in the mouth so that the entire length of the cuspid tooth is centered on the film. The resultant film should not show the cuspid tooth running diagonally across the film surface. Such a result is due to faulty film placement; the lower border of the film was not parallel with the occlusal plane of the maxillary arch. When angulating for the cuspid tooth, one should make no particular effort to go through either the cuspid-lateral or the cuspid–first bicuspid interproximal space; these areas will be demonstrated on the central lateral film and on the bicuspid film. Rather, the ray is directed at the cuspid so that the image of the cuspid will be centered on the film.

When the cuspid film is positioned, particularly if 1.2 film rather than 1.1 film is used, it is sometimes necessary to crease or sharply bend the upper anterior corner of the film in order not to traumatize the patient's palate. This practice may be employed with wider film if necessary, but unbent narrower film is preferable.

Maxillary bicuspid area

An examination of the maxillary bicuspid area requires the use of 1.2 film with the widest dimension placed horizontally. The operator may stand either

---

*A properly diaphragmed, open-end, lead-lined cylinder is recommended.
†Theoretically, the central ray should pass through the tooth apex to satisfy the rules of isometry; modern collimating procedures might cause cone cutting under these circumstances. (See also footnote, p. 93.)

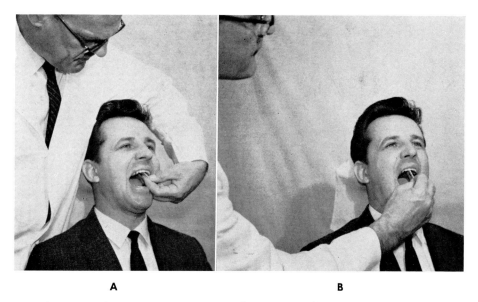

A   B

Fig. 5-21. A, Preferred positioning technic for maxillary bicuspid film placement in the bisecting technic. B, Acceptable but less-preferred procedure.

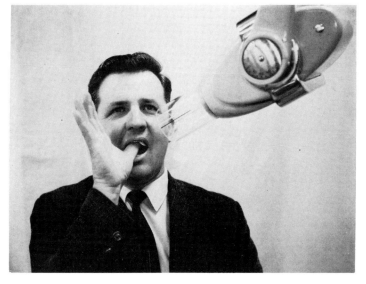

Fig. 5-22. Procedure for retaining maxillary bicuspid films in the bisecting technic. Pad of thumb should contact both the palate and upper film border.

in front of the patient or at his side. The film may be placed with either hand. The technic wherein the operator stands to the right of the patient (to the left of the patient if the operator is left-handed) seems preferable. Much is done by touch rather than by sight. The preferred and the less preferred positions are demonstrated in Fig. 5-21. The preferred film procedure is somewhat more difficult for short people; film positioning from the front of the mouth may have to be used by individuals of short stature. Only the preferred technic is described in detail here.

The middle of the lower film border is grasped by the thumb and index finger. Approximately ⅛ inch of the thumb tip covers the exposure side of the film. The film is carried in a horizontal position into the mouth and touches neither the tongue nor palate until it is sufficiently far distally. The anterior border of the film should be at the midline of the cuspid tooth. At this time the film is rotated upward with a single motion and is held firmly on the palate. The operator's thumb tip should rest on the occlusal surfaces of the bicuspid teeth. It is important, especially if the gag reflex is active, that the film not be moved after it is placed. If the film position is incorrect, the film should be removed from the mouth, and the patient should be allowed to swallow and regain composure before the film is replaced. With the film in this position, the thumb of the patient's hand on the opposite side of the body from that being examined is introduced. This may be done with or without guidance by the operator (Fig. 5-22). The pad of the thumb should contact *the film and the palate at the upper border of the film* while the fingers are extended and rotated out of the visual field. The thumb should *not* contact the middle of the film, because pressure will cause the film to bend and result in image distortion (root elongation).

With the film held by the patient in this position, the line of the film can be seen; the long axis of the tooth is visualized, and the x-ray machine is angulated in accordance with prior instruction. Horizontal angulation should be such that the rays go directly through the interproximal spaces between the cuspid and first bicuspid, the first and second bicuspids, and the second bicuspid and the mesial surface of the first molar. This ordinarily necessitates horizontal angulation that is a little anteroposterior to a line perpendicular to the sagittal plane. As mentioned earlier, visualization of proper horizontal angulation can be enhanced if the beginning operator will insert small pieces of matrix band material between the interproximal surfaces of the teeth being examined. The line of the x-rays should be parallel with the plane of the matrix strip. The matrix material is removed prior to film exposure.

Maxillary molar area

Film placement and angulation procedures for the maxillary molar area are almost identical to those for the maxillary bicuspid area. Two major differences exist: (1) The film must be placed farther distally in the mouth. The molar film must demonstrate the entire third molar area including the upward curvature of the tuberosity. For the film to be placed more distally, the film is grasped by the thumb and forefinger at the lower anterior corner. (2) Horizontal angulation for the molar region differs from that of the bicuspid region in that the rays are directed at right angles or in a slightly posteroanterior direction to the midline of the palate in order that they may go through the interproximal spaces distal to the first and second molars. The difference in horizontal angulation between the bicuspid and molar views is shown in Fig. 5-12. It is pertinent to emphasize again that the operator must observe tooth positioning prior to estimating proper angulation. Previously determined fixed angulations are often unsatisfactory.

Mandibular central lateral area

Fourteen film intraoral periapical surveys ordinarily include one 1.2 film for the midline segment of the mandible and one film of each cuspid. It is preferable to use four 1.1 anterior films, including one of the central lateral area and another of the cuspid area on each side of the mouth. The mandibular anterior films, particularly if the narrow film is employed, are inserted rather easily. The film is placed so that the narrower dimension is horizontal. The upper border of the film rests against the incisal edges of the teeth with approximately ⅛ inch showing above the edge. The lower border of the film is placed on the floor of the mouth under the tongue in as comfortable a position as possible. Using the patient's hand on the opposite side of the arch, the operator places the pad of the index finger across that portion of the film resting just below the incisive edges. The fingertip should not rest on the film; rather, it should rest on the teeth distal to

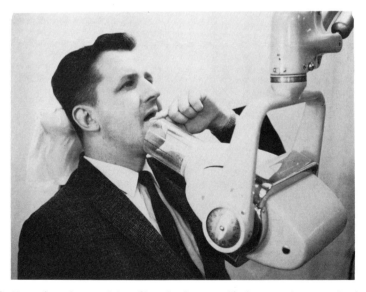

Fig. 5-23. Procedure for retaining films in the mandibular anterior area in the bisecting technic. Note that the pad of the index finger rests on the edges of the teeth. Care must be used **not** to curve the film by finger pressure near the floor of the mouth.

the posterior edge of the film. This method of holding the film is important. It is undesirable for the pad of the fingertip to press the film in such a manner that the film is curved against the lingual tissues. The proper technic for holding mandibular anterior films is demonstrated in Fig. 5-23. The remainder of the fingers and thumb are made into a fist, and the patient's elbow is elevated to remove the fingers from the operator's line of vision.

The rules for vertical angulation previously described are used, and the operator makes certain that the rays are horizontally angulated so as to go through the interproximal space between the central and lateral teeth.

Mandibular cuspid area

Film placement for the mandibular cuspid is identical with the placement for the central lateral area except that the film is placed so that the image of the cuspid will be centered on the film. Care must be taken so that the long axis of the cuspid does not cross the film diagonally. No particular attempt is made to direct the rays through the interproximal spaces on either side of the cuspid tooth since these areas will be shown clearly on the central lateral view and on the bicuspid film.

Mandibular bicuspid area

Mandibular bicuspid and molar films may be placed with the operator standing in front of the patient or at the patient's right side (when the operator is right-handed). The latter is usually preferable. The film is grasped by the upper anterior corner with the left hand when film is placed on the left side of the mandible; the right hand is used when the film is placed on the patient's right side. The index finger of the operator's hand not being used to hold the film is rotated under the tongue between the tongue and the lingual surface of the mandible. It

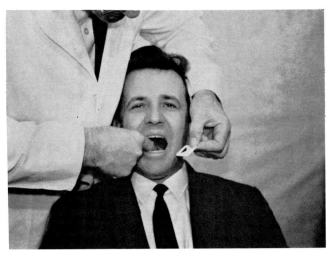

Fig. 5-24. Tongue retraction prior to placing an intraoral film in the mandibular bicuspid area.

is used to retract the tongue and to create a space into which the film may be placed. This procedure is illustrated in Fig. 5-24. Once this space is created, the film is easily inserted so that its anterior border is at the midline of the cuspid tooth and so that its superior border is approximately ⅛ inch above the occlusal surface.

Having positioned the film, the operator momentarily retains it in position, first with the retracting finger and then by placing the pad surface of the thumb of the hand used to insert the film on its superior border. Almost simultaneously, the operator places the index finger of the patient's hand (the patient's right hand is to retain films on the left side of the mandible and vice versa) on the film in such a manner that the film is pressed rather firmly against the mandible. Every effort is made not to curve the film. If the muscle attachments are high so that the lower border of the film is away from the apices of the teeth, it is preferable to hold the film against the lingual surfaces of the tooth crown rather than deeper in the mouth floor. This procedure prevents film curving. With the film positioned in this manner, the rules for horizontal and vertical angulation of the x-ray beam, as discussed earlier, are followed. A film held in this manner is shown in Fig. 5-18.

Mandibular molar area

Film placement for the mandibular molar area is identical with that of the bicuspid area except that the film is placed sufficiently far distally to reveal the entire third molar area and the beginning of the upward inclination of the anterior border of the ramus. Usually, the anterior border of the film is placed somewhat distal to the midline of the second bicuspid. Angulation procedures follow previously emphasized rules.

ALTERNATIVE METHOD FOR X-RAY BEAM ANGULATION

Frequent reference has been made to the central ray. The reader has been instructed to direct the central ray perpendicular to either the long axis of the tooth and to the film plane (paralleling technic) or to the bisector of the angle formed by the long axis of the tooth and the x-ray film (bisecting technic). The reader also has been instructed to direct the central ray through the interproximal spaces of the teeth being examined (both technics).

There is an alternative to use of the central ray as a basis for establishing correct vertical and horizontal angulation. This alternative uses the plane of the opening in the distal end of the cylinder (the end of the cylinder that touches or approximates the face). This plane is perpendicular to the central ray. If one prefers to use this plane to determine x-ray beam angulation, the plane must be made parallel with either the long axis of the tooth and the film plane (paralleling technic) or with the bisector of the angle formed by the long axis of the tooth and the x-ray film (bisecting technic). Concurrently, with either technic, the plane of the cylinder opening must be parallel with an envisioned line that touches the buccal surfaces of all teeth being examined. If necessary, this line can be envisioned readily by placing a tongue blade, swab stick, or similar object on these buccal surfaces. The tongue blade or swab stick is removed before the exposure is made.

This method can be used when angulating for bite-wing films and for views employing the occlusal film. The descriptions of these technics use the central ray as a basis for angulating. Utilization of this alternative method simply employs parallelism of lines and planes rather than perpendicularism. This alternative method may be more useful to some than the procedures emphasized throughout this chapter.

COMPROMISE PROCEDURES COMBINING PARALLELING AND BISECTING TECHNICS

Anatomic considerations sometimes make it extremely difficult to apply all of the principles of the paralleling technic. Extremely high and narrow palatal vaults make film placement for posterior parts of the maxilla relatively easy, but they interfere with film positioning in the anterior part of the mouth. High muscle attachments in the floor of the mouth on the lingual surface of the mandible sometimes make it almost impossible to insert a film deep enough and sufficiently far toward the midline. Other examples of anatomic considerations that make the use of the paralleling technic rather difficult could be cited.

Under adverse circumstances, it is suggested that every effort be made to utilize the basic principles of shadow casting (these are fundamental to the paralleling technic) and yet to compromise when necessary by permitting the film and the long axis of the tooth to be minimally nonparallel. When this lack of parallelism exists, vertical angulation must be increased slightly so that the central ray is perpendicular to a line bisecting the angle formed by the long axis of the tooth and the x-ray film. Even when the operator must compromise, the tooth and film rarely contact. The angle just mentioned is formed by an extension of the tooth and film lines. It is recommended that no change be made in the target-object distance; the use of the extended cylinder is advantageous with both the paralleling and bisecting technics.

Some dental offices are so small that the use of the extended cylinder appears to be prohibited because of room dimensions and the proximity of the dental chair to the x-ray unit. It is inadvisable to employ a short cone or cylinder when the paralleling technic is used. However, in most cases the extended cylinder can be used if the operator rotates the chair and the patient's head as well as the x-ray tube head.

FILM PLACEMENT AND ANGULATION PROCEDURES USING BITE-WING FILMS

Posterior bite-wing films are essential if the bisecting technic is used in order to demonstrate interproximal carious lesions adequately and to visualize the underlying periodontal condition. Bite-wing films are helpful if the paralleling technic is used, particularly if any compromise between the two methods becomes necessary. In the adult mouth it is preferable to use two bite-wing films on each side of the face in preference to one long, narrow film. The 2.3 bite-wing film, measuring approximately $2\frac{1}{8} \times 1\frac{1}{16}$ inches, is too narrow to reveal the periodontal bone level consistently, particularly if there has been substantial bone loss. In addition, this film is not as satisfactory for the detection of interproximal caries, because one horizontal angulation must suffice for at least two different interproximal pathways. Arch configurations pertinent to the last statement are illustrated in Figs. 5-12 and 5-17. Although bicuspid and molar bite-wing films are ordinarily necessary for adult patients having a complete or nearly complete dentition, one bite-wing film on each side is usually sufficient for patients through approximately age 12 years.

Bite-wing films may be purchased from the manufacturer with attached tabs. A more economical method utilizes periapical film inserted into a paper or plastic bite-wing tab. Some available bite-wing film holders are shown in Fig. 5-25.

Bite-wing films are placed in an identical fashion for both the bicuspid and the molar areas. However, the anterior border of the bicuspid bite-wing is expected to reveal the distal surface of the cuspid tooth as well as mesial surface of the first molar. The molar bite-wing film should ordinarily reveal the distal surface of the second bicuspid tooth and all interproximal surfaces distal to this area. This requires that the molar bite-wing film be placed more distally in the mouth.

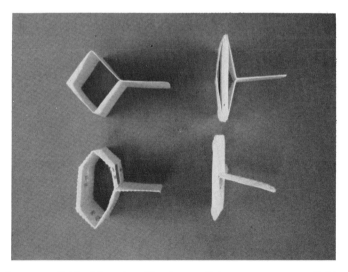

Fig. 5-25. Some available bite-wing film loops. Other types are available. *Upper left,* Most commonly used type; *upper right,* film inserted into the loop; *lower left,* loop adjustable for several film sizes; *lower right,* tab with an adhesive that permits it to be attached directly to the film.

When the bite-wing film is placed, the bite-wing tab is folded upward against the film surface. The film is placed like any mandibular bicuspid or molar film except that it is inserted less deeply into the floor of the mouth. The film tab in the middle of the film should be at the level of the mandibular occlusal surfaces. The film tab is now turned downward onto the mandibular occlusal surfaces; the tab is held in position with the operator's index finger. The film should *not* be held too firmly in contact with the teeth. The patient is asked to close *slowly* on the tab. As the patient slowly closes, a tongue blade is used to push the upper border of the bite-wing film away from the palatal surfaces. This simple maneuver avoids an early contact between the palate and the upper border of the film. If this is not done, the film may be forced too far into the floor of the mouth and/or twisted on the tab so that the occlusal plane is projected diagonally across the film rather than parallel with the upper and lower borders of the film. In Fig. 5-26 the operator is shown holding the bite-wing tab and concurrently pushing the upper border of the film away from the palate as the patient closes on the tab.

A vertical angulation of from 0 to +5° is ordinarily used with a horizontal angle designed to permit the rays to go through the interproximal spaces between the teeth being examined.

ALTERNATIVE FILM-HOLDING DEVICES

An effort has been made thus far in this chapter to present principles of film placement and x-ray beam angulation. Methods used by us have been discussed. It is pertinent to note that various types of film-holding and angulation devices that may be of use to the dental practitioner or his assistant are available. During the past several decades, a variety of such items have come into being, and it is impractical to illustrate and discuss all such equipment. However, it seems useful to illustrate some of the more commonly used devices. Methods that

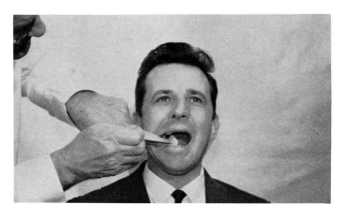

Fig. 5-26. Adjustment of the bite-wing film position performed concurrently with mouth closure.

eliminate the necessity for exposing the patient's hand should be used when feasible. Fig. 5-27 illustrates useful equipment.

Most operators use a variety of film holders for intraoral radiography. Although a particular film holder may work well for an operator in accordance with his particular ability and type of radiographic projections, few holders will satisfy all operators for all projections on all patients. In evaluating film holders or in considering the purchase of one of these devices, one must keep certain factors in mind. Nondisposable film holders made of plastic (for example, the types shown in Figure 5-27, *B*, and *C*) cannot be sterilized in an autoclave and can be used only where cold sterilization technics are acceptable. Bite-block film holders similar to the type shown in Fig. 5-27, *D*, are available in wood, metal, rubber, plastic, and Styrofoam. Some wood, metal, and rubber blocks can be autoclaved, and the Styrofoam type is disposable. Although the Styrofoam block is softer and is better tolerated than the other blocks by patients who have to bite the block on the gingiva, it breaks more easily. The patient must be instructed to bite more gently on Styrofoam blocks. Bite-block film holders need only the closing of the patient's jaws to maintain them in place. This technic is advantageous when the patient has a broken or unsteady arm and cannot assist in holding the film holder in position. However, bite-block holders have the disadvantage of being positioned on the tooth being radiographed and cannot be used where instruments, such as endodontic reamers and files, are protruding from the tooth under examination.

Film holders using an extraoral x-ray beam–positioning extension (for example, the types shown in Fig. 5-27, *A* and *C*) are designed to position the central x-ray beam perpendicular to the film or perpendicular to a plane that is expected to be located at the bisector of the angle formed by the film and long axis of the tooth. Such film holders aid the operator in avoiding "cone cutting" the film. They also assist in identifying the horizontal and vertical x-ray beam direction when the film is placed in the ideal position. However, when the film in the holder cannot be positioned planoparallel to the long axes of the teeth or to the bisectors of the tooth-film angles (as in patients with tori, small oral cavities, and malpositioned teeth), the operator must be aware that the device tends to direct the x-ray beam in a less than optimal direction relative to the teeth and their interproximal spaces.

Some film holders with x-ray beam–positioning extensions have been designed to be used with rectangular collimators. One such device is shown in Fig. 4-3. The rectangular extension of these devices has its greater dimension in the vertical plane for anterior teeth and in the horizontal plane for posterior teeth. This requires use of a matching rectangular collimator, attached to the x-ray machine tube head, that can turn on its base. The operator must make the proper rotation of the rectangular x-ray beam, a procedure not required by circular beams; however, rectangular beams expose less tissue of the patient to primary radiation.

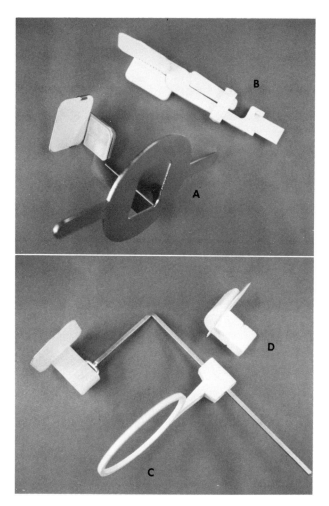

Fig. 5-27. Four types of commercially available intraoral film holders. **A,** The precision x-ray instrument consists of a facial shield attached to an arm that supports the film in a position parallel with the shield. The rectangular hole in the shield is designed to be used at a specific distance from the x-ray tube. It permits passage only of those x-rays that will strike the film. The patient closes on a bite block just in front of the film. The open end of the x-ray machine cylinder is placed in contact with the shield. These instruments are available in sets for all areas of the mouth, for children as well as adults, and for the intraoral technic used by the dentist. **B,** The Snap-A-Ray is designed to hold the film, as illustrated, between two plastic jaws that can be locked in place. Provision is also made for supporting a film on the opposite end of the instrument. The plastic jaws, when closed, serve as a bite plane on which the patient bites after the film has been positioned. **C,** The X-C-P instrument functions similarly to the instrument shown in **A.** The circular area is adjustable; this permits the film to be positioned first and the ring to be brought into contact with the face secondarily. As with **A,** the open end of the x-ray machine cylinder is made to contact the ring. These instruments can be purchased in sets. Different instruments are used for the various intraoral areas, for different mouth sizes, and for each of the two commonly used intraoral technics. *Also note Fig. 4-3 for a modification of the X-C-P instrument.* **D,** A disposable Styrofoam film holder applicable to almost any area of the mouth. The film can be positioned either horizontally or vertically, as illustrated, and the patient closes onto the soft plastic. One such holder usually serves for a complete set of intraoral films. It can be used effectively when taking anterior extraoral tangential views of the maxilla or mandible (see Fig. 6-6, **A**). (**A,** Courtesy Precision X-ray Instrument Co. and Dr. Fred Medwedeff; **B,** Courtesy Rinn Corp. and Dr. William Updegrave; **C,** Courtesy Rinn Corp. and Dr. Harry Greene; **D,** Courtesy Delaware Plastics Co.)

FILM PLACEMENT AND ANGULATION PROCEDURES
USING AN OCCLUSAL FILM

Occlusal films are placed into the oral cavity and hence can be classified as intraoral films. However, they are used generally for the same purposes as extraoral films—to demonstrate an area of greater dimension than is possible on a single periapical film. Occlusal films (3.4) measure approximately $2\frac{1}{4} \times 3$ inches.

The occlusal film is ordinarily inserted with the longest dimension of the film in an anteroposterior position. It is retained by the patient's closing on the film as though he were biting a sandwich (the occlusal film is sometimes referred to as a sandwich film).

In the edentulous arch the film is held against the maxillary ridge by the patient's thumbs and on the mandibular ridge by the forefingers. If the patient is unable to support the film with his hands, the operator must improvise by using cotton rolls or moldable wax. The occlusal film may be used successfully to produce a topographic view of an area or to show the area in cross section.

Topographic occlusal view

A topographic radiograph looks similar to the ordinary periapical film except that it is larger. The film is inserted into the mouth as previously described with the exposure side of the film toward the teeth to be examined. The film must be positioned in such a way that the shadow of the questionable area will be cast onto the film when an exposure is made. Occlusal film placement for the anterior segment of the mouth is shown in Fig. 5-28. Film placement for the posterior area is similar except that the film is positioned more distally and more toward the side being examined.

Angulation rules for topographic projections are identical with those of the bisecting technic. With the film on the horizontal plane, the operator must envision the bisector of the angle made by the long axis of the teeth and the x-ray film. He must then direct the radiation, using either the short cone or cylinder, or the long cylinder, through the apex of the teeth at right angles to the bisector. Concurrently, the rays are expected to pass directly through the interproximal spaces of these teeth. Ordinarily, the horizontal angulation is of less concern than the vertical angulation because the occlusal film is rarely used to better understand caries or the periodontal condition. Fig. 5-28 can be useful for understanding angulation technics. The film must be envisioned in a horizontal plane. Vertical angulation is increased for examination of areas in the distal part of the palate.

Cross-sectional occlusal view

Optimum interpretive results often require bidirectional or multidirectional views of a questionable area. The cross-sectional occlusal projection occasionally can be helpful. This view can be made of a specific area or of an entire dental arch. The occlusal film is placed in the mouth as for the topographic view, but

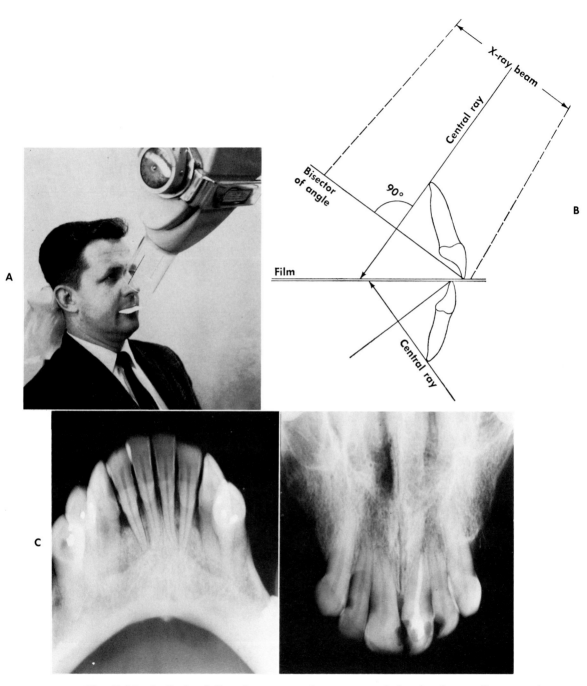

Fig. 5-28. A, Occlusal film placement and correct angulation for the maxillary anterior area. **B,** Diagram illustrating angulation theory for topographic projections. **C,** Typical mandibular and maxillary anterior topographic radiographs.

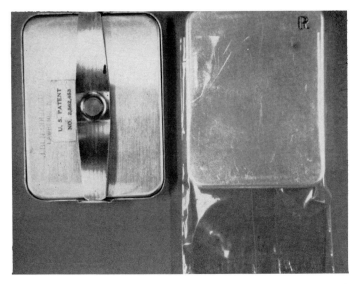

Fig. 5-29. Back and front of an intraoral cassette. The cassette at the right is partially inserted into a plastic envelope.

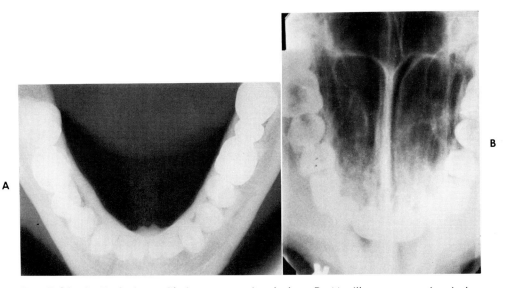

Fig. 5-30. A, Typical mandibular cross-sectional view. **B,** Maxillary cross-sectional view.

the rays are directed through the questionable area and parallel with the long axis of the teeth included in or directly adjacent to the area. Thus, the teeth are observed in the processed film as circular or elliptical areas. When the entire dental arch is to be observed, the central ray is directed perpendicular to the film.

Exposure procedures vary with the type of lesion being examined. For example, the location of an impacted tooth would require a given exposure, whereas an attempt to locate a small salivary stone in a lingual or submaxillary duct would require considerably less exposure. A cross-sectional view of the maxilla requires as much as 5 to 8 seconds of exposure at 10 mA, approximately 65 kVp, and a target-scalp distance of approximately 8 inches. The rays are directed through the top of the head and must penetrate considerable tissue thickness. The use of an intraoral cassette equipped with intensifying screens is recommended in these circumstances. The regular doublepack occlusal film formerly could be removed from its packet and used singly in the intraoral cassette. Occlusal film (3.4) is no longer useful with intensifying screens. If intraoral cassettes are to be used, a film of suitable size must be cut from a larger sheet of x-ray film designed to be used with intensifying screens. An intraoral cassette is pictured in Fig. 5-29. Plastic envelopes are available into which the cassette can be inserted before it is placed into the oral cavity.

The film speed of occlusal film is the same as that of the fastest commonly used periapical film. It has an ANSI* speed rating of D, which gives the operator an approximate idea of the necessary exposure time. The type of films that can be expected from the occlusal cross-sectional technic is shown in Fig. 5-30.

EXPOSURE FACTORS

Exposure factors include film speed, kilovoltage peak, milliamperage, filtration, target-film distance, and exposure time, all of which are discussed in Chapters 1 and 2. Collimation of the beam by the use of a diaphragm has also been mentioned. For purposes of emphasis, it is important to restate that the total filtration should be the equivalent of 1.5 to 2.5 mm. of aluminum (the higher thicknesses are preferable), and the beam diameter at the skin should not exceed 2.75 inches. Collimation and filtration must comply with state laws.

Exposure time will vary with the factors mentioned previously. The determination of proper exposure values is discussed in Chapter 4.

---

*See Table 1-3.

CHAPTER 6

Essential extraoral technics

Intraoral radiographs examine only a portion of the mandible and maxilla—the teeth and their immediate supporting structures. In many instances, periapical films do not show an entire lesion. In addition, the dentist may suspect the existence of other lesions beyond the area examined by regular intraoral radiographs, or he may be unable, for one reason or another, to obtain intraoral radiographs. A complete oral diagnosis often demands the use of radiographs that will depict and localize a lesion in its entirety and detect similar lesions elsewhere in and around the jaws. It is essential that the dental practitioner be proficient in some extraoral radiographic technics.

Extraoral radiography calls for the use of large films. This in turn necessitates the use of film holders, cassettes, and other x-ray accessories. Since extraoral radiography is not a routine procedure for most dental patients, essential extraoral technics, of necessity, must be practical for the average dental office. Filtration, unless otherwise stated, is similar to that recommended for intraoral radiography. The beam size should be limited to adequate coverage of the area of interest. This can be accomplished in most instances with cones and diaphragms used in intraoral radiography. Essential extraoral technics discussed in this text are restricted to those technics that can be accomplished with the use of occlusal and nonscreen films. Additional extraoral procedures requiring somewhat more specialized equipment are discussed in Chapter 7.

Technics using nonscreen film can also be accomplished with screen film used in cassettes equipped with fluorescent screens. The latter method is preferable from a radiation health aspect since the amount of radiation needed to expose the film-screen combination is much less than that needed to expose the nonscreen film; in addition, much shorter exposure times can be used. Cassettes and screens are an additional expense for equipment that may not often be used. Many dental offices may be equipped only with nonscreen film holders; thus this chapter will emphasize those extraoral radiographic procedures that are practical for nonscreen film.

Nonscreen film is usually placed in cardboard film holders, although such film is supplied in individual light-tight packets ready for use. The film holders and individual packets are light in weight and can be supported easily in position by the patient.

Often, more than one extraoral radiograph is needed when a patient is being examined. Since these cardboard film holders are inexpensive, the dentist can have two or more of these films ready for use at any time. The size of nonscreen film most commonly used in dentistry is 5 × 7 inches. Occlusal and 5 × 7 nonscreen film require no additional equipment in the x-ray room or darkroom beyond that needed for intraoral radiography except if the Morlite filter is used for safelighting. A Wratten 6B filter is needed for all extraoral film (see Chapter 9). *Essential* extraoral technics are thus designed around the use of the occlusal and 5 × 7 film.

BASIC NONSCREEN FILM TECHNICS

Nonscreen film is readily available in two sizes, 5 × 7 inches and 8 × 10 inches. The most common size used is 5 × 7 inches. Nonscreen films are used in cardboard film holders. Left (L) and right (R) lead markers must be used on the exposure side of the film holders to identify on the radiograph which side of the patient was examined. All films must be identified as to the patient's name and the date. This can be done by writing on the film in lead pencil or ball-point pen either before or after exposure but before developing. There is another, more easily observable, method of film identification. A small sheet of lead is placed over a part of the film holder to prevent film exposure under a specific area. Patient information is printed on this area photographically. This is done in the darkroom with the use of a film identifier that uses a card with the necessary information written on it. The masked film holder, the identifier, the card, and the reproduced information are shown in Fig. 9-3.

Nonscreen films have thicker emulsions and may require an increase of 50% in the usual processing times; the film manufacturer's processing instructions should be observed. Thicker emulsions need less total radiation to produce the required film density. These thicker emulsions also show an increased contrast range. Although the technics to be described will specify nonscreen film, screen film in cassettes with intensifying screens utilizing shorter exposure times can also be used. The weight of the metal cassettes makes it more difficult for the patient to support the equipment in the proper position. Radiographs produced using intensifying screens have a shorter scale of contrast than do radiographs made with nonscreen film.

Dentists should be capable of examining radiographically the entire maxilla and mandible. Intraoral, including occlusal, radiographs fulfill this assignment to a large extent. However, there are many areas that these radiographs do not cover. Proper use of the 5 × 7 nonscreen film will, to a considerable degree, satisfy this need. Essential projections using nonscreen film can be classified into (1) lateral jaw projections, (2) lateral condyle projections, and (3) lateral sinus projections. For the examination of larger areas or thicker body parts, the use of the more radiosensitive screen film–cassette combination is mandatory.

Lateral oblique projection of the mandible and maxilla

Lateral jaw radiography is the term generally used to describe lateral views of the mandible and/or maxilla. A true lateral projection of an entire side of a jaw is not possible, since the image of the opposite side would be superimposed on it. The lateral jaw projection must be made with some oblique angulation. The beam of radiation can be directed at the area of interest from two basic directions: (1) from underneath the mandible opposite the side under examination and (2) from behind the ramus of the mandible opposite the side under examination. The beam can also be directed from any area between these two basic positions. When the beam is directed underneath the body of the mandible, a large area of the mandible and maxilla can be shown on the film. However, the images

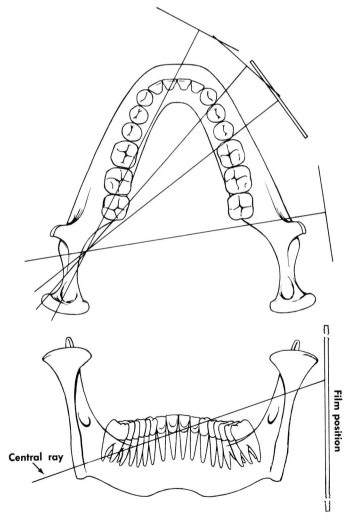

Fig. 6-1. X-ray beam direction for the lateral jaw projection. Rays strike the film obliquely in the vertical plane but should be perpendicular in the horizontal plane.

will suffer from distortion because of the great degree of vertical angulation. When the beam is directed between the ramus and the vertebral column from behind the ramus, distortion of the images is held to a minimum, but the area that can be examined is more limited in size. Beam direction used in this second method is shown in Fig. 6-1. A good survey of an entire side can be made with four films by taking the ramus, molar, bicuspid, and incisor areas separately. Lateral jaw radiographs should be made with the second method whenever possible. The first method and/or a compromise between the two is used only when circumstances make the second method impractical.

Positioning of the patient is important. The patient is seated in an upright position with the teeth in occlusion and the occlusal plane parallel with the floor. The chair headrest is placed fairly high on the head. This allows more freedom of movement for positioning the head of the x-ray machine. The patient is asked to project his chin as far forward as is comfortable in order to separate the mandible from the vertebral column and to prevent contraction of soft tissue posterior to the ramus. This patient position generally will be satisfactory for all projections; however, for the bicuspid and incisor areas, the patient's head can be rotated slightly in the direction away from the x-ray tube. Tipping the patient's head away from the x-ray machine for the ramus and molar projections can be useful.

The machine is used with an 8-inch or greater target-skin distance. The central ray is directed at a point just medial to the ramus and about ½ inch above

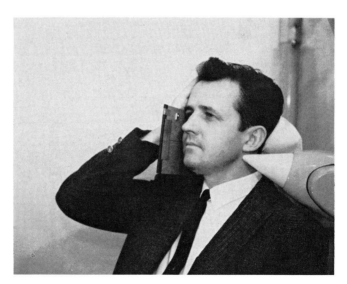

Fig. 6-2. Lateral jaw technic for the mandibular right bicuspid area, demonstrating positions of the x-ray machine, patient, and film. The pointed plastic cone is used in this illustration even though the lead-lined open cone is ordinarily recommended. One of us (L. R. M.-H.) believes that greater accuracy can be obtained using the pointed cone; the desirability of superior radiographs supersedes the need to reduce secondary radiation.

the angle of the mandible on the side of the face nearest the x-ray machine. Simultaneously, the central ray is directed toward the occlusal plane of the teeth at a point just anterior to the area of interest. For example, when the molar area is being examined, the central ray is aimed at the cusps of the maxillary second bicuspid. The x-ray beam thus covers fairly equal segments of the mandible and maxilla. It is more difficult to position for the ramus than for the other three areas, and it may become necessary to direct the central ray from underneath rather than from behind the near mandible.

The film is positioned so that the central ray is as perpendicular as possible to the film in both the horizontal and vertical planes. This can be achieved on the horizontal plane, but perpendicularity with the x-rays in the vertical plane rather widely separates the film from the tissue. Acceptable radiographs can be made with the film held either parallel with the vertical axis of the skull or at right angles to the central ray.

Acceptable film positions for examining the various areas of the jaws can be achieved without using any accessory equipment. The film is held by the patient between the heel of the hand and the malar or zygomatic bone (Fig. 6-2). In the anterior areas the nose assists in horizontal stabilization of the film, and in the posterior areas the zygomatic arch assists in stabilization. In all instances, the patient curves the fingers of the hand holding the film over the top of the film and rests them on the cranium. This position of the hand stabilizes the film in the vertical plane.

Examples of lateral jaw radiographs and film exposure factors are shown in Fig. 6-3. It is obvious that these projections are invaluable when the patient cannot open his mouth. They are also of assistance when the making of intraoral radiographs is impractical, as in very young children, geriatric patients, and patients with an extreme gag reflex. Since large areas of the mandible and maxilla can be examined, lateral jaw radiographs are very useful in showing the boundaries of large lesions and are of value in the evaluation of bone.

Lateral condyle projection

The condyle of the mandible is situated so that the medial border is slightly posterior to the lateral border. A true lateral view of this structure (which would be slightly posteroanterior to the midsaggital plane) cannot be obtained radiographically without superimposition of the vertebral column and/or parts of the cranial base. However, a slightly mesio-oblique lateral view provides a wealth of information about the head and neck of the mandibular condyle and about the zygomatic arch.

For this projection, the nonscreen film in a cardboard film holder is held against the side of the face as in a posterior lateral jaw view. The patient is asked to open the mouth as widely as possible. This moves the condyle under examination out of its socket in a forward and downward direction. Opening the mouth also lowers the coronoid process and sigmoid notch on the side not being examined. The central ray is now directed through the sigmoid notch of the mandible nearest the x-ray source and at the condyle being examined. Approximately an 8-inch target-skin distance is used. This technic and the resultant radiograph are illustrated in Fig. 6-4.

When the patient is unable to open the mouth, the technic is modified. The cone is eliminated except for the threaded end, which is used to retain the dia-

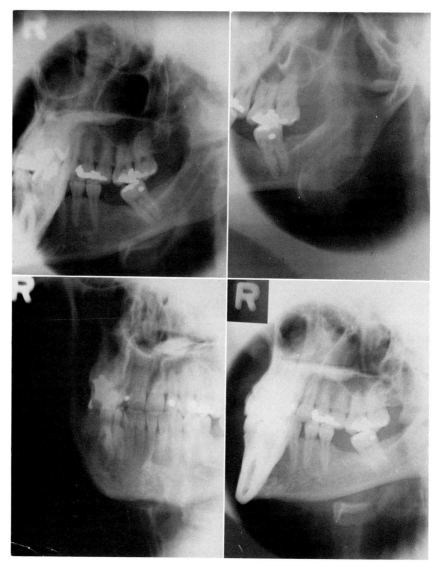

Fig. 6-3. Examples of lateral jaw radiographs. The exposure factors include 65 kVp, 10 mA, an approximately 12-inch target-film distance, 2.25 mm. total aluminum (equivalent) filtration, nonscreen film, a ³/₄-inch diaphragm aperture, and the following exposure factors: molar area, 1¼ seconds; ramus, 1 second; anterior, 2 seconds; and bicuspid, 1½ seconds.

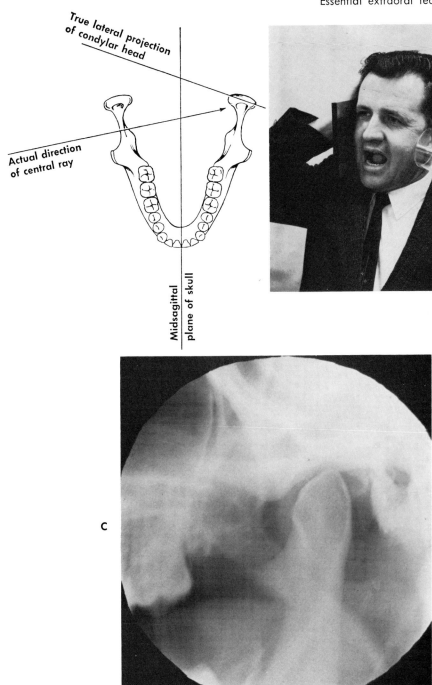

Fig. 6-4. A, Diagram of x-ray beam direction for the lateral condyle projection. **B,** Machine, patient, and film relationships. **C,** Radiographic result. Exposure factors: nonscreen film, 65 kVp, 10 mA, recommended filtration and collimation, an 8-inch target-skin distance, and an average exposure time of 1¼ seconds.

phragm and filter; a 4-inch tube-skin distance results. Because of the nearness of the patient's skin to the tube, the x-ray beam filtration should be increased by 0.5 to 1 mm. of aluminum. The film position remains the same. The x-rays will now have to pass through the ramus of the mandible opposite the condyle being examined. Thus these two structures will be superimposed. However, since the obstructing ramus is near the tube and far from the film, its image on the radiograph will be blurred. Conversely, the image of the condyle under examination will be sharp because of its nearness to the film and its relatively great distance from the x-ray source. This modification can be used even if the patient can open his mouth. Reduction of skin exposure is the reason for suggesting the 8-inch target-skin distance.

The lateral condyle projection is useful in the investigation of the temporomandibular joint and in examining the neck of the condyle and the coronoid process. The shape and position of the condyle is seen clearly, usually without the superimposition of other calcified structures. Erosions on the surface of the condyle and fractures of the neck or coronoid process of the mandible can usually be demonstrated in this projection. If the mouth cannot be opened, the articulating surface of the condylar head is not clearly seen.

Lateral sinus projection

For the lateral sinus projection,* the film is placed planoparallel to the midsagittal plane and is held against the side of the face, as in the posterior lateral jaw projection. The x-ray beam is directed perpendicular to the sagittal plane and film in both horizontal and vertical planes. The central ray enters the face at approximately the apex of the maxillary first molar tooth. The tube-skin distance is approximately 12 inches.

Like the lateral condyle projection, this view of the sinuses examines parts of the face that intraoral and lateral jaw radiographs are unable to show clearly. Lesions involving the superior or posterior areas of the maxilla can be seen in this view. The nasal bones are also shown. A moderate decrease in exposure time often shows the nasal area more effectively. The technic and resultant radiograph are shown in Fig. 6-5.

USE OF OCCLUSAL FILM

Extraoral projections using occlusal film are possible in some instances. The occlusal film can be substituted for a 5 × 7 film when the area to be examined is small, as with very young children. In such instances, the substitution of the occlusal film for 5 × 7 nonscreen film is quite practical. The required exposure is slightly greater than that for identical views taken with nonscreen film.

---

*The more conventional lateral sinus projection utilizing intensifying screens is discussed in Chapter 7.

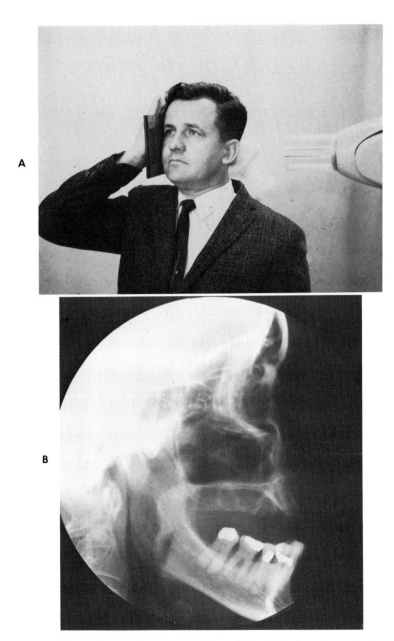

Fig. 6-5. A, Film, patient, and x-ray machine relationships for a lateral sinus projection. **B,** Resultant radiograph. Exposure factors: nonscreen film, 65 kVp, 10 mA, recommended filtration and collimation, an approximately 12-inch target-skin distance, and an average exposure time of 1¼ seconds.

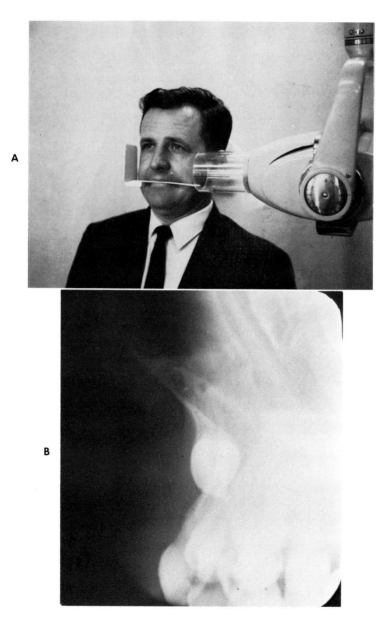

Fig. 6-6. A, Film, patient, and x-ray machine relationships for an occlusal film tangential projection. **B,** Resultant radiograph. Exposure factors: 65 kVp, 10 mA, recommended filtration and collimation, and an average exposure time of ½ second.

Tangential projection

The occlusal film is very useful in obtaining a tangential projection of an anterior tooth or area. For this projection, the film is placed in a groove or slot in a wood or plastic stick. The stick is held between the teeth with the film positioned beyond the area of interest. The central ray is directed in such a manner as to be perpendicular to the film in both horizontal and vertical planes and to form a tangent with the curve of the jaw at the area under examination. This projection is shown in Fig. 6-6, in which an 8-inch tube-skin distance was used. An increased distance also can be employed. Tangential projections are useful in localizing objects in the anterior areas of the mandible and maxilla.

CHAPTER 7

Specialized extraoral technics

INTRODUCTION

Extraoral radiographic procedures are not widely used in dentistry. This is unfortunate because they can be of considerable diagnostic use to the conscientious dentist who has made an effort to understand radiographic findings. Contrary to popular opinion, extraoral procedures are ordinarily less difficult than are intraoral technics.

There are many extraoral radiographic procedures that, in the aggregate, are capable of examining the entire head and neck. Of these, many are highly specialized and are designed to provide specific types of information. Some specialized technics are more useful in dentistry than are others. Those technics that are both useful and practical for the dental practitioner are discussed in this chapter. Technics included under the discussion of *extraoral projections* are useful for both general scanning and specific purposes. The procedures described in the discussion of *special purpose projections* are designed mainly for specific types of information.

STANDARDIZATION

The diagnostic radiograph must portray changes in the object. Since this is a major objective of the diagnostic radiograph, all factors (1) that can create radiographic changes that do not exist in the object and (2) that would tend to confuse the interpreter must be kept constant for any particular projection. It is also advisable that these factors be standardized as much as possible for the majority of the different extraoral projections. To accomplish this, the radiologist must know the role that all factors play in the production of the radiograph. Only when these factors are understood and controlled can the radiologist conclude that variations seen in a radiographic image are the result of changes in the object being examined. The major radiographic variables are briefly discussed here from the standpoint of their standardization or control in specialized extraoral radiography. The reader is referred to earlier chapters, particularly Chapter 2, for a review of the *role* that these variables play in radiogaphy.

Exposure time

Exposure time is the factor most often varied. It is usually changed to adjust for smaller differences in the thickness or density of the object or patient. Variations are necessary if the overall blackness of different radiographs is to be maintained.

Milliamperage

Milliamperage can be varied instead of or in addition to exposure time to compensate for different object thicknesses. However, the mA range (usually 0 to 15) on dental x-ray machines is small, and control of film density by this means is impractical for dental radiography. The most common constant milliamperage setting used is 10 mA.

Kilovoltage

Some radiologists use variable kVp technics to adjust for object thickness. Increased kVp is needed for increased photon penetrability when very thick or dense objects are to be examined. However, to utilize this technic, the diagnostician must be experienced in viewing the different scales of contrast that result from varied kVp. For dental radiography, 65 kVp will usually suffice for both intraoral and extraoral radiography. However, many diagnosticians utilize kilovoltages as high as 100 kVp, which is the upper limit on the dental x-ray machine.

Filtration

Dental x-ray machines should have at least 2 mm. of aluminum (equivalent) total filtration. In some areas of the United States, 2.5 mm. of aluminum filtration is required. This amount of beam filtration is sufficient for almost all dental radiographic technics. However, if the tube-skin distance is less than 8 inches, it is suggested that the filtration be increased by 0.5 to 1 mm. of aluminum over that used at 8 inches or more.

Collimation

The size of the area being examined varies greatly between different extraoral projections. The collimation required for any particular projection must be such that the beam of radiation is of the smallest practical size necessary to cover the area being examined. Since beam size varies with target-object distances, the distance factor can be used to control beam size. Lead collimators with various-size apertures can also be used effectively to control beam diameter; it is the preferable method. The preparation of suitable collimators is discussed in Chapter 2. For purposes of practicality in this text, technics are suggested that employ, whenever possible, the lead-lined, open-end, short cone and the diaphragm ordinarily used with this cone. When feasible, distances are varied to obtain the desired area coverage without changing the diaphragm.

Distance

Target-object distance, according to projective geometry, should be as great as possible. Great distances unfortunately require long exposure times and increase the chance of a blurred image from patient movement. Basically, exposure times not exceeding 3 seconds are quite practical in extraoral radiography; tube-object distance for a particular technic is usually set at a distance that requires an exposure time of less than 3 seconds. Exceptions to this rule for determination of target-object distance include those techniques that are designed to use advantageously two characteristics of the x-ray beam. These characteristics are (1) spreading of the x-ray beam from the focal spot and (2) increased radiographic magnification and unsharpness of objects close to the x-ray tube, for example, the lateral condyle projection used when the patient is unable to open the mouth. Spreading of the x-ray beam can be used to prevent superimposition of two objects situated one behind the other; for example, a short rather than a long target-object distance in the lateral jaw technic allows the examination of a larger area of the mandible and maxilla.

Films and intensifying screens

Generally speaking, extraoral radiography requires the use of screen film and cassettes with intensifying screens. When speed of exposure and/or patient radiation dose reduction is essential, high-speed screens are used. When roentgenographic detail is necessary, low-speed screens are used. In the main, extraoral dental radiography is adequately accomplished with medium- or par-speed screens. Screen film of various sensitivities is also available. If satisfactory image quality can be obtained, the fastest film should be used. In general, the use of slow film results in improved image quality.

Grids

The use of a grid or a Potter-Bucky diaphragm is the exception and not the rule in extraoral radiography. Although these devices assist in producing radiographs of high quality, they are expensive, and reasonably good diagnostic radiographs can be made without them. However, it is desirable that these x-ray accessories be utilized, particularly in offices and clinics where many extraoral projections are made routinely. The quality of the resultant film is definitely enhanced. Considerably greater exposure is necessary when grids are used.

Film processing

It is highly desirable that film processing be standardized for extraoral radiography. A multitude of film faults and artifacts can be produced by improper darkroom technic. Film quality control cannot be obtained with a variable film-processing technic. This subject is discussed in Chapters 1 and 2 and is expanded in Chapter 9.

Film holders

Supports or holders for the cassette that maintain cassette position without patient cooperation are desirable but not essential for extraoral radiography. These devices do not change the tube-object-film relationship for any particular projection. However, they do make it easier and more comfortable for the patient and operator to obtain the necessary tube-object-film relationship.

Constant factors

Extraoral technics described in this chapter are all affected by variable radiographic factors. Some radiographic factors remain the same for all technics. In order to avoid constant repetition of the same values, these factors and their values are stated for all procedures:

1. Milliamperage of 10 mA
2. Kilovoltage of 65 kVp
3. Total beam filtration of 2.5 mm. of aluminum (equivalent)
4. Medium-speed screens
5. Kodak R-P Royal X-Omat* film
6. Nonuse of grids or Potter-Bucky diaphragm
7. Film processing on a time-temperature basis as recommended by the manufacturer of the processing solution
8. Short cylinder with collimator provided by manufacturer unless specified†

Although these standard factors are used in this text, they may be modified to obtain radiographs most satisfactory to the individual dentist.

Nonconstant factors

Nonconstant factors are listed for each projection as the technic is described. These factors include tube-film-patient positioning, tube-film distance, and exposure time. Dental x-ray machines vary considerably in output. The exposure times stated may be incorrect for some machines; under unusual circumstances they may vary by a factor of as much as 2.5. In general, however, they will produce usable films.

EXTRAORAL PROJECTIONS

The radiographic projections shown in Figs. 7-1 to 7-8 are commonly used when a radiographic survey of the skull is indicated. When the x-ray beam is essentially parallel with the sagittal plane of the skull, the x-rays enter posteriorly and emerge anteriorly; that is, the technics are posteroanterior projections.

---

*This mention does not imply endorsement of the product.
†The size of the beam of radiation varies with collimation and distance. X-ray tube–collimator distance varies with different machines. Most modern machines provide an approximately 2.75-inch diameter beam at the end of the short cylinder. Some machines may require special collimators to obtain the desired beam size for extraoral procedures.

Text continued on p. 150.

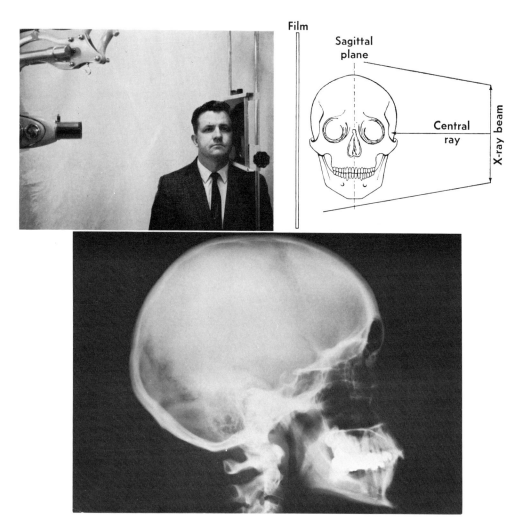

Fig. 7-1. Lateral skull projection. The film is positioned planoparallel with the sagittal plane of the skull. The central ray is directed perpendicular to the film horizontally and vertically. The central ray enters approximately 1 inch above the external auditory meatus. The target-film distance is 36 inches, and the exposure time is approximately ¾ second. X-ray beam coverage must include the entire skull. In the absence of a film holder, the patient supports the cassette on the shoulder and holds the top of the cassette against the side of the head. In the accompanying radiograph, it will be observed that the right and left sides of the skull are superimposed on each other. The side nearer the x-ray tube is magnified slightly more than the side nearer the film. Basically, the radiograph surveys the entire skull. More specifically, it shows the anteroposterior and superoinferior borders of the various anatomic entities. In addition, it demonstrates the anterior, posterior, superior, and inferior relationships of one part to another. Profile views of the soft tissues can be obtained by a 50% reduction in exposure time.

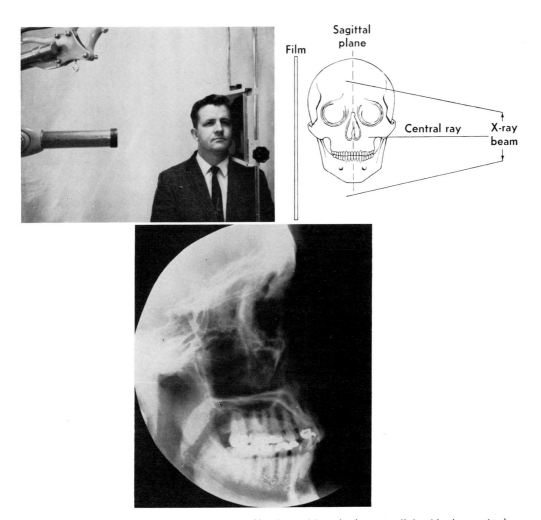

Fig. 7-2. Lateral sinus projection. The film is positioned planoparallel with the sagittal plane of the skull. The central ray is directed perpendicular to the film horizontally and vertically. The central ray enters at the apex of the maxillary first molar tooth. The target-film distance is 36 inches. An exposure time of $2/5$ second is required. In the absence of a film holder, the patient supports the cassette on the shoulder and holds the top of the cassette against the side of the head. The x-ray beam must be collimated to expose only the paranasal sinus area. The collimation ordinarily used with an extended cone is satisfactory. This projection evaluates most of the face from the lateral aspect. Anteroposterior and superoinferior borders of oral structures and lesions affecting the face can be shown clearly in this projection.

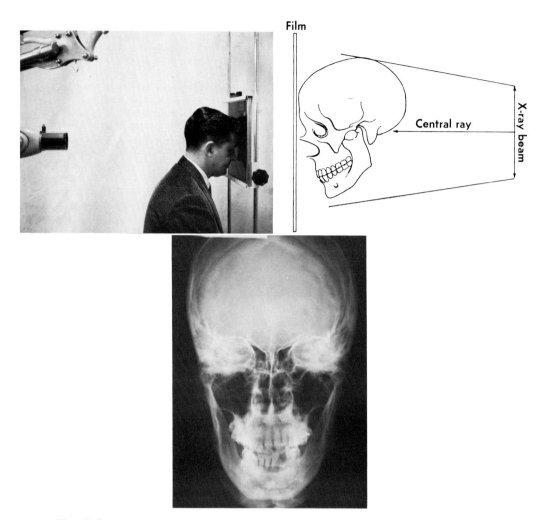

Fig. 7-3. Posteroanterior skull projection. The film is positioned at right angles to the sagittal plane of the skull. The patient rests the forehead on the cassette with the orbito-meatal (canthomeatal) plane (a line or plane drawn from the corner of the eye to the external auditory meatus) perpendicular to the film vertically and horizontally. The central ray is directed through the sagittal plane and parallel with the orbitomeatal plane at the level of the bridge of the nose. An exposure time of approximately 1½ seconds is used with a target-film distance of 36 inches. X-ray beam coverage must include the entire skull. In the absence of a film holder, the cassette can be supported against a wall by the patient's thumb and forefinger of each hand (the thumb is placed under the lower border of the cassette, and the forefinger supports the cassette against the wall by pressing on the front of the cassette). The superior, inferior, medial, and lateral borders of skull parts are shown in this projection. The mediolateral and superoinferior positions of objects or lesions can be identified. The mandibular symphysis is superimposed on the vertical column. The symphysis can be seen without this superimposition by taking right and left lateral jaw radiographs of the incisor area.

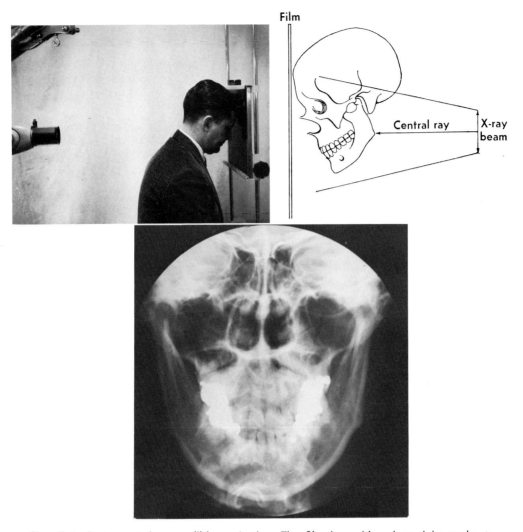

Fig. 7-4. Posteroanterior mandible projection. The film is positioned at right angles to the sagittal plane of the skull. The patient rests the forehead on the cassette. The central ray is directed perpendicular to the film horizontally and vertically through the sagittal plane at the level of the angle of the mandible. The chin is retracted away from the cassette until the central ray bisects the angle of the mandible. The target-film distance is 36 inches, and the exposure time is approximately ³/₄ second. The x-ray beam must be collimated to expose only the mandible. As in the posteroanterior skull projection, the cassette can be wall supported by the patient if a cassette holder is not available. The posteroanterior mandible projection is valuable in showing the mediolateral position of the various parts of the mandible. Lesions affecting the width of the mandible, fractures of the mandible, and radiopaque objects encroaching on the mandible are well portrayed. *The head of the condyle* is observed more clearly in this projection if the patient opens the mouth, causing the condylar head to move downward and forward out of the glenoid fossa. Films exposed using a slight rotation of the patient's head (approximately 5°) often are helpful as supplementary views.

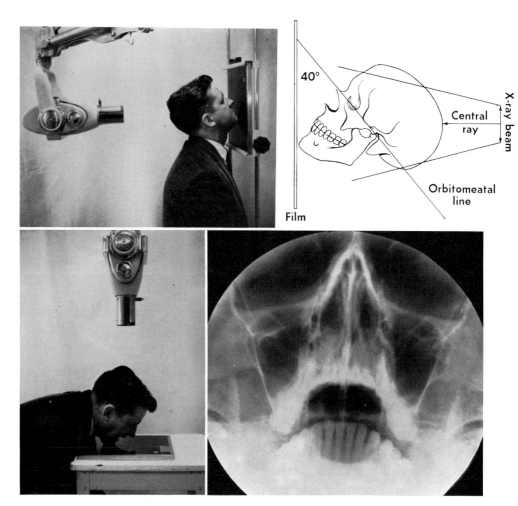

Fig. 7-5. Posteroanterior maxillary sinus projection. The film is positioned at right angles to the sagittal plane of the skull. The film may be placed in either a vertical or horizontal position. In the latter position, care must be exercised to avoid gonadal radiation exposure. The central ray is directed perpendicular to the film horizontally and vertically through the sagittal plane at the level of the middle of the maxillary sinus. The patient's chin rests on the cassette, and the head is tipped backward until the orbitomeatal (canthomeatal) line makes an angle of approximately 40° with the film (under these conditions, the tip of the nose will be ¾ to 1 inch away from the cassette). If the petrous portion of the temporal bone is superimposed on the lower border of the sinus, the patient's head must be tipped farther backward. The target-film distance is 24 inches, and the exposure time is approximately 1 second. When the orbitomeatal line is in the same position but with the mouth open, the image of the sphenoid sinus will appear on the palate. The x-ray beam must be collimated to include only the paranasal sinuses. Basically, this projection is made to demonstrate the maxillary sinuses. The other paranasal sinuses can be observed, particularly the ethmoids. In addition, the orbital and nasal cavities can be observed. In contrast with the horizontal film position, the vertical, or upright, position permits the detection of fluid level in the maxillary sinuses.

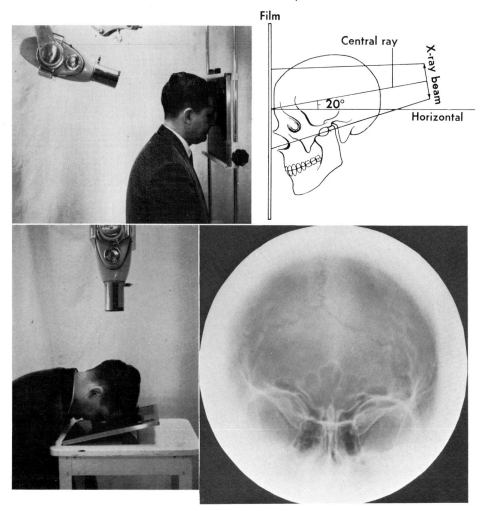

Fig. 7-6. Posteroanterior frontal sinus projection. The film is positioned at right angles to the sagittal plane of the skull. Preferably, it is held in a vertical position. The patient's forehead and nose are made to touch the film. The central ray is directed in the sagittal plane through the frontal sinus at approximately a 20° downward angle. The target-film distance is 24 inches, and the exposure time is approximately ³/₄ second. This sinus view can be made with the film placed on a metal table at an angle of about 20°. Under these circumstances, the x-rays are directed at right angles to the table top. Care must be taken to avoid gonadal exposure. This projection is designed to show the frontal and ethmoidal sinuses. The petrous portion of the temporal bone obscures the maxillary sinuses. Although the frontal and ethmoid sinuses are seen on the maxillary sinus projection, the object-film distance used results in some loss of detail in the frontal and ethmoid sinuses.

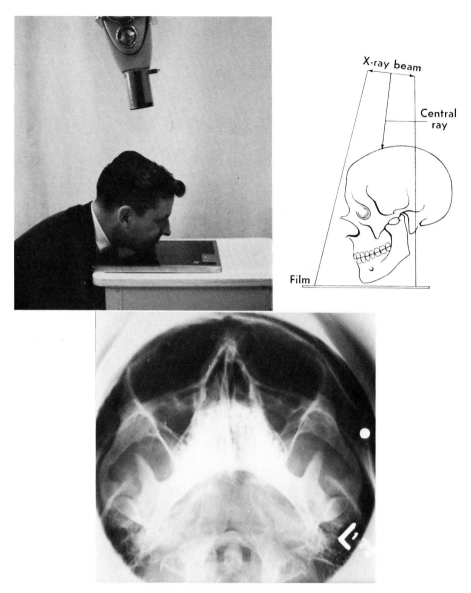

Fig. 7-7. Bregma-mentum projection. The film is placed horizontally on a metal table. The cassette is positioned under the chin with the chin extended as far as possible and comfortable. The border of the cassette nearest the patient should touch the neck in the region of the cricothyroid cartilage in order to allow for sufficient forward extension of the chin. The sagittal plane is perpendicular to the film. The central ray enters at the bregma and exits at the mentum. The target-film distance is 24 inches, and the exposure time is approximately 1½ seconds. Care must be exercised to avoid gonadal radiation exposure. The anterior, posterior, medial, and lateral walls of the maxillary sinus, nasal cavity, and orbits are clearly portrayed. The mediolateral position of parts of the entire mandible is also seen. This projection also shows the mandibular condyle and zygomatic arch as seen from above.

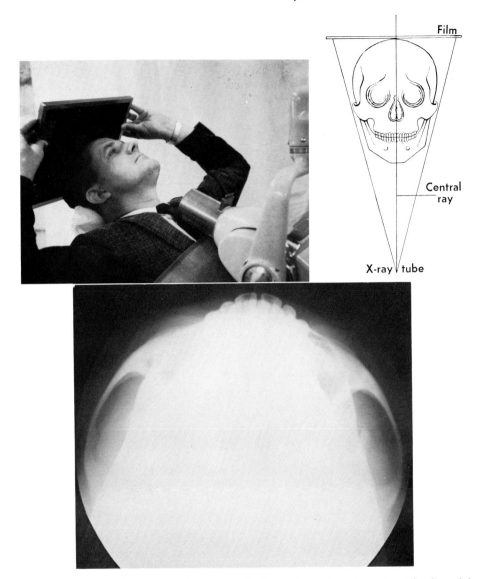

Fig. 7-8. Inferosuperior zygomatic arch projection. The patient is reclined backward in the dental chair. The central ray is directed in the sagittal plane through a point midway between the two zygomatic arches and perpendicular to a cross-sectional plane of the head. The film is positioned on the top of the head as perpendicular as possible to the central ray. The film is usually held by the patient although the film can be stabilized, if necessary, by another individual not ordinarily subjected to man-made ionizing radiation. Care must be used not to subject an assisting individual to primary radiation, and a leaded apron over the chest and gonads of the patient is advocated. The target-object distance is 18 inches, and the exposure time is $\frac{1}{4}$ second. The target–zygomatic arch distance is important; greater or lesser distances tend to superimpose one or both arches on the temporal bones or mandible respectively. Relatively short exposure time is needed because the zygomatic arches are thin bony structures. Changes in one or both zygomatic arches can be observed in this single projection.

Posteroanterior projections of the skull are more useful in dentistry than are anteroposterior projections because the oral structures are closer to the film and appear in the radiograph with maximum image sharpness.

SPECIAL PURPOSE PROJECTIONS

In some instances the need arises to survey radiographically a particular part of the skull to provide a *specific* type of information. Only the more basic special projections that have definite value in dentistry are presented in this chapter.

Temporomandibular joint radiography

The temporomandibular joint is an extremely difficult part of the skull to examine effectively because the joint is closely allied to the dense, petrous portion of the temporal bone. Many technics for examining this joint have been described. We feel that four basic projections provide all the information that is generally needed. Three of the four projections have already been described. These are (1) a lateral view of the mandibular condyle (Chapter 6), (2) a posteroanterior view of the condylar head using an open-mouth posteroanterior mandible projection (Fig. 7-4), and (3) the bregma-mentum projection (Fig. 7-7). A fourth projection for temporomandibular joint radiography is important; this procedure is basically a superior oblique lateral view of the joint. A minimally short tube-film distance and a specially designed localizing and collimating device are used. The use of the localizing device is also applicable to projection (1) above.

The localizer collimator is not available commercially, but it can be made in any metal-working shop at small cost. A localizer is shown in Fig. 7-9. The localizer must be so constructed that, as the space between the collimator and the localizing nuts is changed, the relationship between these parts remains constant except for the change in distance; an opening or closing of the appliance must not change the level of the nuts in their relationship to the central ray. Prior to initial use of the localizer, the nuts must be adjusted and locked so that they are in the exact center of the radiation beam. This is done by trial-and-error film exposures. In Fig. 7-10 is shown the ball (formed from the nuts) in the exact center of such a film. The collimator should give a beam diameter at the film of approximately 2 inches.

The central ray is directed at the joint being examined by placing the localizer ball appropriately on the side of the face. The central ray enters on the opposite side of the skull at a point, in an adult, 2 inches above and $\frac{1}{2}$ inch posterior to the external auditory meatus. The target-film distance is approximately 10 inches and the exposure time, $2\frac{1}{2}$ to 3 seconds. Nonscreen film in a cardboard film holder is placed between the skin and the localizer arm after angulation is completed. This technic allows the x-ray beam to pass just posterior to the sella turcica and just above the petrous portion of the temporal bone on the side being

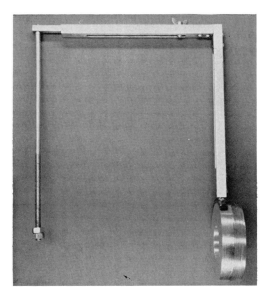

Fig. 7-9. Temporomandibular joint localizer. The portion of the instrument that screws into the head of the x-ray machine provides for inserton of suitable filters and beam collimators. The localizing arm can be extended or retracted according to the width of the patient's head; a wing nut locks these movable parts.

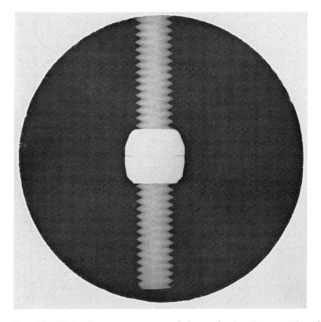

Fig. 7-10. Localizer "ball" in the exact center of the radiation beam. (The "ball" is created by reshaping the locked nuts shown in Fig. 7-9.)

examined. This technic and the resultant radiograph are shown in Fig. 7-11. An oblique view of the glenoid fossa and the head of the condyle is clearly shown in the radiograph.

Serial radiographs using this superior oblique lateral view of the temporomandibular joint are sometimes used to show the relative position of the condyle to the glenoid fossa with the patient's mouth open, closed, and at various positions between these extremes. Such radiographs need a stabilizing device for the patient's head; this device may be positioned vertically or horizontally.* An angle

---

*There is a difference of opinion among radiologists regarding the optimum position of the patient's head. Some feel that it is important to have an even distribution of weight between the two joints. Thus the vertical position is favored.

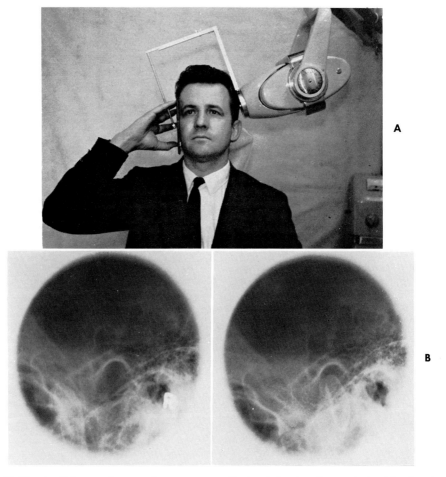

A

B

Fig. 7-11. A, Tube, patient, and temporomandibular joint localizer relationship for the supero-oblique lateral projection of the temporomandibular joint. **B,** Examples of the resultant film.

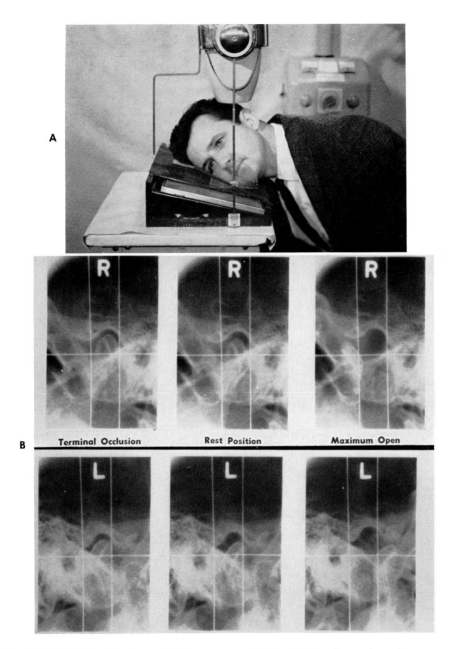

Fig. 7-12. A, Technic for serial temporomandibular joint radiography using an angle board designed by Dr. William Updegrave. **B,** Example of a serial temporomandibular joint radiographic survey. (Courtesy Dr. W. Updegrave.)

board with an earplug attached to it is often used. Calibrated markers attached to the board are used to assist in positioning the x-ray beam and in repositioning the patient's head at some future time. The cassette is usually freely movable in a slot or groove under the angle board. Also, it is shielded completely from the x-ray beam with the exception of that part directly under the temporomandibular joint being examined. By moving the cassette for each exposure, serial radiographs for one side of the patient can be made without changing the patient's head position. This technic and an example of the resultant radiograph are shown in Fig. 7-12.

There is a wide range of opinion among diagnosticians regarding the value of serial radiographs of the temporomandibular joint. Two important points concerning temporomandibular joint radiography must be emphasized: (1) There is no really satisfactory device, such as the orthodontic cephalostat, which permits accurate head positioning, reproducibility, and standardized angulation. (2) No one view of the temporomandibular joint can give satisfactory diagnostic results. Films of the temporomandibular joint should be taken as a survey using *all* views described in the foregoing pages.

A contrast medium injected into the joint spaces has been used to show the size and shape of the compartments above and below the articular disk and the existence of a connection between the compartments. The value of this procedure remains to be evaluated.

Cephalometric radiography

When skull radiographs are used for making skull measurements, there must be some means of registering the head position for purposes of reproduction and standardization. There are available to the dental profession many head-stabilizing devices (cephalostats or craniostats), some of which are calibrated (craniometers or cephalometers). Most of these devices use earplugs to stabilize the patient's head. The x-ray tube must also be fixed in a constant position and in a predetermined relationship to the head positioner. The lateral and posteroanterior skull projections are the most common radiographic views used for skull measurement. Of these two, the lateral skull projection is utilized most frequently. The posteroanterior projection is not widely used. There is a need for further study of cranial growth patterns using a posteroanterior cephalometric procedure.

For the lateral skull projection, the film is positioned planoparallel to the sagittal plane. The central ray passes through both earplugs. The target-film distance is 60 inches or more. Care must be taken to see that the exposure is limited to the skull and jaws. Unless properly collimated, the x-ray beam at a 5-foot distance can cover a large portion of the body. An exposure time of 3 to 6 seconds is required, and suitable intensifying screens must be used. The long target-film distance minimizes the difference in magnification between the two sides of the head. Mathematical tables are sometimes used to reduce further the error from magnification.

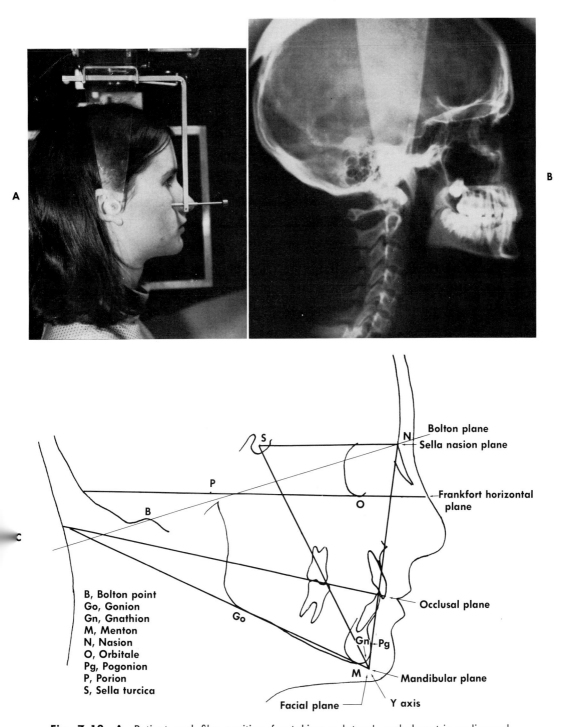

B, Bolton point
Go, Gonion
Gn, Gnathion
M, Menton
N, Nasion
O, Orbitale
Pg, Pogonion
P, Porion
S, Sella turcica

Bolton plane
Sella nasion plane
Frankfort horizontal plane
Occlusal plane
Mandibular plane
Facial plane
Y axis

Fig. 7-13. A, Patient and film position for taking a lateral cephalometric radiograph. **B,** Resultant film. **C,** Line drawing of the same radiograph, showing some basic anthropometric landmarks and planes. (Courtesy Dr. J. Mehta and Dr. H. P. Hitchcock.)

Cephalometric radiographs are used to identify the positions of certain an-thropometric landmarks. The distances between the various landmarks and the angles formed by planes resulting from the joining of certain points give a mathe-matical evaluation of the growth and development of the patient (Fig. 7-13).

Carpal index radiography

Radiographs of the hand and wrist are easily made with screen or nonscreen films. With nonscreen film and a tube-film distance of 36 inches, the average ex-posure time is 1 second. The carpal bones seen on such a radiograph can be compared with any standard text on the development of the hand and wrist.* The technic and an example of the resultant film are shown in Fig. 7-14.

Comparative studies give an accurate estimate of the bone age of the patient. Hand and wrist radiographs can be useful when skull changes suggest the pos-sibility that other bones of the skeleton may be involved. This part of the anatomy is easily radiographed, and the patient is not embarrassed by having this exami-nation done in the dental office.

Lateral velopharyngeal radiography

A lateral projection of the oral pharynx is easily made with a modern dental x-ray machine. The sagittal plane is planoparallel to the film. The central ray is directed perpendicular to the film. With a target-film distance of 24 inches, 90 kVp, and 15 mA, the exposure time is $\frac{1}{10}$ second. An exposure of this duration can be done while the patient is making a prolonged sound. This projection is used to show the relationship of the soft palate or an obturator prosthesis to the posterior pharyngeal wall and pharyngeal tonsils. The technic and resultant film are shown in Fig. 7-15.

Use of contrast media

The diagnostic radiograph is unable to depict very small differences in x-ray absorption between two parts of an object. For example, the radiograph does not adequately show cavities within soft tissues. For these cavities to be visual-ized, radiographic contrast between the cavity and its surrounding tissues must be increased; this can be done in two ways: (1) by reducing the x-ray absorp-tion of the cavity and (2) by increasing the x-ray absorption of the cavity. An example of the first is replacing the fluid in the ventricles of the brain with air. An example of the second is using the radiopaque contrast media widely em-ployed in medical radiography to show much of the digestive, cardiovascular, pulmonary, and renal systems. In oral radiography, the use of a radiopaque ma-terial as the contrast medium is by far the more efficient and practical technic.

The essential part of any radiopaque medium is a heavy element that can absorb most of the x-ray beam. The element must be noninjurious and easily

---

*For example, Gruelich, W. W., and Pyle, S. I.: Radiographic atlas of skeletal development of the hand and wrist, Stanford, Calif., 1959, Stanford University Press.

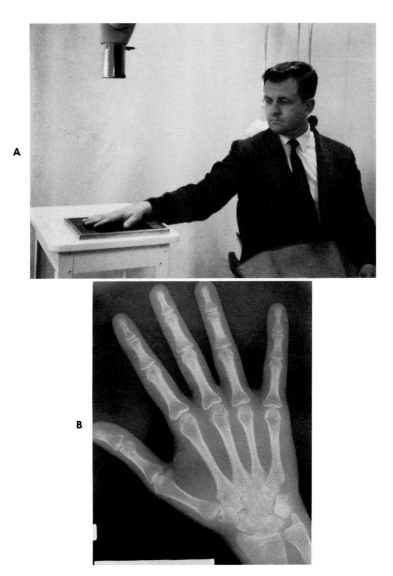

Fig. 7-14. A, Technic for making a hand and wrist radiograph of an adult patient.
B, Example of the resultant film.

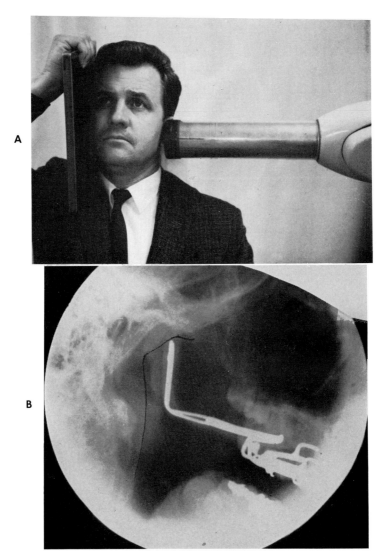

Fig. 7-15. A, Tube, patient, and film relationships for a lateral projection of the velopharynx. **B,** Radiograph shows an obturator prosthesis in relation to the soft tissues. The posterior pharynx is outlined for better visualization.

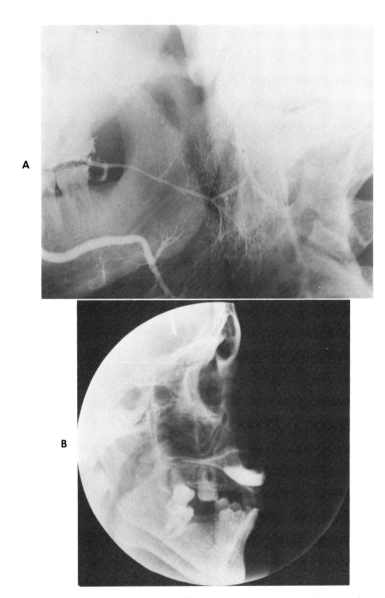

Fig. 7-16. A, Sialogram made with a lateral jaw projection showing the submaxillary and parotid gland. **B,** Radiopaque material injected into a cyst after some of the cyst fluid had been withdrawn. The boundaries of the cyst lying within the soft tissues can now be identified.

eliminated. The essential element most commonly used in dentistry is iodine. Both aqueous and oil suspensions of iodine-containing compounds are available to the dental profession, for example, Lipiodol and Dionosil. Barium sulfate is used in medicine, particularly in the examination of the gastrointestinal tract. It is also useful in dental radiology.

Radiopaque solutions are used in sialography to show the ducts and acini of the salivary glands (Fig. 7-16, *A*). The material is slowly introduced into the duct of the gland with a blunt cannula connected to a plunger type of syringe by plastic tubing. After the material is injected, it can be retained in the gland and duct during radiographic examination by having the patient occlude the tubing. Sialograms are valuable in the diagnosis of duct obstruction, deviation of the ducts because of soft tissue growth, destruction of parts of the gland, and so forth. A liquid contrast medium can also be used to localize the boundaries of soft tissue cysts (Fig. 7-16, *B*). It can be used also to locate the origin of fistulous tracts and to outline such anatomic spaces as the oral cavity, pharynx, and maxillary sinus.

Radiopaque material in the form of pastes has also been used to show periodontal pockets on radiographs. Metal probes can also be classified as contrast media. Such probes have been used to show the position of periodontal pockets and to trace fistulas. The use of the endodontic file in measuring the length of a tooth with radiographs is another example of the utilization of contrast media in oral radiography. Paste or liquid contrast media can also be used in taking lateral head films to outline the soft tissue profile.

Stereoscopic radiography

Stereoscopic radiography is basically a localization technic. It is discussed briefly in Chapter 10. It should be considered also as a special examination method and should be used when needed by the practitioner of dentistry. The procedure involves rigid technical requirements.

CHAPTER 8

Panoramic radiography

Radiographic procedures in the average dental office ordinarily employ technics that utilize a fixed position of the x-ray source, object, and film. The resultant films show segments of the mandible and/or maxilla; used collectively, a series of such radiographs constitute a panoramic view of these structures.

The desirability of being able to cast an image of the maxilla and mandible on a single film is obvious, provided that the quality of the conventional radiograph can be maintained. Indeed, some sacrifice in quality can be tolerated if the film is to be used only for survey purposes rather than for critical interpretation. Survey quality radiographs showing the mandible and maxilla regardless of their curvatures can be made by various means. There are three basic methods: (1) the x-ray source and the film can be made to rotate around the patient; (2) the patient can be rotated between the x-ray source and the film; and (3) the x-ray source can be placed in the patient's mouth with the film wrapped around the face. The former two methods employ the principles of laminagraphy, or body section radiography. The latter method is, in principle, similar to conventional procedures in that the x-ray source, object, and film are stationary; the principal difference between the third method and usual procedures centers around the position of the x-ray tube and its construction.

LAMINAGRAPHY

Laminagraphy, as the term suggests, is a technic designed to study layers or laminae within a volume of tissue. An appropriate analogy is that of examining one slice of bread somewhere within the entire loaf. Laminagraphic studies can be of either a flat or curved plane.

Fig. 8-1 diagrammatically illustrates the concepts of flat plane laminagraphy. The intent is to sharply reproduce all points on or near the plane in which point A is located and to grossly blur all points (represented by X and Y) not in the near vicinity of the plane. Point A is representative of all points on the plane. *Under predetermined conditions designed to accomplish the intended purpose, it is possible to reach this goal.* It will be noted that the shift of the image of point A (and all other points on plane A) on the film (T_1A to T_2A) is exactly

161

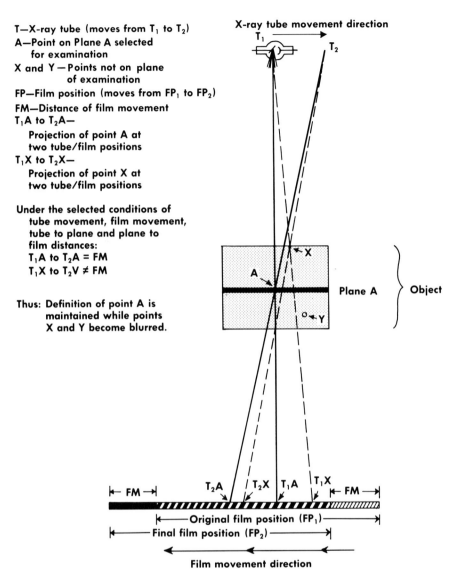

T—X-ray tube (moves from T_1 to T_2)

A—Point on Plane A selected
    for examination

X and Y —Points not on plane
            of examination

FP—Film position (moves from FP_1 to FP_2)

FM—Distance of film movement

T_1A to T_2A—

Projection of point A at
two tube/film positions

T_1X to T_2X—

Projection of point X at
two tube/film positions

Under the selected conditions of
tube movement, film movement,
tube to plane and plane to
film distances:
T_1A to T_2A = FM
T_1X to T_2V ≠ FM

Thus: Definition of point A is
maintained while points
X and Y become blurred.

Fig. 8-1. Flat plane laminagraph. An x-ray beam having an axis of rotation at point A is projected through a mass of tissue. The film is at a predetermined position and is made to move so that the image of point A is projected on the same spot on the film when the x-ray source moves from T_1 to T_2. Under these circumstances, all points on plane A are similarly cast in a constant position on the film. All points in the tissue not on plane A (represented by X and Y) are distorted; because of the geometry involved, it is impossible for other points to be cast in a constant position on the x-ray film.

equal to the shift of the film (FM). The image shift of point X (and hence plane X) is not equal to FM. A projection of point and plane Y would be similarly distorted. Thus only plane A is sharply reproduced. Fig. 8-2 shows a series of laminagrams.

Thus far, the axis of rotation has been through the point or points in the plane being studied (point A in plane A [Fig. 8-1]). This is not essential. The axis could be located at virtually any position, and given points on the same plane could be clearly projected onto a film, provided that the tube movement, the film movement, and the distances from the tube to the object and from the object to the film were predetermined accurately. Under these circumstances, the x-ray beam must be narrowly confined, as opposed to the widely divergent beam spreading from the tube in Fig. 8-1. The procedure now becomes one of scanning a given plane and projecting sequential points onto a film. Fig. 8-3 illustrates this concept.

The above principles can be applied equally well to a curved layer, provided that the curvature of the section to be studied is known. The simplest curve to examine is one that has a constant radius. Two methods for examining a curved

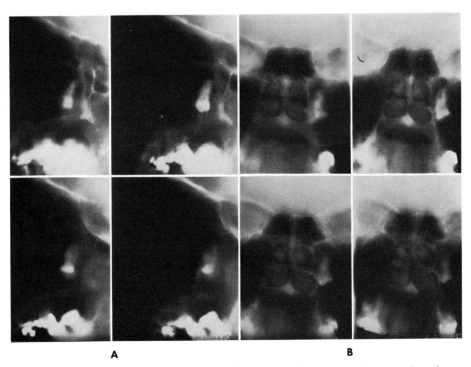

A   B

Fig. 8-2. A laminagraphic series. **A,** Lateral laminagraphic views of the maxilla taken at sequentially increasing depths of 0.5 cm. **B,** Posteroanterior views of the same region using similar procedures. The presence and location of a maxillary tooth in the maxillary sinus can be readily determined.

section are shown in Figs. 8-4 and 8-5. Fig. 8-4 utilizes a flat film; Fig. 8-5 utilizes a curved film. In principle, the two procedures are identical. Diagrammatically, curved surface AB is being examined in both Figs. 8-4 and 8-5. Areas on either side of AB are blurred. If the relationship between beam speed and film speed were changed or if the axis of beam rotation were altered, a curved layer other than AB would be well defined, and areas on either side of it would be blurred.

Consideration can now be given to a curved lamina having more than one radius. A layer within the mandible or maxilla is an example of such a situation. The radii of curvatures of the mandible and maxilla are larger in the posterior areas than in the anterior area. Fig. 8-6 demonstrates diagrammatically the curvatures found in the jaws. Alphabetical designations (that is, A, B, W, X, Y, and Z) are identical to those used in Figs. 8-4 and 8-5. The radii of the posterior segments in Fig. 8-6 are, for practical purposes, equal, but they differ materially from the radius of the anterior segment. In all instances the centers of the circles of beam rotation are in different positions, but the centers of the posterior curvatures tend to be in essentially the same contralateral positions. The principles expressed relative to Figs. 8-1 to 8-5, particularly Figs. 8-4 and 8-5, can now be applied. Panoramic procedures ordinarily used in dental radiology are premised on an "average" curvature for both the mandible and maxilla; the same average is used for all adults, and an alternate average is ordinarily used for children. The quality of the resulting panoramic film depends on how closely the patient's jaw curvature approximates the average curvature selected as a model by the equipment manufacturer.

Panoramic radiographic devices employ the concept of (1) x-ray beam axis shift and (2) alteration in the relative speeds of the film and x-ray beam. Some available equipment uses two centers of rotation and varies the speed of film movement (Panorex) (Fig. 8-7). Other equipment uses three centers of rotation (Orthopantomograph) (Fig. 8-8). Still other equipment uses a single center of rotation and a film curvature designed to approximate the shape of the mandible and maxilla (Rotograph) (Fig. 8-9). The GE-Panelipse (Figs. 8-10 and 8-13) has a continuously moving axis that follows the arc of the mandible and maxilla. In addition, the arc is not of fixed size but can be adjusted for different-size jaws. The shape of the arc is essentially one half of a two-to-one ellipse. Like the Panorex and the Orthopantomograph, the GE-Panelipse places the patient in a stationary position and rotates the tube head cassette holder assembly. As with the other pantomographic machines, the tube head collimator is of the slit type, and the film shield has an opening of a similar shape but different size to permit access of the x-ray beam to the film. Theoretically, it is possible to manufacture a machine capable of continuous axis relocation and film speed adjustment designed to examine specific jaw curvatures on a highly individualized basis. However, the mechanical and electronic components of such a device appear to be economically incompatible with dental practice.

Text continued on p. 173.

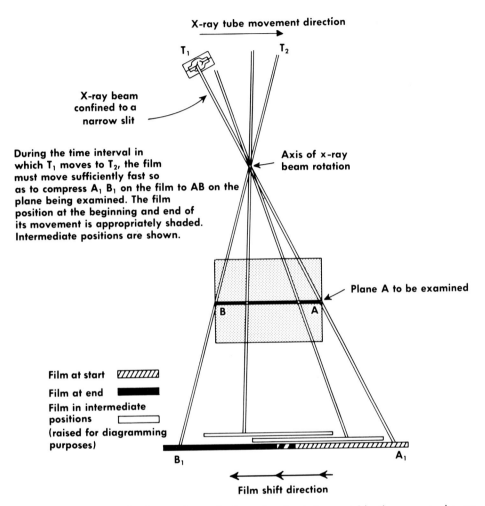

X-ray tube movement direction

T₁   T₂

X-ray beam
confined to a
narrow slit

During the time interval in
which T₁ moves to T₂, the film
must move sufficiently fast so
as to compress A₁ B₁ on the film to AB on the
plane being examined. The film
position at the beginning and end of
its movement is appropriately shaded.
Intermediate positions are shown.

Axis of x-ray
beam rotation

Plane A to be examined

B   A

Film at start

Film at end

Film in intermediate
positions
(raised for diagramming
purposes)

B₁   A₁

Film shift direction

Fig. 8-3. Flat plane laminagraphy with the axis of rotation outside the mass to be examined. A narrow x-ray beam is employed. Using predetermined speed and distance
factors, it is possible to scan a plane at any desired level. As the narrow beam scans
from point A to point B, the x-ray film must move in a coordinated fashion so that the
distance from point A to point B will be represented by this dimension on the resultant
film. Under these circumstances, all points above and below plane A will be distorted.

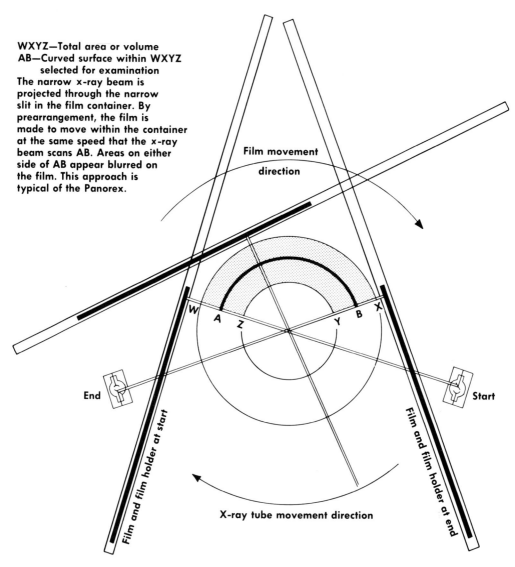

WXYZ—Total area or volume
AB—Curved surface within WXYZ
    selected for examination
The narrow x-ray beam is
projected through the narrow
slit in the film container. By
prearrangement, the film is
made to move within the container
at the same speed that the x-ray
beam scans AB. Areas on either
side of AB appear blurred on
the film. This approach is
typical of the Panorex.

Film movement
direction

End

Start

Film and film holder at start

Film and film holder at end

X-ray tube movement direction

Fig. 8-4. Curved surface laminagraphy. The same principles are used as for flat plane laminagraphy. An axis of rotation is selected, and the narrow x-ray beam scans from *A* to *B*. The film, in its container, moves past the narrow slit in the container at a speed equal to that with which the beam scans the selected layer in tissue *(AB)*.

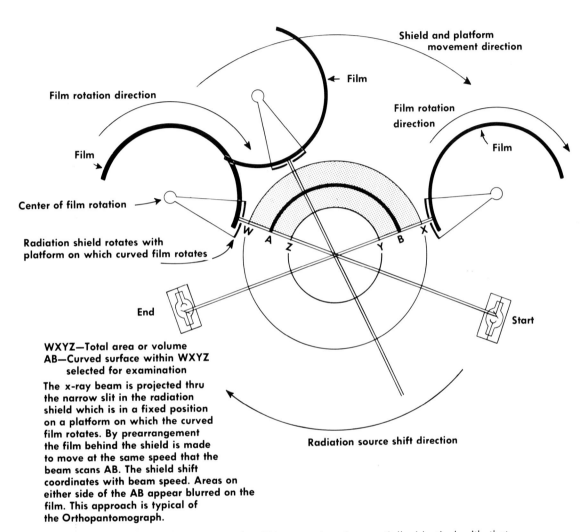

Shield and platform
movement direction

← Film

Film rotation direction

Film rotation
direction

Film →

Film →

Center of film rotation →

Radiation shield rotates with
platform on which curved film rotates

W A Z Y B X

End

Start

WXYZ—Total area or volume
AB—Curved surface within WXYZ
   selected for examination

The x-ray beam is projected thru
the narrow slit in the radiation
shield which is in a fixed position
on a platform on which the curved
film rotates. By prearrangement
the film behind the shield is made
to move at the same speed that the
beam scans AB. The shield shift
coordinates with beam speed. Areas on
either side of the AB appear blurred on the
film. This approach is typical of
the Orthopantomograph.

Radiation source shift direction

Fig. 8-5. Curved surface laminagraphy. This procedure is essentially identical with that shown in Fig. 8-4. The film is curved. It moves past the slit in the radiation shield at a speed equal to that with which the narrow x-ray beam scans the selected tissue layer (*AB*). The shield is attached to a platform on which the film rotates. The shield and the platform maintain a constant relationship to the x-ray beam as both orbit around the structure being examined.

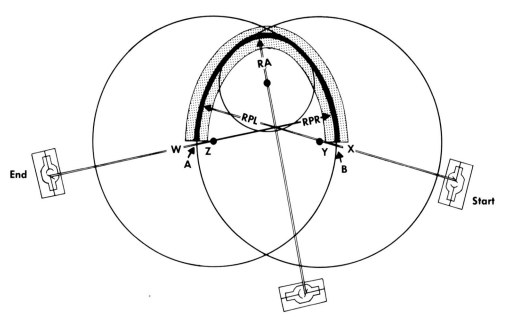

WXYZ—Total area or volume
AB—Curved surface within WXYZ selected for
  examination
RA—Radius of anterior segment curvature
RPL—Radius of posterior left segment
  curvature
RPR—Radius of posterior right segment
  curvature—RPR is approximately
  equal to RPL

● — Axes of beam rotation

Fig. 8-6. Curved surface laminagraphy. In this situation two or more radii of curvature are present. The principles expressed in prior illustrations are used, but provisions must be made to adjust to the variation in curvature. This can be done by changing the axis of rotation, adjusting film speed, or providing a curved film shape essentially identical to the shape of the layer being examined. Each of these three methods can be used individually or in combination.

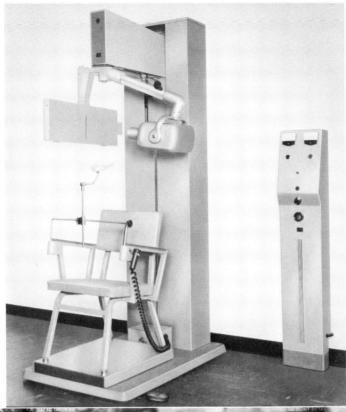

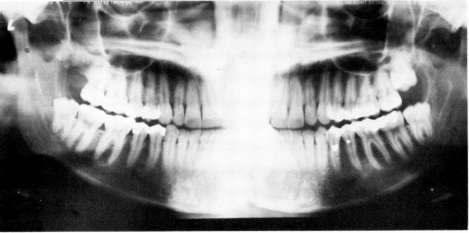

Fig. 8-7. Panorex unit and an example of the panoramic radiograph made with this unit. The x-ray tube and the cassette holder revolve around the patient's head. A thin beam of x-rays emerges from the tube head, passes through the patient, and then enters the slit opening shown in the cassette holder. The cassette in the cassette holder moves behind the slit at the same speed as the jaw is scanned by the x-ray beam. (Courtesy X-Ray Manufacturing Corp. of America, Great Neck, N.Y.)

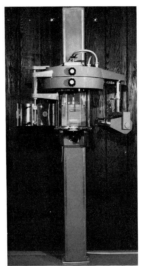

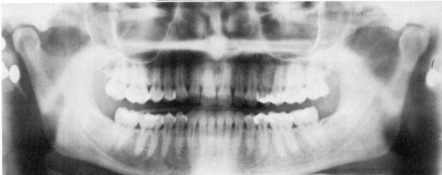

Fig. 8-8. Orthopantomograph-3 and an example of a film taken with this equipment. The x-ray tube head and the curved film rotate around the patient's head. The film rotates concurrently behind a shield in which is located a narrow vertical slit. The narrow slit through which the beam emerges from the tube head can be seen in the upper right illustration. Film rotation and beam movement must be properly coordinated if optimum results are to be obtained. (Courtesy Sieman's Medical of America, Inc., Union, N.J.)

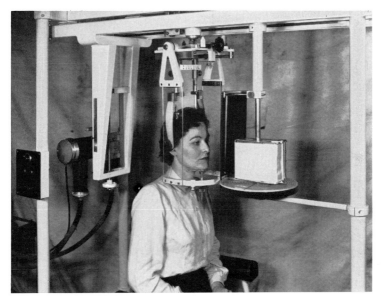

Fig. 8-9. Rotograph. The panoramic view is achieved by rotating the patient and a curved film simultaneously in both directions while a narrow beam of x-rays passes through the area under examination. (Courtesy Watson & Sons, Ltd., London.)

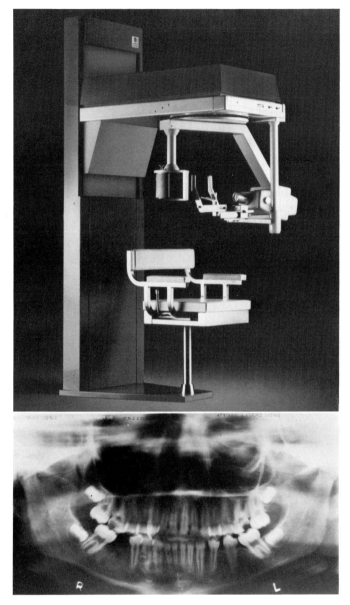

Fig. 8-10. GE-Panelipse panoramic x-ray machine and an example of a radiograph made with this equipment. The film in a flexible cassette moves on a rotating drum around the patient's head in conjunction with the x-ray tube head. The center of rotation of the tube head–film holder assembly moves continuously along the arc of the mandible and maxilla. The size of the arc followed by the center of rotation is adjustable to match the arch size. (Courtesy General Electric Co., Milwaukee, Wis.)

The Panorex, Orthopantomograph, Rotograph, and GE-Panelipse are four examples of equipment that utilize laminagraphic principles. Prior comments and diagrams have explained in some detail the principles used by the Panorex, the Orthopantomograph and the GE-Panelipse. The principles of the Rotograph are similar except that the patient rotates within a fixed, narrow x-ray beam as the film concurrently turns at predetermined rates.

The panoramic radiograph of the jaws made with laminagraphic principles spreads a curved layer of the patient's anatomy on a flat film. The anatomical landmarks seen in this type of radiographic projection are identified in Figs. 13-26, 13-27, and 13-28.

The quality of laminagraphic films is generally not as satisfactory as that of properly taken intraoral films. However, they are excellent for survey purposes. This is especially true because they show a considerably greater area of the mandible and maxilla than do intraoral films. Limited patient exposure and a materially decreased chair time are important considerations, especially for mass population surveys.

In recent years, there has been a proliferation of the type of panoramic machines offered to the dental profession. Many of these machines use different x-ray beam rotation centers, and they can produce panoramic radiographs that vary between the machines. The radiographic factors of some of these machines are shown in Table 8-1. The individual dentist must know exactly what layer of the patient his panoramic machine examines and must be aware that pantomograms made by machines of another make must be interpreted differently.

The design of individual pantomographic machines undergo continual modification. One type of machine (Panex-E) has been constructed as a free-standing model and has also been designed to be built into the wall of the operatory (Fig. 8-11). Many machines can be purchased with attachments for cephalometric radiography. One such machine (Orthopantomograph-3) is shown in Fig. 8-12. Panoramic machines have also been modified to permit a patient in a wheelchair to be radiographed without being removed from his wheelchair (for example, GE-Panelipse) (Fig. 8-13). Recently a machine (Tomorex) has been developed that makes a panoramic radiograph of the dentition with the patient in the supine position (Fig. 8-14).

PANAGRAPHY

Panagraphy suggests another technic designed to study structures in a panoramic fashion. The Panagraph, or Panoramix, is an x-ray machine utilizing an intraoral source of radiation to expose film placed extraorally. The Panagraph (Fig. 8-15) consists of two specialized components unique in dental radiographic apparatus: the constant potential generator and the Panoramix x-ray tube.

The constant potential generator provides a constant potential high voltage supply for the x-ray tube; x-ray photons created by electrons passing through the high, constant potential voltage are of shorter wavelength—hence are more pene-

Text continued on p. 182.

Table 8-1. Panoramic machines and machine factors*

Name	Beam rotation centers	kVp	mA	Exposure time (seconds at 60 Hz)	Film size (cm.)	Focal trough size	Tube focal spot size (mm.)	Patient position	Image magnification ratio	Cassette type	Power requirements
Rotagraph	1	75-80	30-40	12	20×30	Fixed	0.8	Seated	~ 1.3	Flexible	220 V 60 Hz
Panographix	1	50-100	5-100	20	15×30	Fixed	0.5	Standing	~ 1.2	Flexible	110-125V 60 Hz
Panorex	2	50-90	0-10	22	12×30	Fixed	0.8	Seated	Vertical 1.1-1.3 Horizontal 0.8-1.5	Flat Rigid	
Orthopantomograph (Siemens)†	3	55-85	15	15	15×30	Fixed	0.6	Standing	Vertical 1.1-1.4 Horizontal 0.9-1.5	Curved Rigid	110-220V 50-60 Hz
Orthopantomo-N-70 (Hida)	3	70-90	10	20	15×30 20×30	Fixed	1.5	Standing	1.1-1.4	Flexible	100-110V 50-60 Hz
Orthopantomo-R100 (Hida)	3	100	20	20	20×30	Fixed	0.8	Standing	1.1-1.4	Flexible	100-110V 50-60 Hz
Americana PX-900	3	90	10-15	16	12×30	Fixed	1.0	Standing	~ 1.12	Flexible	110V 60 Hz
Panoramax AX-4	3	50-90	0-15	16	12×30 15×30	Fixed	1.5	Standing	1.2-1.3	Flexible	100-110V 50-60 Hz
Panoramax 100-20R	3	50-100	0-20	13	15×30	Fixed	0.8	Standing	1.2-1.3	Flexible	100-200V 50-60 Hz
Panora 40-200	3	50-85	10	20	12×30 15×30	Fixed	1.8	Standing	1.1-1.3	Flexible	115V 50-60 Hz

Machine										
Panora R150	3	60-75	20	15	12×30 15×30	Fixed	1.5	Seated	1.1-1.3	Flexible	115-220V 50-60 Hz
GE-3000 and Panelipse	Moving	40-100	8-15	20	12×30	Variable	1.0	Seated	Vertical 1.1-1.3 Horizontal 0.8-1.4	Flexible	115V 60 Hz
Panex-E	Moving	70-90	0-10	15	12×30 15×30	Fixed	1.5	Standing	1.2-1.3	Flexible	115V 50-60 Hz
Panex-100	Moving	60-100	0-15	20	20×30	Variable	1.5	Seated	~ 1.1	Flexible	100V 50-60 Hz
Panoradix†	1	60-95	3-40		15×30	Fixed	1.8	Seated	~ 1.17	Flexible	100-200V 50-60 Hz
Tanaka		120	60	20	15×30	Fixed	1.0	Seated	1-1.2	Flexible	100-220V 50-60 Hz
Philips AX-4000	3	55-90	10	16	15×30	Fixed	0.8	Seated	1.2-1.4	Rigid	100-220V 50-60 Hz
Toslayer TR-840		63-100	10	18	15×30	Fixed	1.5	Seated	1.1-1.2	Flexible	100V 50-60 Hz
Kinki KR Type	3	60-95	3-40		15×30	Fixed	1.8	Seated	~ 1.25	Flexible	100-220V 50-60 Kz

*From Manson-Hing, L. R.: Panoramic Dental Radiography, courtesy of Charles C Thomas, Publisher, Springfield, Ill.
†Machine also manufactured with rotation anode tubes.

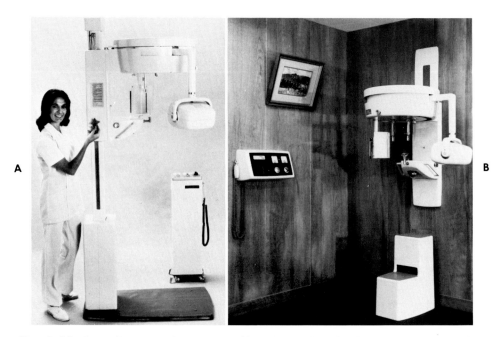

Fig. 8-11. Panex-E panoramic x-ray machine designed to be freestanding or attached directly to the wall with remote movable or wall-attached control panels. Either unit can be raised or lowered: very short patients are provided with a two-step platform. (Courtesy Oratronics, Inc., New York, N.Y.)

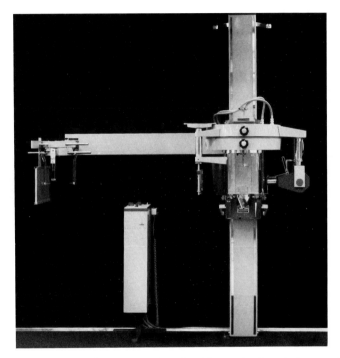

Fig. 8-12. Orthopantomograph-3 panoramic unit with attached cephalometer (Ortho-ceph). The tube head is easily disconnected from the panoramic movement and placed in a stationary, prefixed position by a metal bar that also collimates the x-ray beam to the proper dimensions for cephalometric radiography. (Courtesy Siemens Corp., Iselin, N.J.)

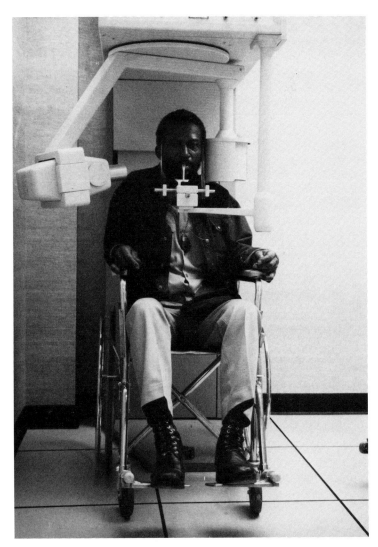

Fig. 8-13. GE-Panelipse: the patient's seat is removed, and a patient in a wheelchair is positioned for panoramic radiography.

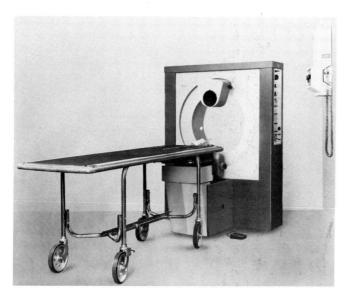

Fig. 8-14. Tomorex machine designed for panoramic radiography with patients in a horizontal position. A conveyor belt in the litter moves the patient into the machine. (Courtesy Medical Products Division, Pennwalt Corp., Philadelphia, Pa.)

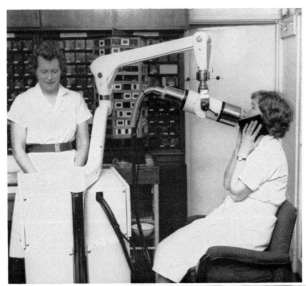

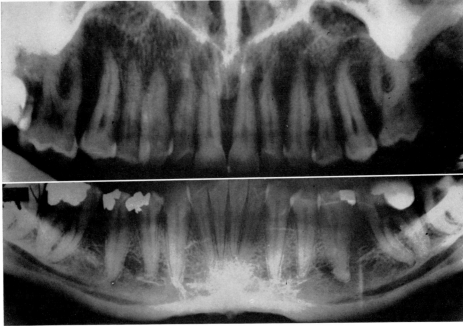

Fig. 8-15. Panagraph and examples of panoramic radigraphs of the maxilla and mandible. The anode of the x-ray tube is encased in the end of a probe that is introduced into the patient's mouth. The film is enclosed in a flexible cassette and is held in place by the patient. (Courtesy Dr. Sidney Blackman.)

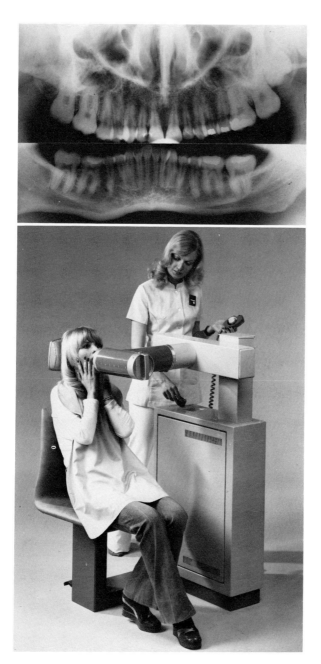

Fig. 8-16. The Status-X machine and examples of maxillary and mandibular radiographs made with this machine. (Courtesy Siemens Corp., Iselin, N.J.)

trating—than x-rays produced by standard dental machines. The increased efficiency and reduced target-film distance result in the use of very short exposure times.

The Panoramix x-ray tube is distinctive, having a long, narrow glass tube projecting from the x-ray bulb. The anode is situated at the end of the tube and consists of a copper cone tipped with a sharp-pointed tungsten target; the focal spot is 0.1 mm. in diameter. Radiation is generated in all directions from the anode and is collimated for dental radiography with special lead shields.

The image produced by the Panagraph extends from third molar to third molar in both the mandible and maxilla; they are usually radiographed separately. Because of the divergence of x-rays from the target, the image is magnified 2 to 2½ times. There are varying degrees of superimposition in the bicuspid and molar regions; vertical, horizontal, and dimensional distortions are present due to the difficulty of adapting the cassette uniformly to the dental arch. Despite these inadequacies, the detail and definition of the magnified image are reasonably good. The main advantages of the Panagraph appear to be that it is relatively portable, is easy to operate, and may be used effectively for mass dental radiography.

The latest development in this radiographic system is seen in the Status-X machine (Fig. 8-16). The tube inserted into the patient's mouth is quite small, thus permitting some flexibility in positioning the source of radiation in different areas of the oral cavity.

CHAPTER 9

The darkroom

Whenever possible, the oral radiography darkroom should be designed when the dental office is planned and should be located conveniently within the office complex. Too often, the darkroom is added as an afterthought, and the result is that this work area is frequently makeshift in nature. An efficient darkroom is necessary if radiographs are to be processed properly. The darkroom should be planned with care for the present and future needs of the dental office. All the care taken in exposing films can be negated if poor quality radiographs result from poor processing technics or facilities. Minimum darkroom facilities are illustrated in Fig. 9-1. Few dentists have a fundamental interest in photography. As a result, they tend to exercise care in the technics of film placement and exposure but neglect proper film-processing procedures.

The following aspects of the darkroom are discussed in this chapter: size and location; construction and design, including the processing equipment; safelighting; darkroom care; and film-processing technics.

SIZE AND LOCATION

The size of the darkroom depends basically on the type and amount of films to be processed. It is obvious that the greater the work load, the larger the darkroom must be. If large films are to be processed, large processing tanks will be needed; hence, a large darkroom becomes a necessity. Extra space must be provided if more than one person is to use the darkroom at the same time. Although it is possible for one person to process dental radiographs in a darkroom with 9 sq. ft. of floor space, it is advisable to have at least 20 sq. ft. of floor space for the average dental office.

The darkroom should be located so that it can be conveniently reached from the room or rooms where the films are to be exposed and examined. Since the temperature of the processing solutions must be kept constant, it is advisable to locate the darkroom in an area of the dental office where the room temperature fluctuates as little as possible. Also, since the best processing is achieved at 68° F. and films have to be stored in a cool place, the room should be located in a cool part of the office. The darkroom should be accessible to plumbing and power lines. Consideration should be given to the humidity of the darkroom area; extreme humidity retards drying of the processed films and damages unused films stored in opened film boxes.

CONSTRUCTION AND DESIGN

The darkroom should be an efficient and pleasant place to work, not just a lighttight room. The room can be made lighttight through the use of a maze or a lighttight door. The maze, a doorless, circuitous corridor, allows people to enter and leave the darkroom without light entering from the outside. The selection of either a maze or door depends mainly on the space available and the work load of the darkroom. If a lighttight door is used, attention must be given to room ventilation. This can be accomplished by one or more lighttight vents constructed of overlapping opaque louvers. Such a vent can be placed in the door. Although not essential, a darkroom fan designed to circulate air from an outside

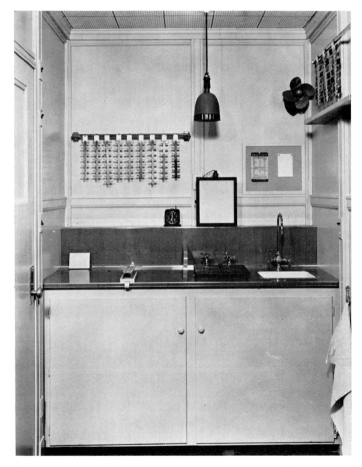

Fig. 9-1. Minimum darkroom facilities. (Courtesy Eastman Kodak Co., Rochester, N.Y.)

source can be helpful. If a maze is used, an auxiliary lighttight door should be constructed for the darkroom because large pieces of equipment cannot be carried in or out of the darkroom through a maze.

The surfaces of the room should be able to resist the processing chemicals. The floor can be waxed to protect it from these chemicals; joints in the darkroom flooring should be very tight. The wall paint should also be able to resist the processing chemicals. The color of the walls should be light enough to reflect the safelight and be pleasant to look at under ordinary illumination. The darkroom does not have to be painted black. If a maze is used, the paint inside the maze should be dull black to assist the maze in trapping light.

The illumination of the room consists of two types, ordinary white light and safelight. A ceiling light to provide ordinary illumination in the darkroom is usually adequate; the switch for this light should be placed high enough on the wall to prevent the operator from accidentally turning it on. The safelight consists of a filtered light beam. This light is safe only when the correct-watt bulb is used and the fixture is placed at or beyond the recommended distance from the work area. The manufacturer's recommendations should be followed; for example, a 10-watt bulb can be used wih a Wratten 6B filter when the fixture is located 4 feet from the work area. When certain intraoral and occlusal films are processed, a Kodak Morlite filter can be employed. Use of this filter provides considerably more safe darkroom light. This filter is unsatisfactory for extraoral film. It is absolutely necessary to have a safelight above the work area, and it is desirable that a second safelight, preferably constructed flush on the wall, be placed directly behind the processing tanks. The second safelight is used by the operator to see when the film has been cleared by the fixer; the radiograph must be cleared before it can be read wet. If wet films are to be viewed in the darkroom, a regular film illuminator or view box should be placed directly behind the *fixer* tank. This arrangement eliminates transportation of dripping films. Placement of the illuminator behind the developer tank results in contamination of developer with fixer. One other light is desirable; this is a red warning light. The warning light is placed outside the entrance to the darkroom; it should be wired so that it is illuminated whenever the safelights are turned on.

The darkroom should be planned to provide a smooth and efficient work area. Film holders or racks should be stored just above or below the workbench, where they can be reached easily. If large films are identified through the use of an electric printing device, this printer should be located on the wall that faces the operator when he is unwrapping films. The workbench should be constructed to provide storage space underneath. The surface of the workbench should be of a material, such as Formica, that resists the processing chemicals and can be cleaned easily. The color of the counter top should contrast with the color of the most commonly used film. Black-and-white checks have been found helpful in dental offices. Special storage boxes should be available for films stored in cabinets above or below the workbench. These boxes should be lead lined or made of steel to prevent stray radiation from fogging the films. Boxes for opened film should be lighttight. The wastebin or basket should be under the workbench. It is very convenient to have this bin directly under a hole cut in the top of the workbench through which the film wrappers can be disposed. A cover for this hole and a chute connecting the hole to the wastebin can be constructed if desired.

Conventional processing equipment

The processing tanks should be situated immediately adjacent and to the right of the film-stripping area, and the developer tank should be nearest to the stripping area. The developer tank is separated from the fixer tank by the water bath. This arrangement allows for the smooth transfer of stripped films from the workbench to the developer, to the water bath, to the fixer, and back to the water bath with the least chance of solution contamination. Note that the developer is alkaline, whereas the fixer is acid; they must not be allowed to contaminate each other. To avoid solution contamination further, one can hang the paddles or stirring rods for the developer and fixer on individual hooks behind the respective tanks when not in use. Tank covers should not be interchanged. A washbasin or sink is convenient in the darkroom. It should be located next to the processing tanks, where it can be used for washing films as well as for cleaning processing tanks.

The processing tanks and all plumbing fixtures must be constructed of materials that will resist corrosion by the processing chemicals. Ideal processing conditions call for both hot and cold water supplies with a vacuum breaker, an automatic blending valve, and a thermometer built into the pipeline supplying the processing tank. The tanks, if possible, should be made of stainless steel* and should consist of a main water tank with smaller insert tanks for the developer, fixer, and possibly stop bath† solutions. Particular attention should be paid to the quality of the waste disposal pipe. Waste disposal should not violate the sanitary codes of the area. If processing chemicals are sent into septic tanks that work on a bacterial principle, these chemicals may cause malfunction of the tanks.

The need of a film dryer depends largely on the number of films that are being processed. The dryer should be placed where the films can be transported to it from the washing tank or sink with a minimum of dripping. If the films are simply hung up to dry, a drip pan should be built under the bar on which the film racks will be hung. Film drying by this method can be accelerated if the

---

*All stainless steel is not suitable. No. 316 or 2S stainless is usually recommended. All joints should be highly polished to prevent corrosion. Stainless steel tanks are not superior to hard rubber tanks unless steel equipment is properly constructed.

†A stop bath is a solution of fixer or weak acetic acid. After development and a very brief water rinse, films are immersed in the stop bath for approximately 5 seconds. Its purpose is to rapidly neutralize any developer on the films before they are placed in the fixing solution.

room air is circulated. Air circulation is also desirable from the standpoint of operator comfort; a fan for this purpose can be located where it will gently blow air on the films being dried.

Automatic processors

Conventional processing equipment continues to be used by most practicing dentists. However, an increasing number of practitioners have purchased or are contemplating the purchase of some type of automated darkroom equipment. Thus it is important to discuss the advantages and disadvantages of darkroom automation.

In the absence of automated processing equipment, it is necessary for a dental office person to remain in the darkroom for certain periods of time; thus this person is unavailable for participation in other office activities. About 4 minutes are required to strip and rack the average complete mouth survey of approximately 18 films. Developing requires $4\frac{1}{2}$ to 5 minutes if recommended time-temperature processing is followed. Rinsing prior to fixing should take another 20 to 30 seconds, and lights (other than safelights) should not be turned on in the darkroom until the film has been in the fixer approximately 2 minutes (until the film has cleared). The auxiliary who processes film usually is unavailable during this approximately 11 to 12 minutes. However, there is no need to remain in the darkroom while the film is developing as long as the cover on the developer tank is lighttight; nor is it necessary to remain in the darkroom while the film is in the fixer. Time required for film stripping will be the same with or without automation, but film-racking time usually is eliminated when automatic film processors are used. Thus some time of the auxiliary is saved when automatic processors are employed. Probably more important, films are processed in a *consistent fashion* (as long as solution strength is maintained); also, with few exceptions, films are available to the dentist *more quickly* and in a *dry state*. Most processors are constructed so that films can be stripped in the darkroom and presented for use, dry, at the end of the processor located outside the darkroom.

Automatic processors function in several different modes. Most have a roller system that conveys the film through the processing cycle. Others use a mechanical conveyer that carries the film (ordinarily on a rack) through the cycle. The rollers may be belt, chain, or gear driven, or a combination may be used. The processing time cycle differs with different processors. Some processors automatically replenish solutions according to amount of use; others are not that automatic, and solutions must be replenished periodically by office personnel. Most processors use higher solution temperatures than that recommended for hand processing; solutions are different from those used for hand processing.

Although it is our opinion that the final product resulting from hand processing is superior to that obtained using automatic processors (when hand processing is done in a recommended time-temperature manner) no *objective* data relating

Text continued on p. 194.

Product and

	All-PRO; Air Techniques, Inc.	*Auveloper, model A; S. S. White Division of Pennwalt Corp.*	*Auveloper, model B; S. S. White Division of Pennwalt Corp.*	*Dentl-D-Veloper; General Electric Co.*
Dimensions: length × width × height (inches); unless otherwise designated, equipment is table mounted	24 × 13¾ × 15⅜; 33½ with daylight loader	31 × 20½ × 16	26 × 12 × 14	26 × 12 × 22¼; all illustrations show this equipment to be wall mounted
Can all American intraoral films be processed?	Yes	Yes[5]	Yes	Yes
Unit usable with a daylight loader hood?	Yes	Yes	Yes	Yes

*All data presented represent information received from the manufacturer or sales representative. Electricity is needed for all processors. "No information" indicates that the manufacturer or

As far as can be ascertained, this table includes all automatic dental x-ray film processors ceived from the Star X-ray Co., the Naca Equipment Corp., and the Adex Corp. These companies ently sold in the United States.

[1]The intent of this inquiry was to determine, exclusive of original cost, the workload necessary fort. Some manufacturers avoided the question, preferring to stress economic advantages in sistant, rapid availability of the diagnostic film, quality control, and so on. These points relate points are important, they do not answer the question: "What is the minimum volume of purchase an automatic processor because maintenance cost (time and expense) would not

[2]Responder was asked to comment only if minimum workload was considered necessary for optimal

[3]Run a panoramic or 8 × 10 "cleaner film" through the processor at least daily. The cleaner film algicide to the washer twice a week.

[4]Clean racks (removable roller racks) weekly with a sponge under warm, running water. Add

[5]Only those designed for automatic processing are recommended.

[6]All temperatures are for a 4½-minute time cycle.

[7]Two orbiting plates using only three gears.

[8]Rate is based on the use of a Panorex (5 × 12) film.

[9]Use care in following daily start-up and shut-down instructions. Change solutions every 2 to 3 maintenance.

[10]Add 2 oz. of developer replenisher and 2 oz. of fixer replenisher after every 100 intraoral

[11]Orbital plate using only three gears.

[12]Manually "top off" chemistry once a day.

[13]Use care in following daily start-up and shut-down instructions. Weekly care (or after the

[14]Litton automatic dental film processors replenish solutions by mechanical means. Instructions of film processed.

[15]Litton states that the P-4 and P-6 processors have 24-volt internal components, which offer

[16]Weekly maintenance involves only removal and cleaning of developer, fixer, and water roller tenance.

[17]Daily care includes changing the water bath, refilling with tempered water (68° to 70°), unit, changing solutions (this can be done biweekly), and cleaning the transport spindle. A mild

[18]Add replenisher daily; no daily cleanup is required. Wash and interchange transport modules fixer roller packs (transport modules). This is said to eliminate chemical cleaning.

[19]This unit is not table mounted. Dimensions will vary depending on how it is installed. The Kodak

Automatic dental film processor, models P-4, P-6, P-10; Litton Medical Systems	Pantomatic; Siemans Corp.	Procomat; Siemans Corp.	Philips 810 automatic x-ray film processor; Dental Systems Division of Philips Medical Systems	RP X-Omat processor model M7A; Eastman Kodak Co.[19]
P-4, P-6: $36\frac{1}{2} \times 19 \times 13\frac{1}{4}$; P-10: $36\frac{1}{2} \times 11\frac{1}{2} \times 11\frac{1}{2}$	$30 \times 19 \times 7\frac{1}{2}$	$18\frac{1}{2} \times 12\frac{3}{4} \times 12\frac{3}{4}$	$30\frac{1}{2} \times 17\frac{3}{8} \times 14\frac{3}{16}$	$29\frac{5}{8} \times 30 \times 27\frac{1}{2}$
Yes	Yes	Yes	Yes[5]	No
Yes	No	Yes	Yes	No

Data do not reflect our experience with the equipment.
supplier has not responded to this question.
available in the United States as of approximately July 1976; no response to inquiries was re-
may produce or distribute automatic film-processing devices. There are foreign processors not pres-

for the equipment to be economically sensible in terms of solution cost and maintenance ef-
terms of time saved, reduction of darkroom tedium, increased availability of the chairside as-
equally to those manufacturers who did try to answer the question directly. Although these
radiographic service (workload) below which a practitioner should probably be advised not to
justify the convenience?"
operation.
cleans the rollers and removes any deposits that might have formed during the idle period. Add

replenisher solutions once a week.

weeks; specified maintenance instructions are given. Additional instructions are given for periodic

films processed.

first 900 intraoral films, whichever occurs first) is required, as is monthly maintenance.
are given for pumping developer and fixer replenishers into tanks according to number and type

a great safety advantage when working in close proximity to water and chemicals.
racks. Additional instructions are given for every-second-week and every-second-month main-

and rinsing the film holder after each use. Weekly maintenance involves cleaning the entire
detergent is recommended.
weekly. Unlike other manufacturers, Philips recommends weekly interchange of developer and

RP X-Omat is useful only when a substantial number of extraoral films are used.

Continued.

Table 9-1. Available automatic dental x-ray film processors: a comparison of their attributes

	All-PRO; Air Techniques, Inc.	*Auveloper, model A; S. S. White Division of Pennwalt Corp.*	*Auveloper, model B; S. S. White Division of Pennwalt Corp.*	*Dental-D-Veloper; General Electric Co.*
Water and waste hookups needed?	Yes	Yes	Yes	No
Condition of processed radiograph	Dry	Dry	Dry	Dry
Total processing time	5 min. (usual); pulley change can reduce time to 3½ min. or to 1½ min.	½ to 8 min.; 4½ min. for intra-oral film	4½ or 7½ min.	5 min.
Equipment temp. (°F) during film processing				
Developer	80	85[6]	80	82
Rinse	—	—	—	—
Fixer	80	80	80	82
Wash	Tapwater	80	80	82
Dry	120	125	125	75 to 85

(For model B: 4½-min. cycle — Developer 80, Fixer 80, Wash 80, Dry 125; 7½-min. cycle — Developer 68, Fixer 68, Wash 68, Dry 125)

	All-PRO; Air Techniques, Inc.	*Auveloper, model A*	*Auveloper, model B*	*Dental-D-Veloper; General Electric Co.*
Maximum film size (inches)				
Width	8	5	3	3
Length	10	Any	Any	Not applicable
Type of drive				
Gear	X	X[7]	X[7]	X[11]
Belt				
Other				
Conveyor system				
Roller	X	X	X	X
Transport arm				
Automatic solution replenishment				
No	Automatic replenishment is under development (4/1/76)		X[10] All replenishment is manual	X[12] All replenishment is manual
If yes, rate of replenishment				
Developer		20 ml. per 12 in. of film[8]		
Rinse		—		
Fixer		40 ml. per 12 in. of film[8]		
Wash		¾ gal. per min.		

manufacturer

Automatic dental film processor, models P-4, P-6 P-10; Litton Medical Systems	Pantomatic; Siemans Corp.	Procomat; Siemans Corp.	Philips 810 automatic x-ray film processor; Dental Systems Division of Philips Medical Systems	RP X-Omat processor model M7A; Eastman Kodak Co.[19]
Yes	Yes	No	Yes, but provision is made for recirculation if necessary	Yes
Dry	Dry	Wet	Dry	Dry
4½ min.	4½ min.	6 min.	40 sec. to 6 min.; 4 min. is usual; 40-sec. rapid process films are not archival in quality	2½ min.
80	86	68 to 72	80	92
—	—		—	—
75	86	68 to 72	80	90
70 to 75	86	68 to 72	60 to 90	40 to 87
100 to 110	113	—	130	110
P-4: 4; P-6: 6; P-10: 10	8	2¼	8	14
P-4: —; P-6: 12; P-10: 12	10	3	Any	36
	X	X	X	
X			Chain	Chain
X	X		X	X
		X		
X Mechanical replenishment[14]		X	X All replenishment is manual	
	30 ml. per min.			75 ml. per 14 × 17 sheet
	—			—
	50 ml. per min.			95 ml. per 14 × 17 sheet
	½ gal. per min.			2½ gal. per min.

Continued.

Table 9-1. Available automatic dental x-ray film processors: a comparison of their attributes

	All-PRO; Air Techniques, Inc.	Auveloper, model A; S. S. White Division of Pennwalt Corp.	Auveloper, model B; S. S. White Division of Pennwalt Corp.	Dental-D-Veloper; General Electric Co.
Frequency of solution change				
Based on 75 intra-oral and 5 panoramic films (if applicable) *per week*	Once a month	Every 3 weeks	After 1,000 intra-oral films or 1 month, whichever comes first	Once a month
Based on 200 intra-oral and 10 panoramic films (if applicable) *per day*	Three times a month	Every 2 weeks	After 1,000 intra-oral films or 1 month, whichever comes first	Once a month
Minimum weekly workload necessary for processor, per se, to be *economically* sensible (estimate)[1]	Information received was non-specific[1]; however, it was estimated that chemistry would cost $200 to $300 a year and electricity, $40 to $80 a year for the "modest user"	1,000 sq. in. per week	200 sq. in. per week	Information received was non-specific[1]
Recommended care				
Daily	Use cleaning film[3]	See Ref. 9	Run 2 or 3 occlusal films thru to clean rollers	See Ref. 13
Weekly	See Ref. 4	See Ref. 9	Rinse transport	See Ref. 13
Is a minimum workload necessary for equipment to function properly?[2]	A cleaning film should be used each morning and whenever the processor has been idle more than 2 hours	Best to use daily		
Retail cost				
1975	$1,995	$3,300	$1,375	$1,750
Estimate 1977	Increase 5% to 7%	$3,300	No information	Same (cost/value analysis)

—cont'd

manufacturer				
Automatic dental film processor, models P-4, P-6, P-10; Litton Medical Systems	Pantomatic; Siemans Corp.	Procomat; Siemans Corp.	Philips 810 automatic x-ray film processor; Dental Systems Division of Philips Medical Systems	RP X-Omat processor model M7A; Eastman Kodak Co.[19]
Twice a month	Twice a month	Twice a month	Twice a month	Once a week
Once a month	Twice a month	Not suitable for this volume of work	Twice a month with daily manual replenishment depending on use	Once a week
P-4 and P-6: 30 intraoral films per day; P-10: designed for high-volume or group practices and where extraoral films are used	No information	No information	150 intraoral; 10 panoramic	50 14 × 17 films or the equivalent in film surface area
See Ref. 9; also see Ref. 15	None	See Ref. 17	See Ref. 18	See. Ref. 9
See Ref. 9; also see Ref. 15	See Ref. 16	See Ref. 17	See Ref. 18	See. Ref. 9
			No	
P-4: $1,095; P-6: $1,340; P-10: $2,840	$3,200	$475	$2,050	$7,337 with 8-gal. tank
No information	$3,200	$550	$2,050	No information

to *diagnostic* superiority is available. The difference, if any, may be discounted in view of other advantages, especially consistency in film-processing procedures.

Table 9-1 is designed to acquaint the reader with data relating to most currently available automatic processors. These data were obtained from equipment manufacturers and do not represent our personal knowledge. Nor have we had a sustained experience with all processors listed in the table. Experience has demonstrated, however, that considerable care must be given to the processors if they are to function properly. Manufacturers' directions must be followed carefully relative to daily and weekly maintenance. Without doubt, some equipment is more trouble free than others. Unfortunately, the literature contains little objective data that provide a comparison of performance among available processors. An article in the September 1975 issue of the Journal of the American Dental Association entitled "Acceptance Program for Rapid Processing Devices for Dental Radiographic Film" is a constructive step. Manufacturers are required to comply with stated specifications and provide information if the product is to be advertised in the Journal.

Because processors can break down, as can any piece of equipment, it is necessary for the dental office to have available a conventional darkroom that will function in times of emergency. This darkroom should be equipped in the most modern fashion if quality standards are to be maintained during times when automated equipment is nonfunctional.

TESTING FOR SAFELIGHTING

The degree of light safety needed for the darkroom depends on the type of film being used and on the length of time films are left unwrapped in the darkroom before being processed. It is best that each dentist determine the safety of his darkroom for his individual needs. This is done in two steps: (1) Turn off all the lights including the safelights; wait a *minimum* of 5 minutes to obtain a fair degree of dark adaption of the eyes; then look for any places where light is getting into the room from the outside. These light leaks should be obliterated. (2) The second step is known as the *penny test*. A film exposed in a normal manner* is taken out of its wrapper in *total* darkness and is placed on the workbench directly under the safelight. A small coin such as a penny is placed on it, and the safelights are turned on. The film is left in this condition for a length of time equal to the maximum time that any unwrapped film of this type may be left in the darkroom before being processed. The film is then processed. If the image or outline of the coin can be seen, the darkroom is not light safe for this film and the safelights should be rectified. Darkroom lighting should be tested for each type of film used in the office unless the operator is certain that a given film is less sensitive to visible light than a film previously tested. Films must be tested for each type of safelight filter used.

---

*Prior exposure is not entirely essential.

CARE OF THE DARKROOM

Cleanliness of the darkroom is of the utmost importance because of x-ray film sensitivity and the desirability of prolonging equipment life. It is imperative that the bench top, tanks, and hangers be kept clean at all times. Tanks should be scrubbed whenever solutions are changed. Abrasive substances, such as steel wool, must not be used. Tanks may be cleaned with a bland soap but must be thoroughly rinsed with water. The fixer tank in addition should be flushed with a weak acetic acid solution followed by a second water rinse. Hangers should be washed and cleaned of residual gelatin in the clips before being stored for future use. This step is especially pertinent for those dentists who wet read and discard some radiographs. Spilt solution should be wiped up immediately, or chemical dust may form. Liquid contaminants and chemical dust can produce artifacts that reduce the diagnostic value of radiographs. Good housekeeping must be maintained if optimum quality radiographs are to be obtained.

Processing solutions

The preparation of processing solutions is important. These solutions are prepared from powders or liquid concentrates; the manufacturers' recommendations should be followed. However, some general precautions are worth mentioning. Water temperature should not exceed manufacturers' specifications. Mixing containers, for example, glass and enamel-surfaced pails, should be corrosion resistant. Powdered chemicals should be added to the water and not vice versa. Separate paddles for mixing the developer and fixer solutions must be used. These paddles should be washed before they are stored. Solutions not currently in use should be stored in brown bottles away from any source of heat.

Processing solutions should be kept at good working strength, and attention should be paid to replenishing the solutions whenever it becomes necessary. The level of processing solutions can be maintained by adding more solution; however, when the developing or fixing time for any particular temperature becomes prolonged, the solutions should be changed. A special replenishing solution can be used to maintain developer level and strength.

The proper developing time for weakened developer solution at the recommended solution temperature can be determined by conducting a simple test. Expose five or six films at the same exposure time,* kVp, mA, and tube-film distance. After unwrapping the films in the darkroom, place all the films on separate racks and insert into the developer at the same time. Remove one film at a time from the developer at intervals of 1 minute, beginning 3 minutes after immersion. Each film is rinsed and fixed after being developed. When the films are examined, it will be seen that film density increases sharply with developing time, up to a certain time. When film density ceases to increase sharply, it

---

*Exposure time should be such that the films are not overexposed. A suggested exposure time for films at cone tip on a tabletop is one tenth of the exposure generally used for a maxillary anterior area.

means that the complete latent image has been developed; this is the proper developing time for the solution.

The fixer solution serves to remove unexposed or undeveloped silver halide crystals; it also hardens the emulsion. The total process requires 10 to 15 minutes. With *fresh* fixer, clearing time (the time required for unexposed or undeveloped areas to become transparent) is approximately 2 minutes; complete removal of the silver halide crystals requires approximately 4 minutes. Emulsion hardening is completed during the remaining period. Excessive fixing tends to fade the radiographic image. When clearing time exceeds 4 minutes, the fixer should be discarded, the tank should be thoroughly cleaned, and the solution should be replaced. Radiographs can be used for diagnostic purposes as soon as they have cleared (they should be rinsed prior to use to prevent accidental spotting of clothing), but they must be returned to the fixing solution prior to washing and drying. Radiographs should be washed in running water for 20 to 30 minutes before they are dried.

The processing tanks should be covered when not in use to prevent oxidation of the developer and fixer. At the beginning of each workday, any observable material or scum on the surface of the solutions should be removed. The solutions should then be stirred with their individual paddles. The water flow must be adjusted or regulated to provide a temperature between 65° and 75° F. This temperature should be maintained throughout the workday.

Removal of fixer stain

Chemical stains, especially fixer stains, are very unsightly on uniforms and clothing. These stains can be easily removed if they are treated before the garments are laundered. Commercially available stain removers such as Fix-Off remove chemical stains with ease.

Care and loading of film holders

Screen cassettes and nonscreen film holders must be kept in good working condition. Screens must be kept clean and free of dust and chemicals, or their ability to project light images onto the film will be impaired. The result of unclean screens is the production of artifacts in the finished radiograph. The actual fluorescent screen can be cleaned with a damp cloth containing a little bland soap.

Cassette and film holders should be kept loaded with film and ready for immediate use. Care must be taken in placing the film in these devices. Screen film is exposed principally by the visible light given off by the fluorescent screens, whereas nonscreen film is exposed by x-rays only. Light-sensitive film is placed between two screens in a screen type of cassette. No paper or other substance should be interposed between the film and screens, and the screens and film must be in firm contact. Nonscreen film, together with its paper wrapper (Fig. 9-2), is placed in a cardboard film holder. The paper wrapper is included as an added precaution against light leaks. It should be noted that the large flap of the cardboard film holder is folded down before the sideflaps and not vice versa. This provides a lighttight seal for the enclosed film.

Film identification

Film identification is of the utmost importance. There is nothing more frustrating to the radiologist than to have a set of good radiographs and not know to whom they relate. Flexible tabs, which can be written on repeatedly in pencil, can be attached to the intraoral film racks. For films larger than intraoral films, the solution of the problem is not as simple. Since large films will ultimately not be mounted in film mounts, it is desirable that the patient's name, date, and other pertinent information be printed directly on the radiograph itself. Also, since there is no way of telling from the radiograph which side of the patient was exposed, there must be some means of identifying the right and the left side.

The best means of identifying which side of the patient was exposed is to place a small R or L lead letter on the exposure side of the cassette or film holder. This letter must be in or very close to the x-ray beam when the exposure is made. This same system can be used for the patient's name and other information. A leaded tape with the information typed* on it can be utilized. However, since this tape is of considerable size, a larger beam of radiation must be used if the tape is not to superimpose its image on some area of diagnostic interest. This system does not lend itself to good radiation protection practice.

---

*That portion of the leaded tape struck by the type is thinned and permits radiation to pass through.

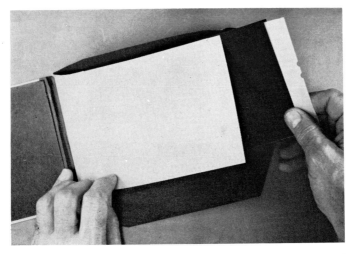

Fig. 9-2. Placement of film in a cardboard film holder. Protective paper is allowed to remain and covers film. The large flap is closed first and then the sides and back of the holder.

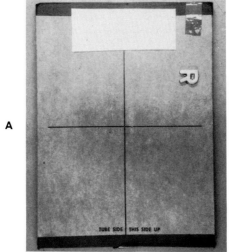

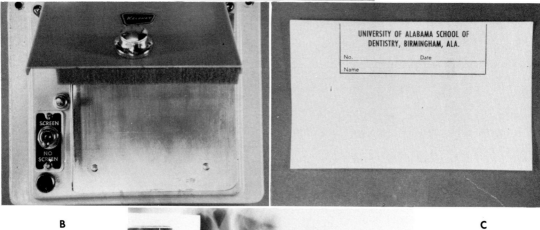

Fig. 9-3. A, Cardboard film holder masked for use with an identification printer. Note also the identifying letter R and the tape above it. Two different colored tapes are used to easily distinguish R's from L's in the cassette storage bin. **B,** Identification printer. **C,** Semitransparent card used for identification purposes. **D,** Information reproduced on the radiograph.

A better system of identification is to cover a small unused part of the cassette with a piece of lead. That part of the film under the lead will be unexposed. When the film is removed in the darkroom, the necessary information can be placed on this unexposed portion by use of a print box and a semitransparent card with the information printed on it. These boxes are available at most x-ray supply stores. A masked film holder, identification printer, card, and reproduced information are shown in Fig. 9-3.

If only an occasional extraoral film is taken, it is probably most practical to write the necessary information on the film border with a pencil or a ball-point pen, using more than usual pressure. The writing can be done either before or after film exposure, but, for permanency, it must be done before developing.

Film and equipment storage

Films are often stored in the darkroom for convenience. It must be remembered that films must be stored away from excessive heat, humidity, and stray radiation. Refrigerators are excellent places to store films if the boxes are unopened; humidity is usually not a problem until the film box is opened. Chemical fumes must not be allowed to come in contact with stored films. If there is any danger of stray radiation reaching films, they should be stored in a lead-lined or steel box. Films must be kept away from hot pipes and radiators. Objects should not be placed on top of stored films, because pressure can cause film artifacts. Films should be arranged in the storage area so that the oldest are used first.

When a darkroom is planned, it should be remembered that the operator must work in limited illumination. Efficiency is therefore greatly dependent on having everything in the darkroom in its proper place. Efficiency is also increased if each piece of equipment is used only for its specific purpose.

FILM-PROCESSING TECHNICS

Film processing requires the film to be carefully removed from its paper packet, cardboard holder, or cassette. The film will show static electric discharges if forcibly removed from its packet or cassette. Care should be taken not to crimp, scratch, or otherwise damage the film. The film should be handled at the edges to prevent finger marks on the emulsion; it is important that the operator's hands be clean and free of chemicals. The film is attached to the film rack or hanger and is checked to see that it is securely fastened. While the film is out of its packet, proper safelight illumination is required, or fogging of the film can occur.

Films ordinarily should be processed using standard solutions that require a developing time of approximately 4½ minutes at 68° F. (Manufacturers' instructions should be followed; variations from this time-temperature combination may be recommended.) Speed developers are available, and their use is indicated under certain circumstances. Film-processing technics are discussed under Routine film processing and Rapid film processing.

Routine film processing

Film processing should be done on a time-temperature basis (see Chapter 1). Proper developing time varies with the temperature of the developer; the temperature of the developer must be taken before processing is begun. With proper-strength developer, the developing time for a range of temperatures is determined from charts supplied by the manufacturer of the developer; optimum developing time and temperature are usually $4\frac{1}{2}$ minutes at 68° F. If the operator is unsure which solution is the developer, he can identify the developer by dipping his fingers in the solution and rubbing them together. The developer has a soapy feel, which is unlike the feel of the acid fixer.

The film is placed in the developer for the predetermined time. Here, a timing device is essential. Note that nonscreen films or films with thicker emulsions may need increased processing times. While the film is being developed, the operator should shake or agitate the film rack two or three times to release any air bubbles attached to the film and to bathe the emulsion in fresh developing solution. The use of sight developing, instead of the time-temperature system, is often associated with overexposure of films and patient and with underdevelopment of the films to give proper radiographic density. Sight-developed radiographs are often of poor diagnostic quality.

After developing, the film is rinsed in running water for 20 to 30 seconds to remove the excess developer. This is necessary since the developer is alkaline and the fixer is acid. The film is then placed in the fixer; when it becomes clear, it can be read while wet. The clear film, when rinsed, can be used in this manner for an hour or more but should not be permitted to dry and must be returned to the fixer for permanent fixing. Total fixing time should be 10 to 15 minutes, depending on fixer strength. If the film is left excessively long in the fixer solution, some of the silver that forms the radiographic image will be removed, and the radiograph will lose density.

To remove the fixer solution from the film, the film must be washed for 20 minutes in *running* water. A film that is not properly washed will have residual fixer chemicals in the emulsion and will become discolored in time. When the temperatures of the various processing solutions vary greatly, the film emulsion is subjected to quick changes in temperature; the emulsion may contract if plunged from warm to cold solution and form a lacelike pattern called reticulation. Passing a film from cold to warm solution is not harmful except that excessively warm solutions cause the emulsion to melt. Overly soft emulsions can slide off the film base.

After washing, the film is dried in a dust-free area before it is mounted. Large films are usually not mounted but stored in envelopes; they often have sharp corners, and these corners should be trimmed to prevent films in the same envelope from scratching each other. Curved corners can be made with a pair of scissors or a commercially available film-cutting device.

Many artifacts can result from improper darkroom technic. Some examples of such artifacts are shown in Chapter 3. Film fog can occur from a multitude of causes—for example, excessive temperature where the films are stored, improper light sealing of the darkroom, and the turning on of lights or lighting of cigarettes in the darkroom before the films have been fixed. Treelike, black linear images can result from static electricity created when the film packet is opened too aggressively. Dark lines can occur from bending the film prior to development. Chemical stains can occur from the contamination of processing solutions, film racks, workbench, or fingers; fluoride is definitely injurious to film. Whenever poor quality radiographs are produced, the dentist would do well to examine first the darkroom and his darkroom technic.

Rapid film processing

Until recently, dental practitioners accomplished a reduction in film processing time by overexposing the film and reducing the time necessary for developing the film. Although the resultant radiograph was not as diagnostically useful as a properly exposed and processed radiograph, a judgment in this matter was left entirely to the individual. Recognition of radiation hazards and the need to limit patient exposure now places such procedures in the malpractice category.

Rapid processing solutions are now marketed and appear to have a place in dental practice, particularly in endodontics and oral surgery, when rapid location of a specific object is required. Rapid processing is also helpful following the placement of a restoration when it becomes necessary to use a radiograph to confirm the nonexistence of an overhang. (Use of a radiograph for this purpose should not be necessary routinely. There are usually other means for detecting overextended restorations.) Solution temperatures as high as 92° F, with developing time reductions to as low as 4 seconds, are being recommended by some manufacturers.

It is the purpose of this text to advise rather than recommend specific products. It is our opinion that rapid processing developers should not be used routinely in the production of general purpose radiographs. Rapid processing at high temperatures tends to produce increased film fog, loss of image density, and alterations in contrast. Some products produce more satisfactory radiographs than do others. The reader is referred to the list of suggested readings for information about specific products. One simple test that can be used to compare a selected rapid processing developer with a standard developer is to process *unexposed* films in the respective developers according to the manufacturer's time and temperature instructions and to compare, after fixing, washing, and drying, these films on the basis of fog (the amount of blackness accumulated by the emulsion due entirely to the action of the developer on the emulsion). This test gives no information about image density loss or contrast changes, but radiographs with a high fog level are usually less diagnostically useful than are those with minimum fog.

CHAPTER 10

Radiographic surveys

ROLE OF THE RADIOGRAPH IN DIAGNOSIS

Earlier chapters of this text deal with technical and physical considerations. The remaining chapters are largely devoted to the interpretation of radiographs. It is important at the outset to consider the role that the radiograph plays in diagnosis.

Diagnosis is defined as the art or act of recognizing disease from signs and symptoms. Symptoms are elicited from the patient. Signs can be categorized as clinical, clinical laboratory, histopathologic, and radiographic. Many disease processes can be diagnosed from symptoms and clinical signs without the assistance of clinical laboratory tests, biopsy reports, or radiographs. Less frequently, a diagnosis can be made from one of the latter three as the sole basis for information. Usually, one or more of these three are combined with clinical signs to arrive at a diagnosis when the patient presents nondefinitive symptoms.

In dentistry, radiographs are used routinely with symptoms and clinical signs to arrive at a diagnosis. A diagnosis almost never should be made on the basis of the radiograph per se; the radiograph should be used in an adjunctive capacity. Conversely, failure to use radiographic information when it is needed is as serious an error as using radiographic data without other supporting evidence.

Radiographs are most important in understanding changes in calcified structures and can be useful in evaluating alterations in noncalcified organs and tissue not visible clinically. Unlike medicine, dental use of the radiograph is confined largely to the former. There is no reason why radiographic interpretation of soft tissue changes cannot be used in dentistry; special equipment and technics are needed for this purpose. Cinefluoroscopy used in evaluation of speech, mastication, and swallowing habits is an example of a special soft tissue radiographic technic. Sialography is another such example; in this case an opaque contrast medium is used to delineate glandular tissue from ducts and their tributaries.

An evaluation of hard structures is mandatory in dental treatment. These hard tissues, other than the crown of the tooth, are overlaid with soft tissue and cannot be observed clinically. Bone alterations in the maxilla and mandible not directly associated with the teeth are usually first detected radiographically unless they have progressed sufficiently to demonstrate gross changes. The radiograph often assists in differentiating one type of change from another.

Although the presence of infection at the apex of the tooth root can become known through acute symptoms, the extent of the destruction is often not determinable through clinical means. Apical disease is found more often in the chronic state than in the acute state and frequently presents vague clinical symptoms. The use of radiography in finding chronic apical disease, residual foreign bodies, and asymptomatic bone lesions classically demonstrates its importance in diagnosis.

Pathologic changes in the supporting structures of the teeth can involve the hard and/or soft tissue; usually changes occur in both. Soft tissue modifications can be seen clinically, and an estimate of bone loss can be attempted through clinical methods. However, the radiograph is the only satisfactory means for determining the height of remaining bone. Incipient periodontal changes are often detected first through careful radiographic examination. Bone characteristics in more advanced lesions assist in evaluating the prognosis and the success of treatment.

Dental caries occur in regions that can be seen clinically; yet the radiograph materially assists in caries detection. Interproximal surfaces are difficult to observe unless contacting surfaces are widely separated; the dentist is reluctant to separate the teeth because of the time involved and the trauma created. Studies have shown that radiography is more efficient than clinical examination in detecting early interproximal carious lesions. Even occlusal caries, because of its configuration, sometimes is observed first radiographically at the dentoenamel junction.

Growth patterns of the face and jaws can be observed clinically, but the most definitive information is often obtained through specialized radiographic procedures. Alterations in temporomandibular joint movement and osseous changes in the condylar head and articular fossa are usually observed best radiographically. Fractures of the facial bones must be observed in order to reduce the fracture most effectively. It is clear that the radiograph plays a most essential role in diagnosis.

Although the importance of the radiograph in diagnosis is emphasized, it is essential to state its shortcomings; mistakes in judgment can be made through overdependence on radiographic findings. Perhaps the most serious deficiency of the radiograph is that it may not show the full extent of the process. This is especially true in acute, fulminating, rampant conditions. Radiographic evidence of changes in hard structures depends on alterations in the mineral content of the part being examined. A disease process can proceed into a calcified structure without immediately altering the structure sufficiently to make it observable radiographically. The radiograph fails to demonstrate soft tissue changes unless special technics are used.

The ordinary radiograph represents a single plane image of a three-dimensional object. The shortcomings of such a situation are obvious, and care must be taken, when necessary, to separate structures superimposed on one another.

From a technical standpoint, the appearance of the same structure varies, and its appearance depends on factors employed. As stated in earlier chapters, film density, contrast, definition, magnification, and distortion are related to kilovoltage, milliampere seconds, filtration, film emulsions, intensifying screens, beam direction, object-film relationships, darkroom procedures, and viewing conditions. All such factors play a role in varying the appearance of a structure viewed radiographically. Technical factors can be controlled by the operator; biologic and anatomic considerations often are noncontrollable.

When can the radiograph be used as the basic source of information? When can it be considered definitive and be used for diagnostic purposes without the support of clinical observations, clinical laboratory tests, and/or histopathologic information? Basically, the radiograph should never be used in this manner, but experience in correlating clinical and radiographic findings justifies limited use of the radiograph for such purposes. For example, interproximal caries seen radiographically is invariably present; care must be taken to differentiate caries from enamel imperfections such as hypoplasia. Crestal interproximal bone loss observed in the radiograph is ordinarily representative of the minimum amount of existing destruction. Foreign bodies located *with certainty* in or around the mandible or maxilla are present. If the radiograph is used as the definitive basis for a diagnosis, extreme care must be taken to verify the accuracy of the findings.

Although using the radiograph in the manner just described may be permissible, a plan of treatment should never be arranged on the basis of the radiograph per se. Many factors that are not determinable radiographically enter into a treatment plan. For example, a cardiac condition could contraindicate tooth removal; uncontrolled diabetes might preclude periodontal therapy. Many such examples could be given.

PEOPLE MANAGEMENT

People management encompasses two quite different frequently encountered problems. The first relates to recalcitrant patients who, for one or more of several possible reasons, refuse radiographic services. The second has to do with the actual management of individuals who, for anatomic, physiologic, psychologic, or other factors beyond their control, simply are difficult to handle. Solutions to all such circumstances are the practitioner's responsibility; it may be helpful to consider some fairly typical situations with the realization that identical dental office circumstances rarely are repeated.

The recalcitrant patient

Radiographs are essential for diagnosis and treatment planning. Failure to adequately examine a patient radiographically can be considered an act of malpractice except in isolated instances. An oral diagnosis ordinarily is incomplete, and treatment should not be started in the absence of a satisfactory radiographic survey. The adequacy of the examination is left to the practitioner's judgment; both the adequacy and the judgment can be questioned legally. For these reasons and primarily because the practitioner desires to render the finest possible dental service, *radiographs must be made when needed.* The intelligent dentist will refuse treatment if necessary. The patient usually can be persuaded to accept a radiographic service. The paragraphs to follow examine problem situations in greater detail.

Fear of radiation exposure. The public is aware of environmental contamination of which radiation exposure is a part; some individuals are more conscious and more concerned than others. Some pregnant women fear for their unborn child. A few people have received substantial therapeutic radiation exposure, and a distinct minority have been occupationally exposed.

One must acknowledge that such people have reason for concern. All ionizing radiation is harmful; it should be used with discretion. Diagnostic gains for health purposes must exceed the health risks; the diagnostic yield from radiation use must be high. Chapter 4 covers radiation hazards and protection. Each dentist and dental auxiliary should be thoroughly familiar with this chapter and, in general, with the suggested readings on this subject found on pp. 477 to 480. Each dentist must follow recommended radiation protection methods. Having done so, the dentist can assure his patient that the planned specific skin area of exposure (in contrast to whole-body exposure) will be as small as possible. Thus the dose delivered to the tissues beneath the skin will be correspondingly small, and the dose received by the reproductive organs (and fetus in the pregnant woman) will be almost infinitesimal. The gains will far outbalance the risks. Under no circumstances should the dentist give the impression that the patient's concerns are ridiculous, speculative, or without scientific merit. To do so would betray the dentist's ignorance and give the patient further reason for continued concern. The intelligent patient's reasons for avoiding radiation exposure are usually good; it is a matter of putting them in proper perspective.

Economic considerations. Health care is expensive. Radiographs cost money. Some people, perhaps more in rural and economically deprived areas, have had dental services in the past without benefit of diagnostic radiographs. Possibly, a prior dentist was permissive and allowed the patient to elect (dictate) policy. All of this can compound into an *initial* refusal of radiographic service.

The dentist has no choice. He must examine radiographically when his judgment dictates. He does have some alternatives in the way he handles his patients and in the way he thinks about the health services he renders. *Service* is the product sold by the dentist—service or *time* needed to perform the service. The dentist does not (or should not) sell radiographs per se (unless he restricts his practice to radiography and produces radiographs to be used diagnostically by others). If this is the dentist's philosophy, he will have no difficulty avoiding a fixed fee for one or more radiographs; he will charge only for the total, completed service.

Patient education should be an integral part of all dental practices. It should take many forms. Patients are entitled to know why radiographs are necessary. If a dentist and/or his auxiliaries cannot convincingly explain why, there is reason to question the dentist's competency. Economic considerations, though important to a patient, lose their importance when the patient becomes convinced that the recommended health care item is essential to his well-being. If the patient genuinely cannot afford a radiographic service, he probably cannot afford any other health service. Health care is no longer a privilege; it has become a right. A discussion about the responsibility for providing this service is not within the province of this text. Refusal to compromise one's professional ethics may result in the loss of a patient. Such a loss could have widespread beneficial results; it almost never will be detrimental to practice building.

Patient management

Most patients present no substantial obstacle to the creation of high-quality intraoral radiographs. Consequently, all dentists and auxiliary personnel should find it possible to produce optimal radiographs routinely. A small minority of patients offer a wide variety of situations that interfere with the production of satisfactory intraoral radiographs. Although many such difficulties must be solved through the ingenuity of the operator, it may be helpful to discuss some of the more common situations and suggest at least a partial solution.

Gagging. The gag reflex is common to all people, but it is more active in some than in others. Intraoral films are placed in oral areas specifically related to the initiation of this reflex. Film placement is at times uncomfortable, and attempts by the patient to relieve the discomfort may stimulate the reflex. Some patients may deliberately or unconsciously activate the reflex as a defense against anticipated unpleasantness. Most gagging can be controlled.

In our opinion, the best method of controlling gagging is through technical expertise and authoritarianism tempered with compassion. The creation of patient confidence through demonstrated ability and the development of a nonpermissive approach in interpersonal relationships greatly minimizes gagging. This can be observed readily in a school clinic situation. A student who has trouble with a gagging patient is often surprised at the ease with which the instructor obtains patient cooperation. The operator must know what he is doing and must do it expeditiously.

All gagging is not so easily solved; at times there is no way to eliminate the difficulty. Extraoral films supplemented with all possible intraoral radiographs may be the only solution. Before or in conjunction with such technics, one can employ various gag-inhibiting methods. Swabbing the soft palate with a topical anesthetic is often helpful. The application of salt on the palate is said to be useful. We ask some patients to breathe deeply and rapidly through the nose and others to hold their breath (the latter requires speed on the part of the operator). Although the success of such methods may be physiologically related, they probably best serve by diverting the patient's concentration away from the gag reflex.

Neuromuscular problems. Patient inability to remain immobile during intraoral film placement, angulation, and exposure procedures constitutes a challenge to the dentist and his auxiliaries. Diagnostically useful radiographs usually cannot be made if the patient moves excessively. Uncontrollable movement takes many forms ranging from a tongue musculature that is unable to relax through the involuntary tremors of the aged to the symptoms of muscular dystrophy and cerebral palsy. It is not possible to discuss separately radiographic technic directly applicable to specific symptoms. Suggestions of a general nature should be helpful to the concerned practitioner.

Speed is essential whenever movement exists. The operator must have technical expertise and be able to execute rapidly whatever radiographic procedures are needed. Minimization of the exposure interval is especially important. This can be accomplished through use of fast film emulsions, shortened radiation source–object distance (hence shortened source–film distance), maximally high kilovoltage, and the highest milliamperage (most dental x-ray machines may not be operated above 15 mA). For example, if high-speed film (D speed) is currently in use (thus the film speed cannot be increased), a change in kilovoltage from 65 to 90, milliamperage from 10 to 15, and distance from 16 to 8 inches will reduce the needed exposure to approximately $\frac{1}{18}$ of that previously used. Intraoral cassettes equipped with intensifying screens for occlusal (3.4) film can be helpful; however, there are problems associated with the use of such cassettes (see pp. 125 and 126).

Extraoral films, particularly lateral oblique projections of the mandible and maxilla, and panoramic views, can be especially useful. These should be supplemented by intraoral views when possible. It is usually easier for the neuromuscularly involved patient to remain immobile when films are placed extraorally. The long exposure time necessary for panoramic films may contraindicate their use. When absolutely necessary, the film holder can be stabilized by another person but not by dental office staff. Every effort must be made to use the services of a person beyond the age of reproduction and to avoid excessive primary beam exposure.

Beyond these suggestions, little can be done toward improving the radiographic service of such disabled individuals. Patience and empathy are extremely important. Fear and lack of understanding must be overcome. Sedation is often indicated. When necessary and under suitable circumstances, radiography, like other facets of clinical dentistry, can be performed under anesthesia.

The child patient. Radiography for the child patient does not differ technically from that for the adult. Management of the child does vary, although many
of the concepts already suggested for adults are applicable to the child. Non-
permissiveness tempered with patience and empathy are essential. The young
patient is apt to be unaccustomed to his surroundings, hence fearful. His mouth
is smaller than that of the adult, yet the radiographic area of interest may be
just as large. Radiographic equipment and particularly the placement of an intraoral film may be entirely foreign to him. His preadolescent reaction to a dental
office will probably relate directly to what he has heard at home.

Several random introductory thoughts are important. One cannot struggle
with a child and expect to get satisfactory radiographic results. One should
not compromise by using conveniently small intraoral films that offer no possibility of demonstrating a reasonably large area of coverage. In our opinion, the
1.1 film is the smallest film that can be used with any expectation of an adequate
diagnostic yield (amount of diagnostic information obtained per unit of radiation absorbed). Extraoral films have a definite place in radiography for the
child. The child is apt to respond to the challenge for cooperation more readily
than the adolescent or adult.

Hopefully, the child's initial experience in the dental office will not be of an
emergency nature. The child's introduction to radiography should be during his
initial visit, at which time he becomes acquainted with his new surroundings.
This activity should not be hurried, nor should the child be apprised of any
negative possibilities such as "it might hurt a bit" or "you might gag a little."
He should be allowed to handle film and encouraged to place the packet in his
mouth. The x-ray machine should be appropriately positioned near his face but
without an intraoral film in place; do not try to make the young child adjust to
two or more new circumstances simultaneously. Acquaint the child with the
sound he may hear in the tube head when the tube is energized; reassure him
without fostering a questioning attitude that could lead to fear. Show him a
radiograph of another child's teeth. Let him observe film placement and angulation procedures on another member of his family, preferably a child. Practice
film placement; start in the anterior regions. Solicit the child's assistance and
praise him for cooperating. A mirror enabling the child to observe may be helpful. All or most of this educational program can be done by the *trained* auxiliary,
but the dentist should have a role; if he does not, he will be the unknown stranger
if his help is ever required.

There will be occasions when a complete mouth intraoral radiographic survey cannot be obtained. Don't waste radiation trying to do the impossible. As
with older patients who are unable to cooperate, use extraoral methods and supplement these with such intraoral films as can be obtained. Bite-wing films of
the posterior teeth and single or multiple maxillary and mandibular films often
can be made even for difficult child patients. As with all patients, do not treat
unless or until a diagnosis is made. Radiographic information generally is essential diagnostically.

RADIOGRAPHIC SURVEY DEFINED

A *survey* is an examination of a part or an area designed to determine whether any abnormal change exists within the part or area. Such a survey (1) can be a routine scanning procedure that may be followed by special films to examine the same or other parts for the purpose of observing the area in question more clearly or examining other areas for associated lesions or (2) can be a specific purpose survey in which one or more films are used to examine a specific area or to fulfill a specific purpose.

Examples of the routine scanning survey include the ordinary complete mouth intraoral series and any single or group of extraoral films used for purposes of general information. The specific purpose survey is illustrated by the orthodontic cephalometric film, designed to study growth patterns, or by the temporomandibular joint film series, used for studying the articulation of this joint.

The surveys discussed in this chapter are confined largely to the routine scanning procedures. They are considered generally as follows: surveys of the teeth and supporting structures, surveys of the face and skull, and localization procedures. The operator must use his judgment in designing specific purpose surveys most suitable for his needs. The discussion related to surveys of extraoral structures has a specific purpose connotation, and the chapters on technic, particularly Chapter 7, give assistance in this regard.

SURVEYS OF THE TEETH AND SUPPORTING STRUCTURES

The practitioner's ability to interpret dental films is limited by the quality of the film he or his assistant has produced. One cannot interpret findings that are partially or totally obscured due to unsatisfactory technics or that are lacking because of inadequate film coverage. It is important to reemphasize that faulty darkroom procedures as well as film placement, angulation, and exposure can impede interpretation.

It is notable how often films are referred for interpretation with an accompanying apology for the film quality. Ordinarily, these apologies are related more to film fog and improper density than to inadequacies of film placement and angulation. Many times, however, the apology should include the latter aspects as well. In view of the present emphasis on the need for reducing exposure to ionizing radiation, it becomes increasingly important that technical excellence be encouraged. It is unlikely that the general practitioner will be restricted legally in his use of ionizing radiation, but if this should occur, it will be because the patient is not receiving sufficient diagnostic value per unit of radiation exposure. The radiation exposure *yield* will be the determining factor.

What is a usable film? Quality assessment for complete mouth surveys is discussed earlier in the text (see p. 89). Much of this is applicable to the single film. Each intraoral film, whether included in a complete mouth survey or used as a single film, should show no film fog other than that inherent in the film base itself and no stain or discoloration resulting from inadequate darkroom procedures. Film density varies with personal preference, but excessively dark or light films are unacceptable. The position of the identifying dot (see pp. 22 and 23) is marked on the back side of the film packet. When the film is placed, the dot must be toward the occlusal plane. Such positioning will avoid superimposing important structures on the dot. The film should be placed so that the incisal edges or cusps of the teeth are approximately ⅛ inch from the film margin. Each single film should show a suitable reproduction of the area being examined; each tooth's image should be neither elongated nor foreshortened (reduced in length); the interproximal surfaces for the teeth should not overlap. Each film should show the interproximal bone crest without superimposition of adjacent teeth. It is necessary that approximately ⅛ to ¼ inch of alveolar bone be observable beyond the apex of the tooth. Excessive tooth length sometimes makes the inclusion of this amount of bone difficult. Certainly, the entire apex must be demonstrated, and it is preferable that a reasonably large amount of surrounding bone be seen. Occasionally, two films of the same tooth are needed to show all areas. Criteria of excellence for extraoral films are largely similar to those for intraoral films. Care must be taken to restrict the exposure area to structures that will be usefully and accurately represented on the radiograph.

Surveys of the teeth and supporting structures are discussed as follows: surveys for adults, surveys for children, surveys for edentulous patients, panoramic radiography, alternate uses of intraoral periapical film, and supplemental films.

Surveys for adults

Routine. The complete mouth survey is designed to examine completely the teeth and tooth-bearing areas. The number of films included in a survey must be decided by the practitioner; some use as many as 28 or 30 films, whereas others are content with 10 or less. A minimum of 14 and a maximum of 17 periapical films accompanied by a minimum of 2 and maximum of 4 posterior bite-wing films are necessary for adequate interpretation of oral conditions in people with a full or nearly complete complement of teeth. The use of bite-wing films in the anterior segments of the mouth is ordinarily not necessary. The 17-film periapical series is preferred. The taking of duplicate films (this is not to be confused with the use of double-packet films) on a routine basis is not recommended, but supplemental films taken after the original series has been observed may be necessary. Although every effort should be made to minimize the amount of ionizing radiation received by the patient, it is unwise to compromise cost and the small additional amount of patient exposure with incomplete diagnostic information. Bite-wing films are unnecessary if the extended cone–paralleling technic has been used properly. Posterior bite-wing films are essential if the bisecting technic is used and may be helpful if the paralleling technic is employed. Bite-wing films 2.2* are manufactured with tabs; 1.2 films placed in suitable preformed holders are equally satisfactory.

---

*American National Standards Institute numbers for film sizes are used (see p. 24).

The preferred 17-film periapical survey consists of 2 horizontal 1.2 films in each quadrant, demonstrating the molar and bicuspid teeth, plus 5 vertically placed 1.1 films in the maxillary anterior area and 4 vertically placed 1.1 films in the mandibular anterior area. The 17-film periapical survey, accompanied by 4 bite-wing films, is shown in Fig. 10-1. The minimum 14-film periapical series consists of, in each quadrant, a horizontally placed film exposing the molar region, a second film similarly placed exposing the bicuspid area, a vertically placed film showing the cuspid and the distal surface of the lateral tooth, and a single midline film demonstrating the central teeth. All films used are 1.2.

The time interval between complete mouth surveys and between bite-wing examinations must be left to the judgment of the dentist. Ordinarily, a new complete survey is not necessary for a period of at least 5 years unless considerable dental work has been done by another dentist in the intervening period. New bite-wing films are often necessary every 6 months and perhaps even more frequently. Single films of questionable areas are also indicated more often than is the complete survey.

Alternate. There is no real substitute for an optimum quality intraoral survey. However, there are a few situations in which an intraoral survey cannot be obtained on an adult—for instance, patients with trismus or those having an extreme gag reflex that the dentist may not wish to suppress. In such cases, the use of lateral jaw projections posteriorly, occlusal films in the anterior segment of the mouth, and suitable bite-wing films can provide an alternate survey.

The area covered by intraoral films may be insufficient to demonstrate an entire pathologic area. An extraoral projection, particularly the lateral jaw film and the topographic occlusal film, can be used to supplement the findings of the periapical survey. A second directional view of an area may be necessary; in such cases the occlusal film or a regular periapical film may be used to provide a cross-sectional projection.

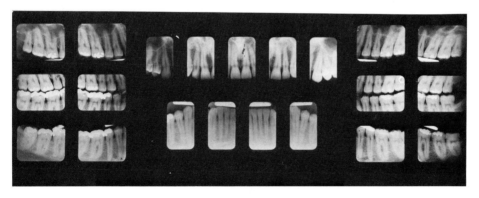

Fig. 10-1. Adult complete mouth periapical survey.

Surveys for children

A complete radiographic survey should be made of a child's mouth on or as soon as possible after his initial visit to the dental office for complete dental care. Although it is ordinarily not necessary to repeat this complete survey more than once every 5 years, growth patterns may make a reduced time interval desirable. In addition to the routine survey, it is recommended that bite-wing films be taken as often as needed. Children whose caries rate is minimum need a bite-wing survey considerably less frequently than do those who develop caries rapidly.

Routine. The number and type of film used in examining children varies according to age, size of the child's mouth, and cooperation of the child. At approximately 10 to 12 years of age, the survey should be basically identical to that of an adult. From age 2 years through approximately 7 years, a survey is recommended that is similar to that of the adult, but 1.1 film is used throughout. The exact number of films used must be left to the practitioner's judgment. A minimum of ten periapical films and two bite-wing films should be used. Additional films are necessary as the child's age increases. The minimum series of ten films plus two bite-wing films is illustrated in Fig. 10-2. The 1.1 film can be tolerated by children of almost any age, provided that they have the desire or can be persuaded to cooperate. Smaller films, such as the 1.0 and 1.00, are not recommended; they are smaller than necessary and do not show a sufficient amount of tooth and bone structure to warrant the expenditure of the necessary x-radiation. Regardless of age, when the child can tolerate 1.2 films, these films should be used in the posterior areas. The 1.1 film in a vertical position is always preferable in the anterior segment. Often only one bite-wing film on each side is needed; whether one or two films are used will depend on the number of posterior teeth present.

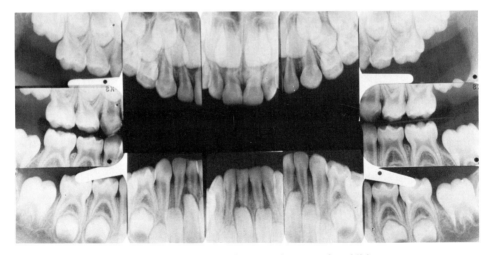

Fig. 10-2. Routine complete mouth survey for children.

Alternate. A quite acceptable alternate for the routine intraoral survey, especially for young and for uncooperative children, is composed of a 5 × 7 lateral jaw film of each side, anterior films of both the mandible and maxilla, and a bite-wing film of the right and left molar regions.

The lateral jaw film, if properly placed and angulated, will demonstrate the region distal to the cuspid tooth; it will show the bone adjacent to the tooth better than will the periapical film, but the interproximal spaces will tend to be overlapped. Bite-wing films are essential if all interproximal caries are to be detected.

The anterior films preferably should be composed of three maxillary and three mandibular projections, using 1.1 film. As an alternate to the use of three films, one occlusal film, 3.4, centered in the midline can be used; in very small mouths a 1.2 film can be substituted for the occlusal film. The occlusal topographic angulation technic is used under these circumstances.

Surveys for edentulous patients

The purpose of surveying the jaws of edentulous people is that of detecting residual infection, foreign bodies, and osseous alterations that might detract from the patient's health and interfere with or contraindicate artificial dentures. Bite-wing films are not used, and ordinarily the bisecting technic is preferred to the paralleling procedure. Film placement in these patients is easier when the bisecting technic is used. The patient's fingers rather than a film holder can be used to support the film. The need for accurate anatomic reproduction is usually less in edentulous patients.

Routine. A 14-film survey (Fig. 10-3) with 1.2 film is recommended; molar and bicuspid films are placed horizontally; the three anterior films in the mandible and maxilla are positioned vertically. When films are placed, care must be taken to have the areas of film coverage overlap. It is more difficult in the edentulous film series to be certain that all areas have been covered than it is in a film series when teeth are present. Care also must be used to place the molar films sufficiently far distally; the maxillary molar film should show the entire tuberosity, and the mandibular molar films should demonstrate the areas slightly distal to the anterior border of the ramus. Reexamination of edentulous areas ordinarily is done less frequently than when teeth are present. The time interval between examinations must be left to the dentist's judgment.

Alternate. Lateral jaw films of each side, plus topographic occlusal films of the anterior mandible and maxilla are useful as alternates to the 14-film series. The lateral jaw film can demonstrate the maxillary and mandibular regions posterior to and often including the cuspid area. One properly placed and angulated occlusal film in the mandible and two in the maxilla will show the entire anterior segment. This alternative is illustrated in Fig. 10-4. If only one occlusal film is used, it is advisable to have the greatest film dimension extend between the corners of the mouth whenever possible. Regular 1.2 films, preferably three for each jaw, can be used instead of the occlusal film.

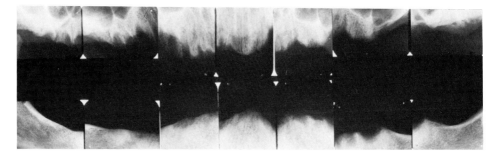

Fig. 10-3. Fourteen-film edentulous radiographic survey.

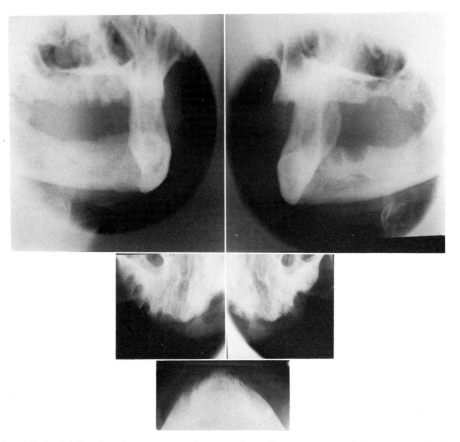

Fig. 10-4. Adult edentulous survey using two lateral jaw views and three occlusal films.

Panoramic radiography

Technics designed to show a continuous view of one or both arches from third molar to third molar have been used with varying degrees of success. The source of radiation has been placed both intraorally and extraorally; thus far, the most usable radiographs have been obtained when the radiation source rotated around the outside of the face.

A panoramic view of the maxilla and mandible can be very useful as a routine scanning procedure. It can be done quickly, but it cannot, thus far, provide the detailed information available from conventional intraoral and extraoral films. Conventional films must be used in a supplementary fashion in order to observe more critically entities uncovered by the panoramic survey.

Panoramic surveys are especially useful in research activities designed to show the presence or absence of teeth, foreign bodies, large areas of osseous change, and so forth. They could be of value to the general practitioner or oral surgeon who has a large emergency service clientele; such people often resist the intraoral survey but might be more willing to accept less time-consuming panoramic surveys. Panoramic radiography is discussed in detail in Chapter 8.

Alternate uses of intraoral periapical film

Intraoral films, particularly the 1.2 film, can be used in other than the conventional manner. Some of these procedures are mentioned earlier in this chapter but are repeated briefly here.

The intraoral film can be used instead of the occlusal film (3.4) to obtain both topographic and cross-sectional views. Naturally, the smaller film will not demonstrate as large an anatomic area, but such a film is easier to place than is the occlusal film; the technic of film placement and angulation is identical. This projection is useful in very young children.

The 1.2 film can also be appropriately bent and used in small mouths as a reduced dimension periapical film or as a bite-wing film. The film, used with the long dimension in a vertical position and with approximately ⅜ inch of the occlusal portion of the film bent at right angles to the remaining film plane, can be used to examine single teeth. The bent portion of the film is held between the teeth like a bite-wing tab. This technic is useful in some gagging patients and in patients who cannot hold the film steady by conventional means. The bite-wing procedure is particularly useful when there are no teeth in the opposing arch; the bent portion of the film rests on the occlusal surfaces and is held by the patient's thumb or index finger, and the remainder of the film is parallel with the long axis of the tooth.

Supplemental films

Additional intraoral or extraoral views of an area are often necessary to confirm or negate a finding. Retakes because of improper or careless technics are generally inexcusable and are not in the category of supplemental films. Supplemental films taken for localization purposes are discussed separately.

Supplemental films taken as part of the original survey because they may prove useful are generally not justified in view of the efforts being made to minimize patient exposure. The number of supplemental films to be taken must be left to the judgment of the operator; circumstances continually alter the situation.

SURVEYS OF THE FACE AND SKULL

Films of extraoral structures are sometimes taken as a routine scanning procedure. For example, when Paget's disease is suspected, skull views are taken. More often in dentistry, extraoral films are exposed with specific purposes in mind. The specific purpose survey must be carried far enough; a sufficient number of different views must be taken to provide complete visualization of a part or area. In Table 10-1 are presented specific purpose extraoral surveys common to dentistry and the films useful for carrying out such surveys. The technical factors are discussed in earlier chapters. Particularly in the case of the temporomandibular joint, functional studies may necessitate several exposures with the same projection. No attempt has been made to tabulate surveys for localization purposes. The surveys included in the table are limited to facial areas.

LOCALIZATION PROCEDURES

The radiograph presents a two-dimensional image of a three-dimensional object. There is often a need for determining spatial relationships. Technics for doing this are discussed as follows: (1) right-angle procedures, (2) tube shift technic, (3) stereoradiography, and (4) use of radiopaque media.

Right-angle procedures

The right-angle localization procedure involves the use of at least two films taken at right angles to each other. For example, a lateral skull projection demonstrates the anteroposterior and superoinferior positions of an object within the skull. In order to locate the object, a view must be taken to show the mediolateral position of the object. Such a projection must be taken at right angles to the first film; in this instance a posteroanterior or superoinferior view of the skull is needed. Sometimes a second projection at right angles to the first projection is difficult or impossible, and oblique projections are used. In such cases more than two projections are usually necessary. This principle applied to intraoral films is shown in Fig. 10-5.

Tube shift technic

The tube shift technic employs the concepts expressed by the so-called Clark's rule. There appears to be no specifically worded Clark's rule. Rather, the concepts of a technic are expressed in an article by Clark.* Bosworth† has

---

*Clark, C. A.: Method of ascertaining the relative position of unerupted teeth by means of film radiographs, Proc. Roy. Soc. Med. (odont. sec.) 3:87, 1909-1910.
†Bosworth, L. L.: Multiple sectional x-ray exposures on the same film, Dent. Cosmos. 76:589, 1934.

Table 10-1. Projections

Specific purpose extraoral survey	Lateral jaw positioned for specific region of mandible or maxilla	Postero-anterior mandible	Lateral skull	Postero-anterior maxillary sinus	Postero-anterior frontal sinus	Lateral sinuses	Temporo-mandibular joint, trans-cranial lateral oblique	Temporo-mandibular joint, lateral through coronoid notch	Bregma-mentum	Submento-vertex
Mandibular body	x	x							x	x
Mandibular ramus	x	x						x		
Mandibular coronoid process	x	x		x				x	x	
Mandibular condylar neck	x	x						x	x	
Mandibular condylar head	x	x					x	x	x	
Maxilla, anterior	x	x		x		x			x	
Maxilla, posterior	x	x				x			x	
Malar bone and orbit		x		x		x			x	
Zygomatic arch	x					x*			x	x
Nasal bones		x		x	x				x	
Temporomandibular joint		x					x	x	x	
Maxillary sinus				x		x				
Frontal sinus					x	x				
Ethmoid sinus				x	x	x				
Sphenoid sinus				x		x				
Soft tissues of neck	x*	x*	x*							
Salivary glands (sialography)	x	x	x							

*Minimum exposure necessary.

added to this concept. This technic is most useful in edentulous mouths for locating small root tips, especially in the maxilla, where an occlusal cross-sectional view taken through the top of the head tends to cause a small object to be obscured by the superimposed structures. After the area in question is anesthetized, a small hypodermic needle is inserted in a vertical position into the mucobuccal fold over the area of the suspected root tip. Periapical technics are used, and the x-rays are directed as nearly at right angles as possible to the plane of the bone surface. The hypodermic needle is retained in position while the film is being processed. The needle should be superimposed directly over the area in question. If it is determined from the radiograph not to be properly placed, the needle is moved so that it is superimposed over the area. It is sometimes desirable to insert a second needle into the lingual or palatal tissues in the same relative position as the buccal needle. Either the shape of the needle hub or the thickness of the second needle should make it distinctive from the first needle.

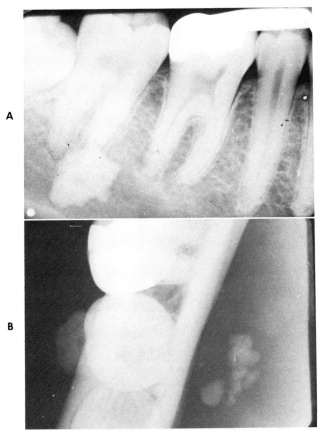

Fig. 10-5. Right-angle projection, **B,** of a typical periapical film, **A,** shows an apparent intraosseous opacity to be located in the soft tissues.

At this time two additional intraoral films are made with the horizontal angle changed (1) so that the rays pass anteroposteriorly and (2) so that the rays pass posteroanteriorly through the area in question. When the two oblique views are used, one can now determine whether the object is more bucally or more lingually (or palatally) placed. If the area in question continues to be close to or superimposed on the buccal needle, the lesion must be buccally positioned. If the distance between the object and the two needles is equal, the lesion is halfway between the two needles. If the area appears widely separated from the buccal needle and hence quite close to the lingual needle, it can be concluded that the object is more lingual or palatal than it is buccal or labial. These observations are based on the fact that two entities in contact cannot have their shadows separated.

When the object in question is close to a tooth or some structure of known position, for example, the metal framework of a partial denture, there is no need

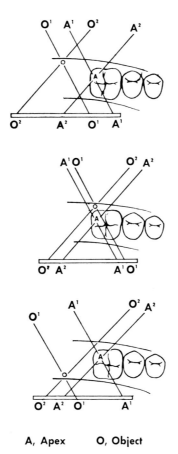

A, Apex   O, Object

Fig. 10-6. Tube shift technic. Object is envisioned in various relationships to the apex of the molar tooth root.

for inserting buccal or lingual needles. In this instance, the shift method will locate the position of the unknown object relative to the position of the known object. For example, a foreign body distal and lingual to a first molar root apex will be superimposed on the apex when the x-rays are directed in an anteroposterior direction and will be separated from the apex when the rays are directed in a posteroanterior direction. Several positions of a foreign object are diagrammatically shown in Fig. 10-6.

Stereoradiography

Stereoradiography is not a widely used technic, principally because it is time consuming. It does, however, have certain advantages and is worth discussing briefly. It is important to point out that films taken with a stereoradiographic technic ordinarily require a special viewing device. However, the operator can train himself to examine films without such a device.

Stereoradiographic films are taken in the following manner. A small paper envelope is made so that an intraoral periapical film can be inserted and easily removed. The film *in its envelope* is placed in the mouth in the proper position, and by the use of wax or some similar material, is held in position; the wax is applied against the envelope and the lingual or palatal surfaces of the adjacent teeth. The wax must not impinge on the film itself; the film must be removable from the envelope. An exposure is now made using a horizontal angulation that is 10° to one side or the other of a true perpendicular projection. The film is removed, and a second film is placed; the second exposure is made using the same vertical angulation but a horizontal angulation that is 10° to the other side of the perpendicular. The two films are processed in the darkroom simultaneously in order that the film density may be identical. These films, properly viewed, will give depth perception and will assist the operator in making a judgment.

Use of radiopaque media

Radiopaque media, such as barium sulfate, Lipiodol, and Dionosil, can be used to demarcate cavernous areas within hard and soft structures (Fig. 7-16). Such materials are also used occasionally to outline soft tissue peripheries such as the profile of the face and neck. The placement of a radiopaque medium is followed by the exposure of radiographic film using a selected specific purpose projection. The use of radiopaque media is discussed in Chapter 7 as a special purpose survey; however, contrast media also can be considered a localizing procedure.

CHAPTER 11

Viewing the radiographic image

In order for films to be properly interpreted, the clinician must have an understanding of the normal radiographic appearance of anatomic structures and must be familiar with the changes that can take place as a result of various types of pathologic disorders. To recognize the normal and abnormal, the dentist must also be familiar with factors and procedures specifically related to film viewing. Without such knowledge, radiographic information could be misleading.

The radiographic film is a single plane representation of a three-dimensional object; thus superimposition exists. Because the x-rays are diverging, magnification and distortion also occur. In addition, certain optical illusions are invariably present. Viewing equipment plays a significant role in the operator's ability to evaluate radiographic results accurately. Of extreme importance are the viewing technics used to extract information from the radiographic films. These considerations are stressed in this chapter. Practical use of these and other factors is further demonstrated in Chapter 15.

IMAGE QUALITY AND PROJECTIVE GEOMETRY

The diagnostic value of a film is related to four film qualities. These qualities are discussed earlier in this text, but a brief review is in order. To be useful, a film must be of the proper density, have a satisfactory degree of contrast, possess good definition, and show minimum distortion of the object. The last quality can be subdivided into magnification and changes in shape. Factors relating to density and contrast are not discussed further in this chapter except as they relate directly to definition and distortion.

As mentioned previously, the resultant radiographic image is similar to shadow casting when a light source is used. Utopia in shadow casting consists of reproducing the object's anatomy on the film in its exact dimensions. Physical circumstances prevent such accuracy. The radiation source is not a point; rather, it is an area of approximately 1 sq. mm. The target-object distance is less than infinite, and the object-film distance is not minimally small. In addition, parallelism between object and film, and a concurrent perpendicular relationship of the x-ray beam to both film and object are not usually possible. The three-dimensional quality of the object would prevent obtaining utopian results even if it were possible to observe fully the basic rules for accurate shadow casting.

The sources of image unsharpness, distortion, and magnification are discussed in Chapters 2 and 3. These image qualities are increased or decreased, depending on the radiographic technic used.

Some aspects of magnification and distortion as related to the radiography of teeth are shown in Figs. 11-1 and 11-2. The diagrams illustrate intraoral structures, but the same principles relate to all radiographic technics.

The x-ray beam direction and the shape of the object greatly affect the film density of various parts of the image, even though the object's mass may be of uniform density. The effect of object shape and ray direction on film density is demonstrated in Fig. 11-3.

These considerations are extremely important from an interpretive standpoint. The periodontal bone level, for example, can look quite different in films of the same area; its appearance depends on whether the rays have gone from buccal to lingual along the crest of the bone or whether the rays have angulated diagonally across the crest of the bone. Two films of the same individual taken within seconds of one another can create delusions and result in diagnostic errors. Facts such as these are covered in Chapter 15, in which radiographic interpretation of common diseases of the teeth and supporting structures are discussed.

OPTICAL ILLUSIONS

The radiologist reads radiographs with his eyes. These visual organs are not infallible, and the viewer must be aware of visual phenomena that can introduce errors in the reading of radiographs. One such phenomena is the *Mach band* effect. When many uniform areas of different density levels are viewed all at the same time, each area no longer seems to be of uniform density. Any area of uniform density appears to the eye to be slightly lighter toward an adjacent area of darker density and slightly darker toward an area of lighter density. This effect is seen if one looks critically at the image of a step wedge (Fig. 1-15). The density of each step is uniform but does not appear to be so when all the steps of the wedge are viewed at the same time.

Visual contrast effects appear mainly where there is a rather well-defined area of very low density in a radiograph, in other words, where there is a bright spot in the radiograph. Such bright spots appear to have rather dark borders around them. This optical illusion is seen most often in dental radiographs where the images of the enamel of two teeth overlap each other. This condition is shown in Fig. 11-4; it is similar to but not identical with the Mach band effect.

Contrast and Mach band effects tend to produce illusions of dark lines where osseous structures overlap. The viewer must be very careful in evaluating such lines, since they can be misinterpreted as sutures, fractures, or even early caries

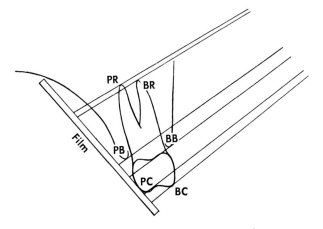

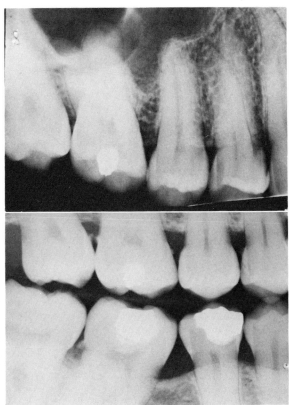

Fig. 11-1. Anatomic inaccuracies inherent in the bisecting technic. The position on the film of the palatal cusp, PC, palatal root apex, PR, and palatal bone crest, PB, vary from the position of the buccal cusp, BC, buccal root, BR, and buccal bone crest, BB, even though the corresponding entities are at the same anatomic level. The radiographs show a periapical film and a bite-wing projection of the same region. Note how angulation in the periapical film has caused the buccal cusps to be longer than the palatal cusps, and observe particularly how the buccal interproximal bone has been cast onto the tooth crown. The parallelism of the tooth and film and the right angle relationship of the beam to both tooth and film in the bite-wing projection give an accurate relationship of anatomic entities.

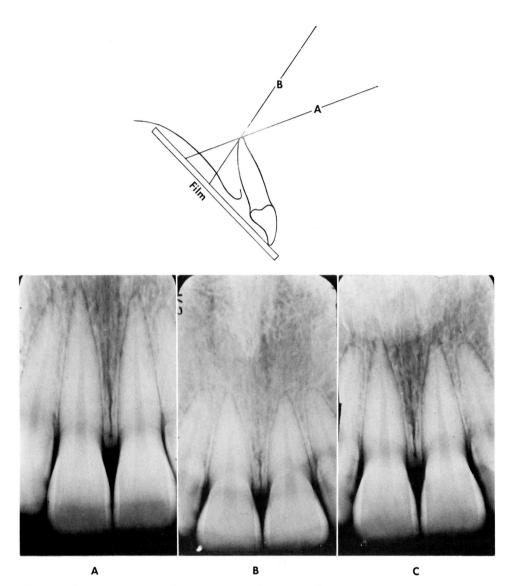

Fig. 11-2. Elongation and foreshortening. Elongation of the tooth occurs when the rays do not have enough vertical angulation, as demonstrated by line *A* and radiograph **A.** Foreshortening of the tooth occurs when the rays are overangulated, as demonstrated by line *B* and radiograph **B.** Radiograph **C** demonstrates proper tooth length.

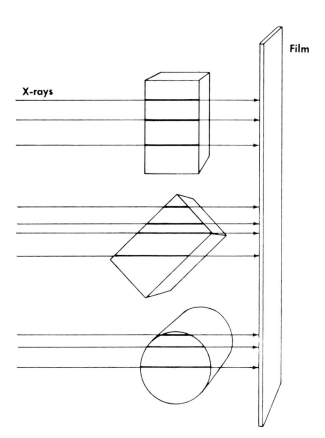

Fig. 11-3. Diagram illustrating the effect of object shape and ray direction on the amount of absorbing material in the path of the x-ray beam. The block (top) absorbs equal amounts of radiation; the same block when tipped (center) absorbs varying amounts of radiation in different parts. The cylinder (bottom), because of its shape, absorbs various amounts of radiation.

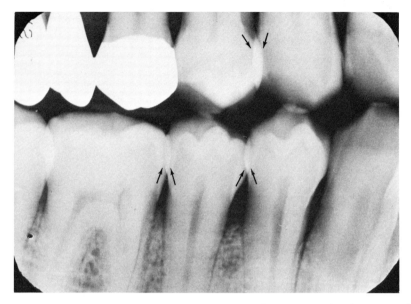

Fig. 11-4. Radiograph shows overlapping of second bicuspids and adjacent teeth. The overlapped area appears to be surrounded by a dark band. This is an optical illusion; the area of apparent increased density is not measurable.

on interproximal tooth surfaces in the area where supportive bone is superimposed radiographically on enamel.

VIEWING EQUIPMENT AND MOUNTS

Viewing equipment in dental offices varies from the use of sunlight coming through the window to rather elaborate equipment designed to produce maximum intensity light that can be restricted in intensity as well as in surface area. The average dental office is equipped with some type of viewer for intraoral dental films, but little attention has been given to such matters by either the profession or the manufacturers. The quality of viewing equipment can make a considerable difference in the interpretative results obtained.

Radiographs are viewed with transillumination. The human eye sees slight differences in film density much better when the background or surrounding illumination is minimal. Radiographs should be viewed in a darkened room or darkened area of a room whenever possible. The human eye detects differences in illumination in relation to the overall background illumination. In order for a density difference between two areas of a radiograph to be detected, the difference in light intensity coming from the two areas must be at least 1% of the amount of background or overall illumination. This visual phenomenon is sometimes referred to as Webber's law and produces a situation where areas of low density in radiographs need to be examined with low-intensity illumination if the eye is to perceive slight differences in the radiographic images. If the same radiograph is brightly illuminated, the background illumination may be so great that a relatively large film density difference is needed before the observer's eye can detect any difference between two areas in the radiograph; therefore, slight density differences will not be visible under the bright illumination condition. The radiologist must also be aware of the limitations of his own visual capacity.

When there is a large area of very low density in a radiograph or when the radiograph does not fully cover the illuminator or view box, the light areas in or around the radiograph should be covered or masked before the darker areas are read. If this is not done, glare is created by the light areas. Such glare prevents the viewer from optically seeing the structures shown in the dark areas.

Masking of complete mouth radiographs is best done by using a film mount that covers the entire illuminator. The film mount should be made of a material that will not allow the transmission of light and will not permit reflection of room light to any appreciable degree. Fig. 11-5, *C*, demonstrates the masking of a small radiograph.

Masking for the examination of small radiographs or small areas on large radiographs can also be accomplished by allowing the eyes to see only the desired area. This can be done through the use of an eye mask, as shown in Fig. 11-5, *D*.

Eye masks can be made of different materials and can have other viewing accessories built in. One commercially available mask is made of plastic and has a magnifying lens built in (Fig. 11-5, *E*). Another mask has a magnifying lens plus an iris diaphragm that adjusts the visual field to the area of the radiograph under examination.

View boxes for extraoral films ordinarily should be larger than those used for intraoral films. An illuminator 10 × 12 inches or larger is useful in the dental office. Several black cardboard masks having cutout areas the size of the extraoral films used in the dental office should be available for the purpose of eliminating peripheral light.

The dental view box or illuminator should give a diffuse light of uniform intensity, and there should be some means of varying the viewing area and light intensity (Fig. 11-6). Many view boxes, although they provide for the diffusion of light, do not give the same light intensity over the entire useful viewing area and/or do not provide a mechanism for changing the level of illumination. Radiographs cannot always be made of identical average density. Radiographs of low density need less viewing light during the reading process, whereas radiographs of high density need more light. It is for this reason that dental view boxes should provide a range of illumination levels. A high-intensity illuminator is especially useful in viewing *very* dark areas on large films or small films that were inadvertently or intentionally overexposed.

The color of light used in view boxes is of interest. Although most colors are satisfactory, red apparently is not suitable for the viewing of radiographs. Red

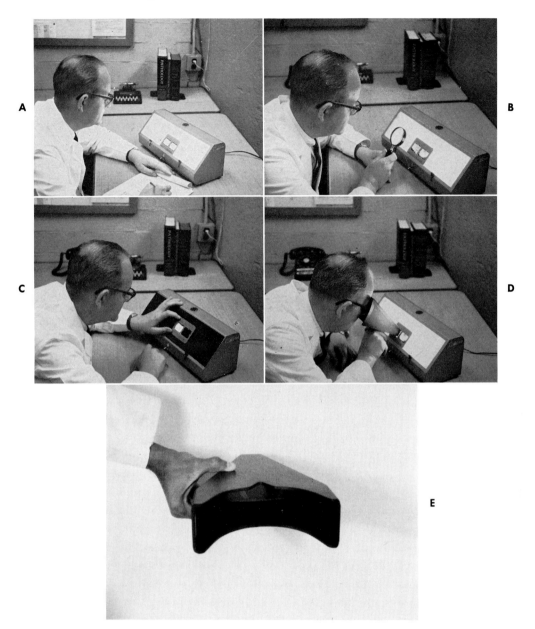

Fig. 11-5. Dental radiograms are usually viewed in a lighted room. **A,** Frequently single films are observed without extraneous peripheral light being eliminated. **B,** Use of a magnifying glass is almost a necessity if films are to be interpreted accurately. **C,** However, a magnifying glass does not eliminate the need for masking all light other than that being transmitted through the radiogram. Optimally, all room lighting should be turned off to eliminate light reflection from the film surface and to permit accommodation for illuminator light only. **D,** Masking of the film and elimination of room lighting can be accomplished by use of an eye mask. **E,** Opaque plastic eye mask designed for dental radiography and incorporating a magnifying lens. (**E,** Courtesy X-Produkter Johansson Och Co., Malmö, Sweden.)

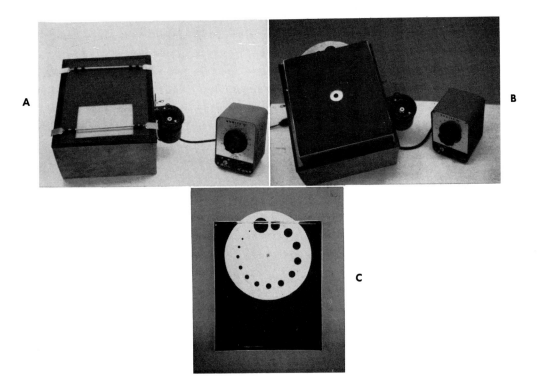

Fig. 11-6. Illuminator with a variable light intensity and viewing area. **A,** View box with five photoflood bulbs for illumination, a fan for eliminating heat, and a control for varying light intensity. The viewing surface is masked for a 5 × 7 film exposed in a horizontal position. Other masks for viewing 5 × 7, 8 × 10, and properly mounted complete mouth intraoral radiograms also are available. **B,** Mechanism for further restricting the viewing area. A box completely covers the illuminator surface. In the center of the superimposed box is a hole that permits a maximum viewing diameter of 2 inches. The viewing area may be reduced from a diameter of 2 inches to ¼ inch by turning the disk at the top of the box. (Note: The illuminator was not on when the photograph was made, and hence the viewing area appears black, whereas the 2-inch diameter hole appears light.) **C,** Underside of the box shown in **B.** The disk with various aperatures revolves so that each hole is centered on the 2-inch opening in **B.**

is unsuitable because the eyes cannot distinguish detail or fine structures as well as when light of another color is used. The use of a magnifying lens is of value in the observation of fine detail and should be included in the viewing equipment.

VIEWING TECHNICS

There is no infallible manner of viewing radiographs so that the reader becomes mentally aware of all that the radiographic image shows. Many factors affect the clinician's ability to extract information from the radiograph. One such group of factors involves viewing technics.

The way in which a person scans a radiograph with his eyes is important. The viewer should not allow his attention to skip from area to area but should scan the radiograph in a systematic manner in order not to miss or overlook any area. Likewise, the observer should, whenever possible, scan the radiograph or group of radiographs for one type of change at a time. In other words, he should scan a complete mouth series of radiographs for carious lesions, then for periodontal changes, then for apical disease, and so forth. There is some evidence in the field of psychologic optics that scanning is best performed by a horizontal movement over the visual field. This suggests that a complete mouth radiographic survey may be more efficiently scanned when mounted in a manner that facilitates the horizontal movement of the eyes. For circular objects (the entire skull, maxillary sinus, large cysts, and so forth), it appears that clockwise scanning is less tiring and less annoying than other methods.

The distance at which radiographs are viewed is important. In order to see a lesion radiographically, the diagnostician must view an area larger than the lesion. In other words, the field of vision must encompass the lesion. It is impossible not to view the surrounding area when very small lesions are observed. The observer will generally use a short viewing distance and may even magnify the image. For a large lesion, the opposite is true. The observer should either stand away from the radiograph or train himself to expand his field of vision while standing close to the film. This is very important when large lesions that show only slight film density changes from their surrounding areas are examined. Demagnification is sometimes employed when extra-large medical films are used.

Optimally, radiographs should be viewed in a darkened room and in the absence of distraction. Under such conditions the examiner must allow his eyes to become adapted to the lower level of illumination before beginning to read the radiographs. Radiographic data should be combined later with clinical findings, at which time questionable radiographic shadows can be verified or negated. It is quite common for the clinician to view films concurrently with the clinical examination; this is done for practical reasons.

When radiographs are being read in conjunction with the clinical examination of the patient, the diagnostician must minimize the number of movements of his eyes from the patient to the x-ray view box. The reason is that the patient's oral cavity is usually under a high degree of illumination, and the observer's eyes are accommodated to this high intensity of light. Since radiographs show lower levels of illumination, time must be allowed for visual adaptation when the diagnostician looks away from the patient and views the radiograph. Failure to allow for visual adaptation results in the observer's being unable to see all the changes shown in the radiograph.

CHAPTER 12

Skull osteology

If one is to utilize effectively the technical information given in the preceding chapters concerned with extraoral technics, and if one is to interpret accurately the normal anatomic landmarks as well as the pathologic changes found on extraoral films, one must be familiar with the bone formations found in the skull and facial skeleton. This same philosophy applies to the interpretation of changes that may be found on the intraoral film. It is impossible in a text of this nature to consider the osteology of the skull completely; space does not allow extensive discussion. For this reason, illustrations designed to point out anatomic entities are used in this chapter. Descriptions are limited to what can be observed on Figs. 12-1 to 12-7. No effort is made to describe anatomic detail, nor is any effort made to relate function to bone structure. We hope that the illustrations together with the associated descriptions will enable the reader to apply this review of skull osteology to the findings that he observes on the radiographic film. Comments relate to the adult skull; growth patterns are discussed in Chapter 14. We encourage the use of a good quality dry skull for assistance in identifying the various landmarks and interpreting radiographic findings. It is expected that this chapter will be used in close association with Chapter 13, which is designed to acquaint the reader with normal intraoral and extraoral radiographic anatomy. The italicized titles of illustrations in this chapter correspond with specific radiographic landmarks mentioned in Chapter 13.

(Figs. 12-1 to 12-7 follow.)

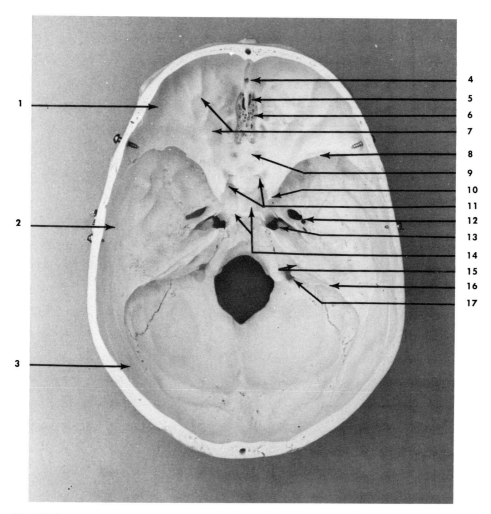

Fig. 12-1. Superior view of the skull base.

1. Anterior cranial fossa
2. Middle cranial fossa
3. Posterior cranial fossa
4. Foramen caecum
5. Crista galli
6. Cribriform plate of the ethmoid bone
7. Floor of the anterior cranial fossa lateral to the midline and roof of the orbit
8. Lesser wing of the sphenoid bone
9. Floor of the anterior cranial fossa in the midline
10. Anterior clinoid process (The foramen rotundum and the superior orbital fissure are hidden under the process and under the beginning of the lesser wing of the sphenoid.)
11. Optic foramen (right arrow) and carotid groove (left arrow)
12. Foramen ovale (medial and anterior) and foramen spinosum (lateral and distal); on the left side, the two openings have joined
13. Foramen lacerum
14. Sella turcica or hypophyseal fossa (right arrow) and posterior clinoid process (left arrow)
15. Internal auditory (acoustic) meatus
16. Crest of the petrous portion of the temporal bone
17. Jugular foramen

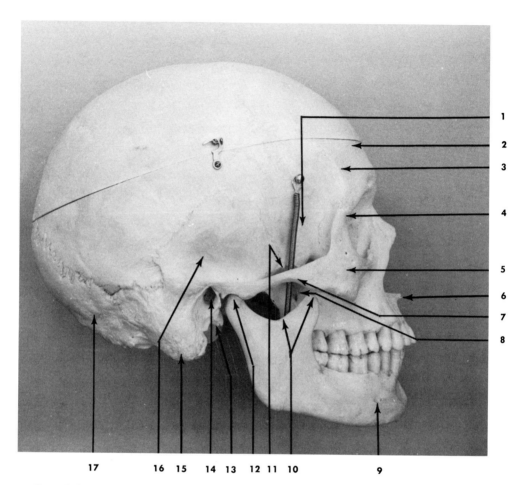

Fig. 12-2. Lateral view of the skull.

1. Sphenoid bone (temporal surface of the greater wing)
2. Frontal bone
3. Anterior border of the temporal fossa
4. Lateral border of the orbit (zygomatic bone)
5. Zygomatic or malar bone
6. Anterior nasal spine
7. Zygomatic process (arch) of the temporal bone
8. Pterygomaxillary fissure
9. Mental foramen

10. Sigmoid or mandibular notch (left) and coronoid process (right) of the mandible
11. Infratemporal crest of the sphenoid bone
12. Mandibular condyle
13. Area of the styloid process (The process in this skull is diminutive and not visible in this photograph.)
14. External auditory (acoustic) meatus
15. Mastoid process of the temporal bone
16. Squamous portion of the temporal bone
17. Occipital bone

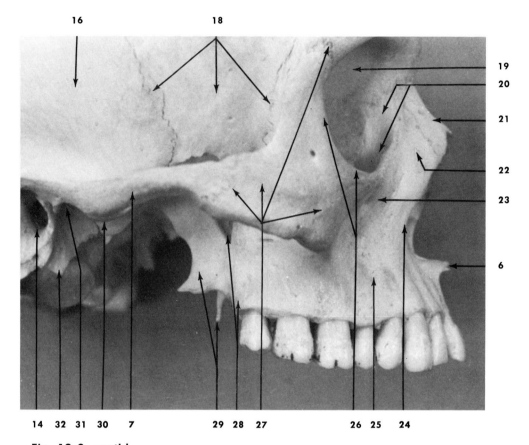

Fig. 12-2, cont'd

18. Temporal surface of the sphenoid bone, the sphenotemporal suture, and the sphenozygomatic suture
19. Ethmoid bone (medial surface of the orbit)
20. Lacrimal bone and lacrimal gland sulcus
21. *Nasal bone*
22. Nasal process of the maxilla
23. *Infraorbital foramen*
24. Lateral border of the nose
25. Maxilla
26. *Lateral* (left) and *inferior* (right) *borders of the orbit*

27. Zygomatic bone and the zygomaticotemporal, zygomaticofrontal, and zygomaticomaxillary sutures
28. Maxillary tuberosity (below) and the pterygomaxillary fissure (above); the largest portion of the fissure is hidden by the zygomatic bone
29. *Lateral pterygoid plate* (left) *and the hamular process of the medial pterygoid plate* (below)
30. *Articular eminence*
31. *Articular fossa*
32. Vaginal process of the temporal bone

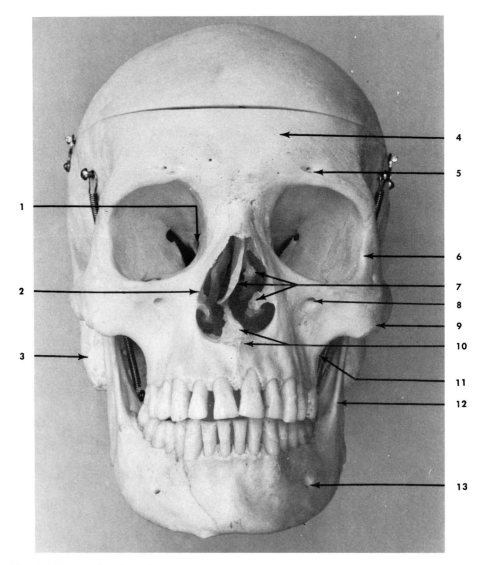

Fig. 12-3. Anterior view of the skull.

1. Optic foramen
2. *Lateral wall of the nose*
3. *Mastoid process of the temporal bone*
4. Frontal bone
5. *Supraorbital foramen* (This is frequently just a notch in the superior border of the orbit.)
6. *Outer or lateral border of the orbit (zygomatic bone)*
7. Nasal septum, middle, and inferior concha
8. *Infraorbital foramen*
9. *Junction of the maxillary and zygomatic (malar) bones*
10. Nasal crest (above) and anterior nasal spine (below)
11. A ridge, sometimes called the jugal ridge, extending upward from the first molar tooth
12. *External oblique line*
13. *Mental foramen*

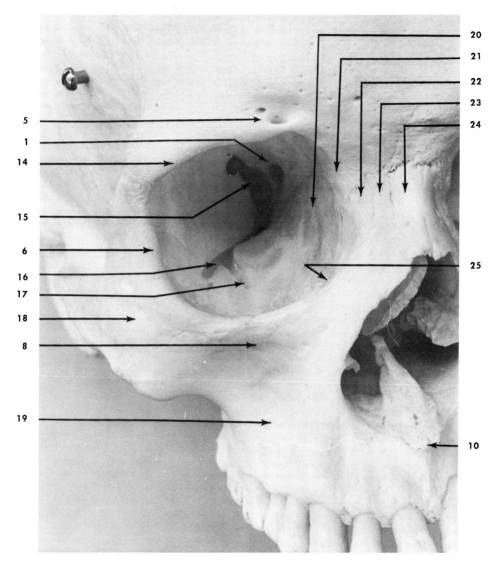

Fig. 12-3, cont'd

14. *Superior border of the orbit (frontal bone)*
15. *Superior orbital fissure*
16. *Inferior orbital fissure*
17. *Infraorbital groove (connecting anteriorly with the infraorbital canal and foramen)*
18. *Zygomatic or malar bone*
19. *Maxilla*
20. *Ethmoid bone*

21. *Medial border of the orbit (Note: The fragility of the bones comprising the medial border (nos. 20, 22, and 23) explains its lack of radiographic opacity, that is, as compared with the other borders.)*
22. *Lacrimal bone*
23. *Frontal process of the maxilla*
24. *Nasal bone*
25. *Lacrimal gland fossa and foramen for lacrimal duct*

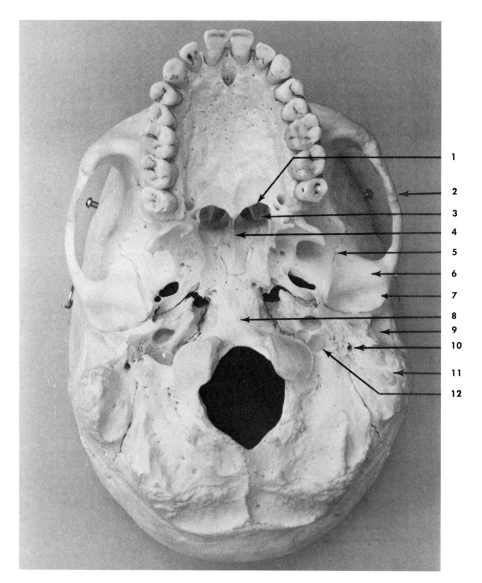

Fig. 12-4. Basilar view of the skull.

1. Posterior border of the hard palate
2. *Zygomatic process (arch) of the temporal bone*
3. Distal aspect of the middle concha (The distal portion of the inferior concha also shows in the enlargement at the right.)
4. *Vomer*
5. Suture between the sphenoid and temporal bones
6. *Articular eminence or tubercle*
7. *Articular or mandibular fossa*
8. *Basilar part of the occipital bone*
9. External auditory (acoustic) meatus
10. Stylomastoid foramen
11. Mastoid process of the temporal bone
12. Jugular fossa
13. Incisive foramen (often divided into the foramina of Scarpa and foramina of Stensen)
14. Median suture (The suture is closed in this photograph, but it frequently appears as a narrow slit.)
15. Approximate junction of the zygomatic (malar) and maxillary bones to form the anterior aspect of the zygomatic arch

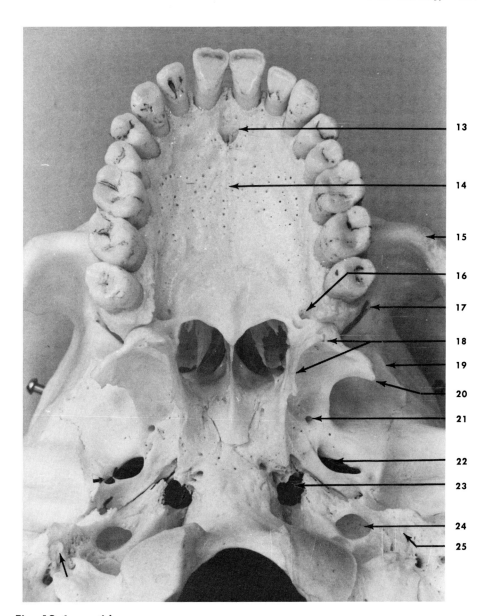

Fig. 12-4, cont'd

16. Greater and lesser palatine foramina
17. *Inferior orbital fissure* (The pterygomaxillary fissure connects with this fissure just behind the lateral pterygoid plate.)
18. *Hamular process* (above) and the *medial pterygoid plate* (below) of the sphenoid bone
19. *Infratemporal crest of the sphenoid bone*
20. *Lateral pterygoid plate of the sphenoid bone*
21. Pterygoid canal with the pterygoid fossa anteriorly between the medial and lateral pterygoid plates

22. *Foramen ovale joined with the foramen spinosum* (The identical area on the opposite side shows a separation of the foramina; the arrow points to the foramen spinosum.)
23. *Foramen lacerum*
24. Carotid canal
25. Area of the styloid process (The process in this skull is diminutive and not easily visible; the arrow on the left side points to the styloid process.)

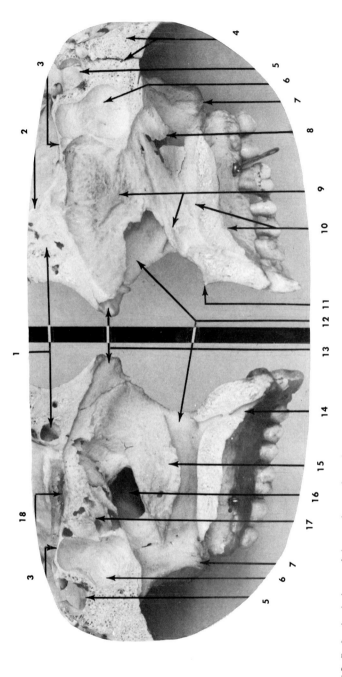

Fig. 12-5. Sagittal views of the oral, nasal, and paranasal areas.

1. Midline union between the frontal sinus on the right and left sides
2. Crista galli
3. Floor of the anterior cranial fossa in the midline
4. Body of the sphenoid bone (The arrow to the left points to a fracture line that coincidentally is in the approximate area of junction between the sphenoid and occipital bones.)
5. Sella turcica or hypophyseal fossa

6. Sphenoid sinus
7. Medial pterygoid plate with the lateral pterygoid plate just behind and slightly distal
8. The vomer (partially shattered in sectioning)
9. Nasal septum
10. Floor of the nose (above) and roof of the palate (below)
11. Anterior nasal spine
12. Lateral wall of the nose

13. Nasal bones
14. Incisive foramen and incisive canal
15. Inferior concha (Note: The middle concha was lost in sectioning; the superior concha partially remains in association with the ethmoid air cells.)
16. Orifice of the maxillary sinus; such orifices vary in size and number
17. Ethmoid sinus (posterior)
18. Cribriform plate of the ethmoid

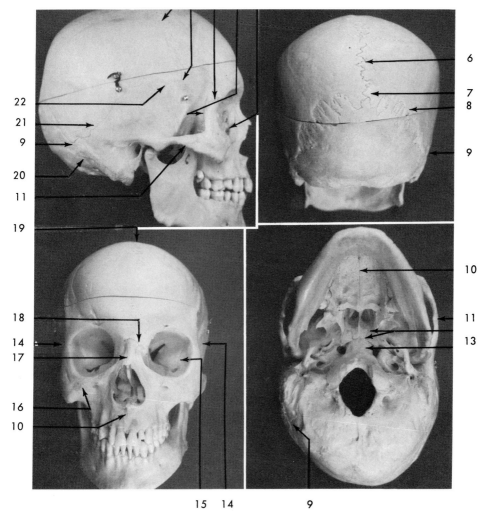

Fig. 12-6. Sutures of the skull. Many sutures are illustrated; some are difficult to see clearly because of suture closure in the adult skull.

1. Coronal suture
2. Junction of the coronal, sphenoparietal, and sphenofrontal sutures
3. Zygomaticofrontal suture
4. Sphenozygomatic suture (located just behind the posterior aspect of the zygomatic bone)
5. Lacrimomaxillary suture—the opening below the arrow tip is the lacrimal fossa plus some destruction of the fine lacrimal bone lamina
6. Sagittal suture
7. Lambda, the junction of the lambdoidal and sagittal sutures and the location of the occipital fontanel in the newborn
8. Lambdoidal suture
9. Junction of the lambdoidal, squamosal, and occipitomastoid sutures
10. Median palatine suture
11. Zygomaticotemporal suture
12. Junction of the vomer with the inferior surface of the sphenoid bone

13. Region of the spheno-occipital suture or synchondrosis—fusion of the sphenoid and occipital bones takes place between 18 and 25 years of age
14. Zygomaticofrontal suture
15. Sphenozygomatic suture
16. Zygomaticomaxillary suture
17. Internasal suture
18. Junction of the frontonasal, frontomaxillary, and nasomaxillary sutures
19. Bregma, the junction of the coronal and sagittal sutures and the location of the frontal fontanel in the newborn (*Note:* The suture-like markings below and anterior to the arrow tip are not suture lines.)
20. Occipitomastoid suture
21. Squamosal suture
22. Junction of the squamosal, sphenoparietal, and coronal sutures

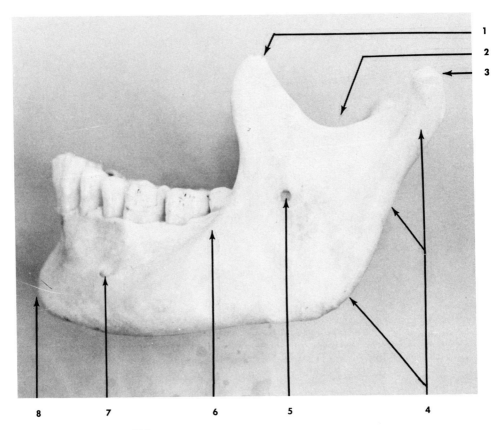

Fig. 12-7. The mandible.

1. Coronoid process
2. Sigmoid or mandibular notch
3. Condyle
4. Condylar neck, posterior border of the ramus, and angle of the mandible (in descending order)
5. Artifact in the ramus (hole drilled in the bone)
6. External oblique line or ridge
7. Mental foramen
8. Mentum
9. Mandibular foramen (left) and lingula (right)
10. Midline—genial tubercles are visible throughout focus
11. Cortical bone on lower border of the mandible
12. Mylohyoid ridge
13. Submaxillary (submandibular) gland fossa
14. Internal oblique line or ridge
15. Mylohyoid groove

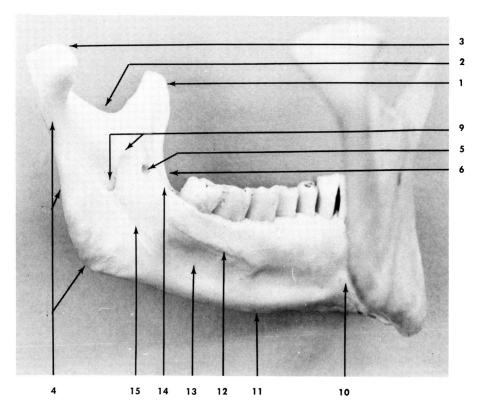

Fig. 12-7, cont'd. For legend see opposite page.

CHAPTER 13

Normal radiographic anatomy

A thorough knowledge of radiographic anatomy is essential before one can attempt to interpret radiograms. In evaluating normal radiographic images, the viewer must use his knowledge of all the variable factors that affect the radiographic image; in addition, he must have a thorough knowledge of anatomy, particularly osteology. It must be remembered that superimposition, magnification, and distortion create major problems in the reading of radiograms and that some objects, such as thin bone, fissures, and septa, are seen only at certain angles or projections. Although dental materials cannot be considered normal anatomy, the radiographic appearance of these materials will be demonstrated in this chapter. Radiographic anatomic landmarks are discussed in two groups: (1) intraoral landmarks and (2) extraoral landmarks.

INTRAORAL LANDMARKS

In a radiogram of average density, the radiographic images of dental structures or parts of these structures can be divided into two groups: (1) radiopaque images and (2) radiolucent images. In Table 13-1 the more common landmarks are grouped under these headings. In Figs. 13-1 to 13-18 each landmark is illustrated at least once; the figure legends clarify the illustrations. Chapter 12 on skull osteology should be used freely in studying normal radiographic landmarks.

EXTRAORAL LANDMARKS

In order to utilize effectively the extraoral technics discussed in Chapters 6 and 7, particularly the latter, it is essential that the practitioner have an understanding of the anatomic landmarks seen on extraoral films. The extraoral landmarks discussed in this chapter are related to three extraoral projections: (1) the lateral skull, (2) the open mouth maxillary sinus, and (3) the bregma-mentum. These projections are basically at right angles to each other and thus provide a three-dimensional study. Several other extraoral technics are also discussed in Chapters 6 and 7. Space does not permit a detailed evaluation of the numerous extraoral landmarks on all of the projections mentioned or on other possible projections available to the radiologist.

Text continued on p. 266.

Table 13-1. Radiopaque and radiolucent structures seen in intraoral radiograms

Radiopaque structures	Radiolucent structures
Anatomic	**Anatomic**
Enamel	Maxillary sinus
Dentin	Nasal cavity
Bone plates	Soft tissues
Lamina dura	Pulp
Septa in maxillary sinus	Enamel organ
Wall of maxillary sinus	Dental papillae
Lower border of mandible	Bone marrow
Lower border of mandibular canal	Gingivae
Lower border of nasal cavity	Periodontal membrane
Cortical plates	Foramina
Nasal septum	Mental
Bone ridges and prominences	Incisive
Internal oblique line	Accessory, e.g., lingual
External oblique line	Canals
Mental prominence	Incisive
Canine prominence	Mandibular
Coronoid process	Nutrient
Hamulus	Sutures
Maxillary tuberosity	Median alveolar
Zygomatic arch	Median palatine
Anterior nasal spine	Bone depressions
Genial tubercles	Lateral fossa
	Submandibular fossa
	Mental fossa
Restorative materials	**Restorative materials**
Gold	Acrylic
Silver amalgam	Silicates
Zinc oxide–eugenol	Calcium hydroxide pastes*
Zinc phosphate cement	Porcelain
Gutta-percha	
Silver points	
Metal bands and crowns	
Metal wires	

*Commercially available products vary in radiolucency. Some pastes are now quite opaque because of the addition of radiopaque material.

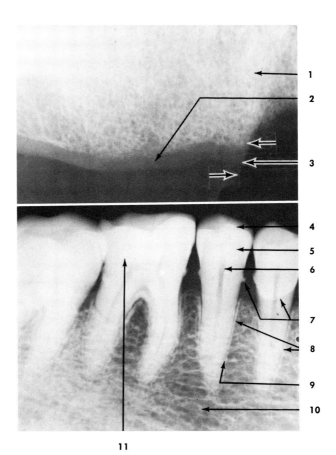

Fig. 13-1. Radiograms demonstrating bone patterns, soft tissues, and other common anatomic entities. The size and number of bone trabeculae vary greatly within the normal range. The maxillary bone tends to show fine trabeculae arranged in a lacelike pattern. The mandibular bone tends to show fewer, coarser trabeculae with wider marrow spaces. The mandibular trabeculae tend to run horizontally. The outlines of soft tissues are sometimes seen in dental radiograms. Primary and secondary dentin have equal radiographic density.

1. Typical maxillary bone
2. Gingiva (soft tissue)
3. Cheek line (three arrows)
4. Enamel
5. Dentin
6. Pulp canal (The pulp chamber has been largely obliterated.)
7. Calculus deposits (Such deposits are sometimes confused with normal crown outline.)
8. Lamina dura
9. Periodontal membrane space
10. Typical mandibular bone
11. Secondary dentin

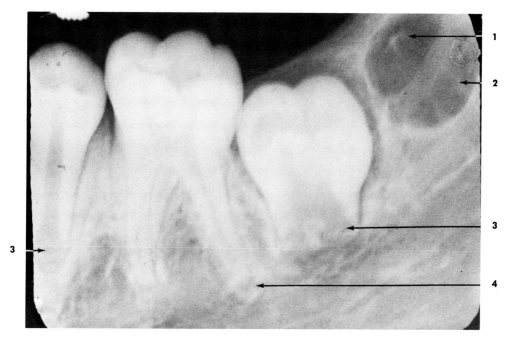

Fig. 13-2. Radiogram of developing teeth. The tooth follicle appears as a spherical radiolucent area within the bone. The beginning calcification of a cusp can be seen within the tooth follicle shown in this radiogram. The size of the enamel organ and dental papilla depend on the stage of tooth development. The incomplete root shows a flaring of the pulp chamber at the root apex. The nearly completed root shows a widened periodontal space of even width around the apex of the tooth.

1. Enamel organ
2. Tooth follicle
3. Incomplete tooth apex

4. Almost complete tooth apex. (The thickened periodontal space tends to persist for 6 months or more after the tooth apex appears complete.)

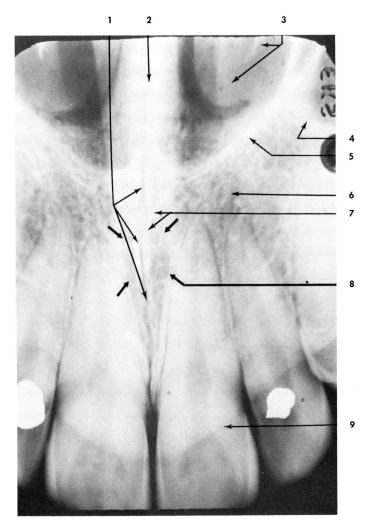

Fig. 13-3. Radiogram of the maxillary midline area. Many structures are superimposed on each other in the midline. The median suture appears as a thin radiolucent line. The incisive foramen is usually oval in shape and may be indistinct in the dentulous patient; the walls of the incisive canal sometimes may be seen connected to this foramen. The anterior nasal spine appears as a V-shaped radiopaque structure situated in the midline above the incisive foramen. A depression in the surface of the bone over the lateral incisor (lateral fossa) may produce an ill-defined area of increased radiolucency at the apex of this tooth.

1. Median suture
2. Nasal septum
3. Anterior aspect of the inferior concha (upper arrow) and soft tissue of the inferior turbinate (lower arrow)
4. Anterior wall of the maxillary sinus

5. Anterior aspect of the nasal cavity
6. Lateral fossa
7. Anterior nasal spine
8. Incisive foramen (four arrows)
9. Border of soft tissue of the nose or of a heavy lip

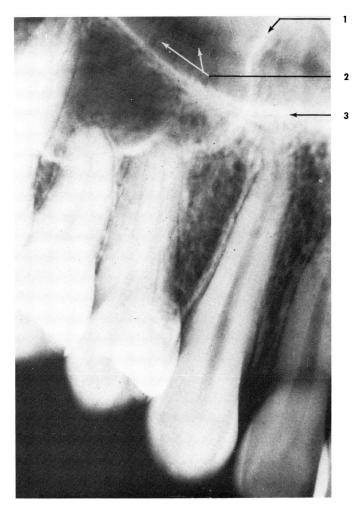

Fig. 13-4. Radiogram of the maxillary cuspid area. The images of the walls of the maxillary sinus and the nasal cavity cross each other in the area of the canine apex. Nutrient vessels may run in canals within the bone or in grooves in the wall of the maxillary sinus. These vessels appear as radiolucent bands of even width.

1. Anterior wall of the maxillary sinus
2. Nutrient canal or groove
3. Outline of the nasal cavity

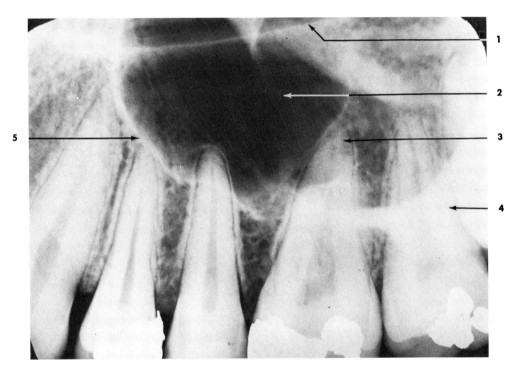

Fig. 13-5. Radiogram of the upper bicuspid area. The floor of the nasal cavity extends anteriorly in the horizontal plane past the upper cuspid tooth. The anterior wall of the maxillary sinus is usually situated just distal to the upper cuspid. The floor of the nasal cavity is only seen when great vertical angulation is used. In such instances the buccal roots of the teeth are usually foreshortened and the shadow of the zygomatic arch is cast coronally on the upper molar teeth.

1. Junction of the lateral wall and the floor of the nasal cavity
2. Radiolucent maxillary sinus
3. Palatal root of the first molar
4. Zygoma and zygomatic process of the maxilla
5. Border of the maxillary sinus

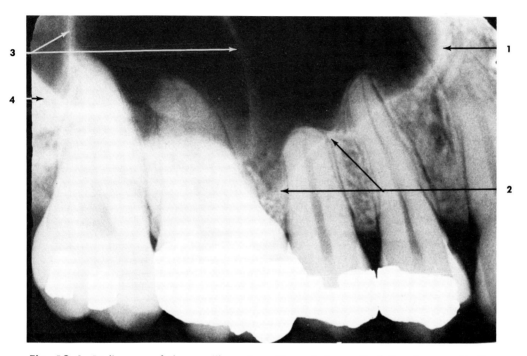

Fig. 13-6. Radiogram of the maxillary sinus. The anterior wall of the sinus usually lies in the area of the cuspid tooth; the posterior wall usually lies in the area of the maxillary tuberosity. Depending on the degree of pneumatization, the floor of the sinus may lie above the apices of the teeth or dip between the various tooth roots. Septa may traverse the sinus; a septum is seen only when the x-ray beam is directed in the plane of the septum.

1. Anterior wall of the sinus
2. Floor of the sinus
3. Sinus septum
4. Zygoma and zygomatic process of the maxilla

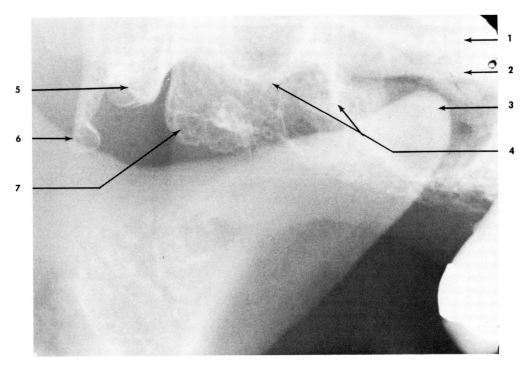

Fig. 13-7. Radiograms of the maxillary molar area. The posterior wall of the maxillary sinus is seen in this projection along with the maxillary tuberosity. Distal to the tuberosity is seen the hamular process and sometimes the pterygoid plates. Depending on the radiographic technic used, the coronoid process of the mandible may or may not be superimposed on this area. The zygomatic arch extends laterally from the maxilla, showing a typical U-shaped radiopacity in the first molar area. The zygomatic arch curves distally, producing a radiopaque image, the lower border of which may or may not be sharply defined.

1. Junction of the lateral wall and the floor of the nasal cavity
2. Lower border of the zygomatic arch
3. Coronoid process of the mandible
4. Floor of the maxillary sinus
5. Pterygoid plate
6. Hamular process
7. Tuberosity of the maxilla
8. Zygomatic arch
9. Maxillary sinus
10. Zygoma

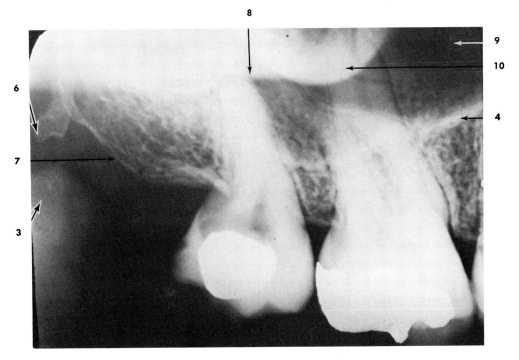

Fig. 13-7, cont'd. For legend see opposite page.

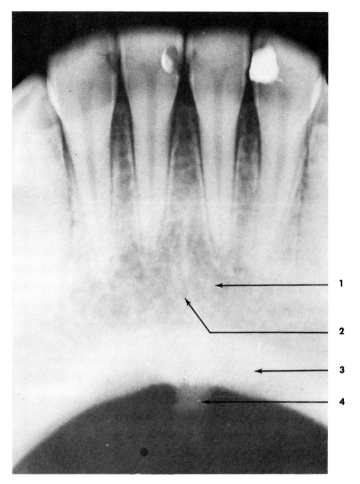

Fig. 13-8. Radiograms of the lower anterior area. The lingual foramen is commonly seen as a single foramen situated in the midline. It appears as a small radiolucency surrounded by a radiopaque border. With increasing vertical angulation, the genial tubercles and lower border of the mandible may appear. In some cases there may be a definite depression or mental fossa on the anterior surface of the mandible; this area will be rather radiolucent.

1. Mental fossa
2. Lingual foramen (The foramen shows clearly in the right photograph; its definition is rather unclear in the left photograph.)

3. Cortical plate
4. Genial tubercle
5. Mental ridge

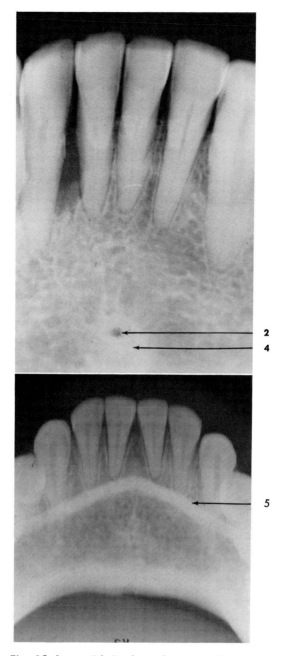

2

4

5

Fig. 13-8, cont'd. For legend see opposite page.

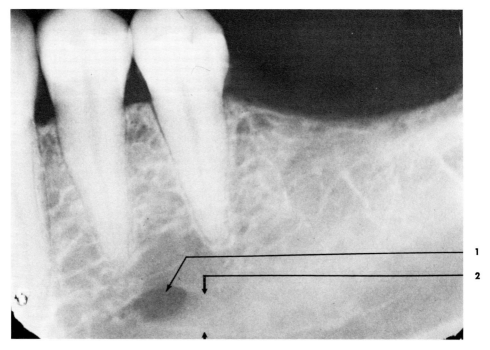

Fig. 13-9. Radiogram of the mandibular bicuspid area. The mental foramen appears as an oval radiolucent area; it is usually situated just below and slightly distal to the apex of the lower first bicuspid. The mental foramen is connected to the mandibular canal.

1. Mental foramen
2. Wall of the mandibular canal (two arrows)

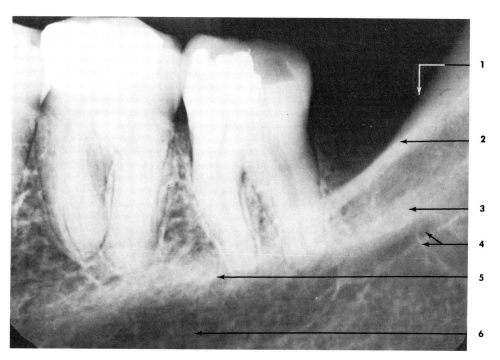

Fig. 13-10. Radiograms of the lower molar area. The anterior border of the ramus blends into the external oblique line, which descends sharply in the third molar area. The internal oblique or mylohyoid line is situated in a more horizontal position in the body of the mandible. Below the internal oblique line is an area of increased radiolucency produced by the submaxillary gland fossa. The mandibular canal appears as a radiolucent band of even width; it may or may not show a continuous or broken calcified border.

1. Anterior border of the ramus
2. External oblique line
3. Internal oblique line
4. Border of the mandibular canal (lower arrow) and the mandibular canal (upper arrow)
5. Mylohyoid line or ridge
6. Submandibular fossa

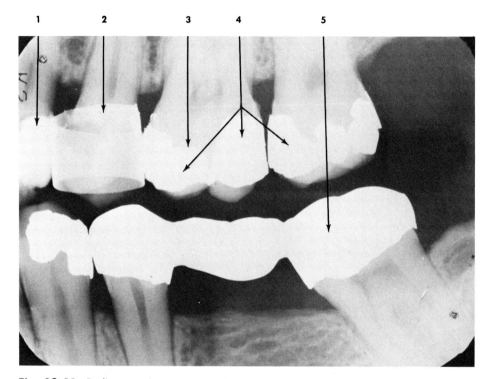

Fig. 13-11. Radiogram demonstrating the relative radiopacity of the following:

1. Zinc oxide—eugenol
2. Copper band
3. Zinc phosphate cement
4. Silver amalgam
5. Gold

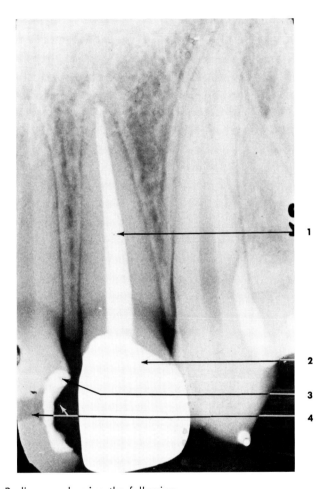

Fig. 13-12. Radiogram showing the following:

1. Gutta-percha
2. Gold

3. Zinc phosphate cement
4. Acrylic

A small amount of gold is radiopaque; thus the margins of gold restorations are sharply defined. It takes relatively large amounts of gutta-percha or zinc phosphate cement to produce totally radiopaque images.

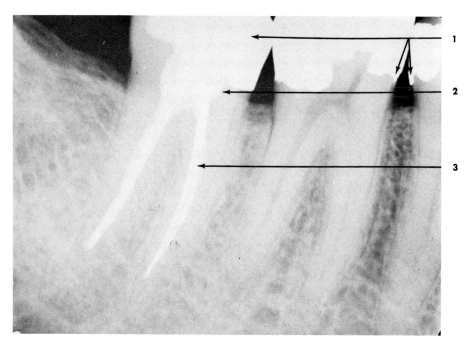

Fig. 13-13. Radiogram showing the appearance of the following:

1. Amalgam
2. Gutta-percha
3. Silver points

The outlines of silver points are usually clearly seen in radiograms. Amalgam is very radiopaque since it is composed primarily of two heavy metals. The arrows on the mesial of the first molar and the distal of the second bicuspid point to typical amalgam overhangs below the margin of the proximal step of the cavity preparation.

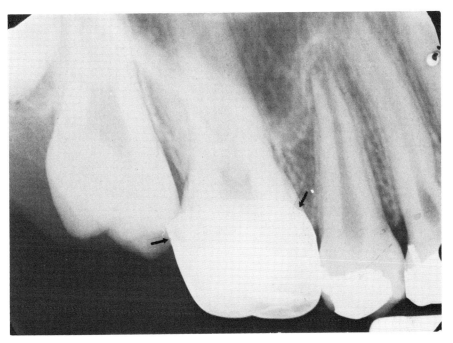

Fig. 13-14. Radiogram showing a temporary aluminum crown. The crown is faintly radiopaque because of the relatively low atomic weight of the metal and the thinness of the crown. Other structures can be seen through the metal crown.

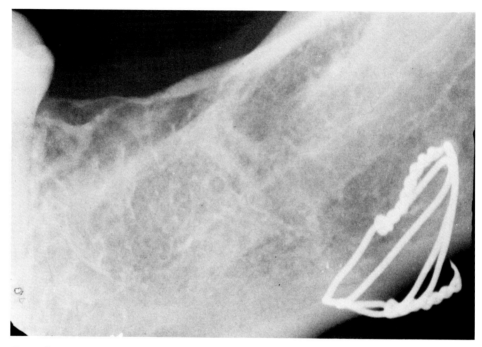

Fig. 13-15. Radiogram of fracture wires. Fracture wires require great strength and are usually made of heavy metal, thus producing a radiopaque image.

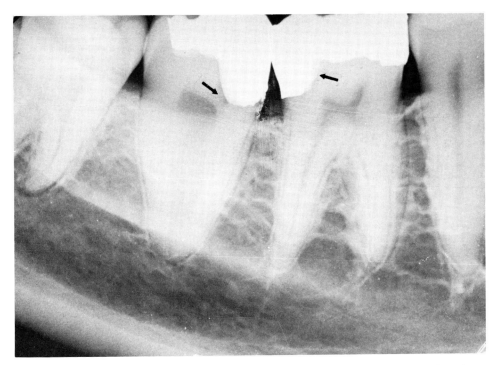

Fig. 13-16. Radiogram showing calcium hydroxide between sound dentin and a zinc phosphate base in the second mandibular molar. The arrow in the first molar points to a zinc phospate base, which can be compared with the radiographic density of a metallic restoration and sound dentin. The percentage of calcium in the total calcium hydroxide mixture is small; therefore, the resultant image is radiolucent. However, commercial products containing calcium hydroxide vary considerably in their radiographic appearance.

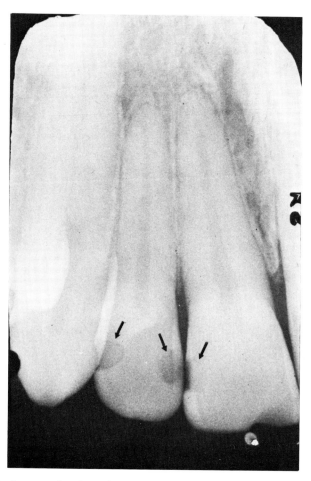

Fig. 13-17. Radiogram showing silicate restorations. Silicate restorations appear to be less dense than dentin; however, it is sometimes difficult to see this difference. The restorations shown here do not possess cement bases; such bases are clearly seen radiographically.

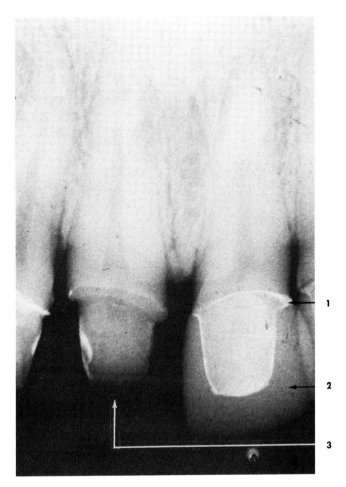

Fig .13-18. Radiographic appearance of the following:

1. Zinc phosphate cement
2. Porcelain jacket crown
3. Acrylic jacket crown

Acrylic is made of elements of low atomic weight and is thus extremely radiolucent, showing no image in the average dental radiogram. Porcelain shows a density similar to dentin. Zinc phosphate cement is radiopaque, and relatively small amounts of this cement can usually be identified.

An understanding of extraoral anatomic landmarks is accomplished by two alternative methods. In the first method, certain anatomic landmarks are outlined by the use of opaque media. The position of these specific landmarks is shown in each of the projections just mentioned (Figs. 13-19 to 13-23). The opaque media are located on the right side of the skull. Corresponding landmarks can be seen in many instances on the unmarked left side. In this manner, the reader can observe how each landmark changes its radiographic position as a result of alterations in the relative positions of the film, skull, and x-ray beam. An anatomic landmark that can be seen clearly in one projection often is indistinct or nonobservable in another projection. This approach is designed to encourage the student to utilize a dry skull in order to evaluate anatomic landmarks that he may observe on a radiographic film. As long as the observer understands the technic—the relationship of x-ray beam, object, and film—he can, if he has a skull at his disposal, make an accurate evaluation of extraoral anatomic landmarks. It must be remembered that the same landmarks in different individuals have a rather constant position but, in some instances, may vary considerably in shape and size.

Text continued on p. 284.

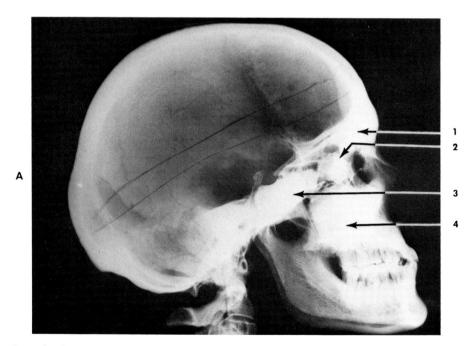

Fig. 13-19. Extraoral landmarks, **A,** Lateral view. **B,** Maxillary sinus view. **C,** Bregma-mentum view.

1. Frontal sinus
2. Ethmoid sinus

3. Sphenoid sinus
4. Maxillary sinus

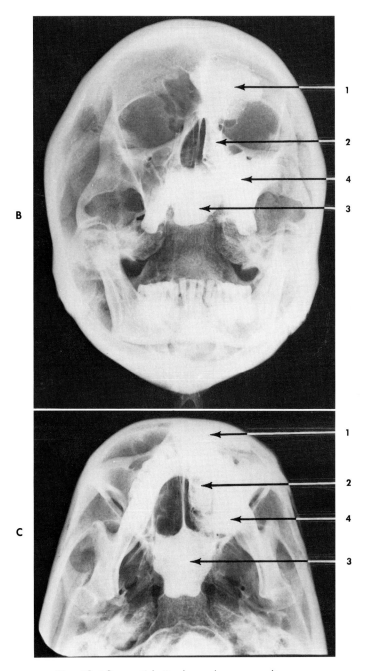

Fig. 13-19, cont'd. For legend see opposite page.

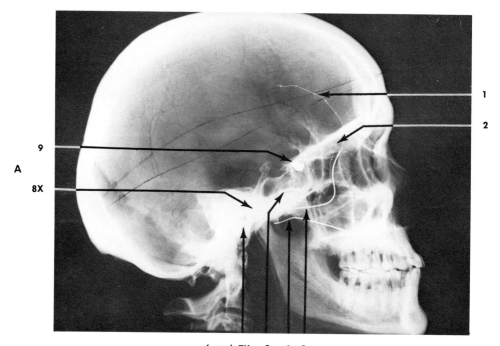

Fig. 13-20. Extraoral landmarks. **A,** Lateral view. **B,** Maxillary sinus view. **C,** Bregmamentum view.

1. Anterior border of the temporal fossa
2. Floor of the temporal fossa from the infratemporal crest of the sphenoid along the anterior aspect of the temporal fossa upward to the lateral aspect of the frontal bone
3. Superior border of the zygomatic arch

4. Inferior border of the zygomatic arch
5. Foramen rotundum
6. External auditory meatus
7. Internal auditory meatus
8. Foramen ovale
9. Optic nerve canal

X. Approximate location—opaque outline of the landmark cannot be seen.

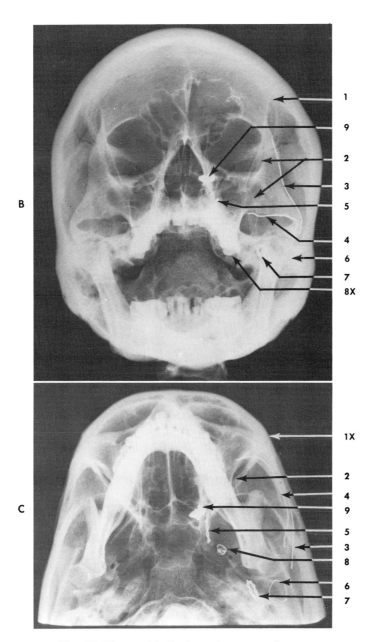

B

C

1
9
2
3
5
4
6
7
8X

1X

2
4
9
5
3
8
6
7

Fig. 13-20, cont'd. For legend see opposite page.

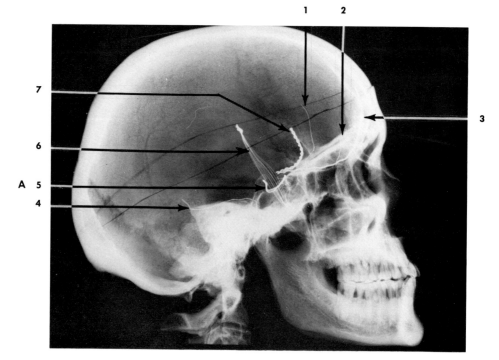

Fig. 13-21. Extraoral landmarks. **A,** Lateral view. **B,** Maxillary sinus view. **C,** Bregma-mentum view.

1. Floor of the anterior cranial fossa lateral to the midline
2. Crista galli
3. Floor and anterior aspect of the anterior cranial fossa in the midline
4. Superior border of the petrous potion of the temporal bone
5. Sella turcica
6. Lateral wall of the middle cranial fossa
7. Posterior border of the lesser wing of the sphenoid

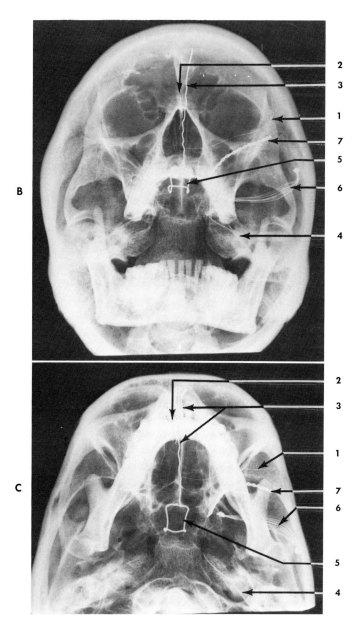

Fig. 13-21, cont'd. For legend see opposite page.

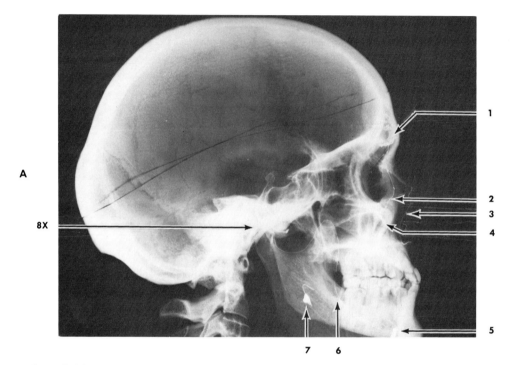

Fig. 13-22. Extraoral landmarks. **A,** Lateral view. **B,** Maxillary sinus view. **C,** Bregmamentum view.

1. Supraorbital canal
2. Rim of the orbit
3. Rim of the nasal cavity
4. Infraorbital foramen
5. Mental foramen

6. External oblique line, anterior border of the ramus, coronoid process, sigmoid notch, and condylar head
7. Lingula and mandibular foramen
8. Articular fossa

X. Approximate location—opaque outline of the landmark cannot be seen.

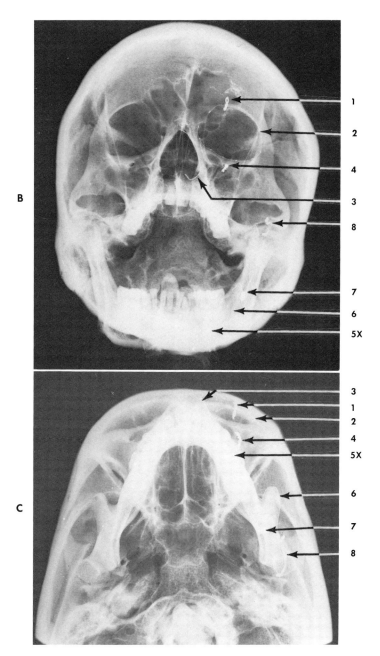

B

1
2
4
3
8
7
6
5X

C

3
1
2
4
5X
6
7
8

Fig. 13-22, cont'd. For legend see opposite page.

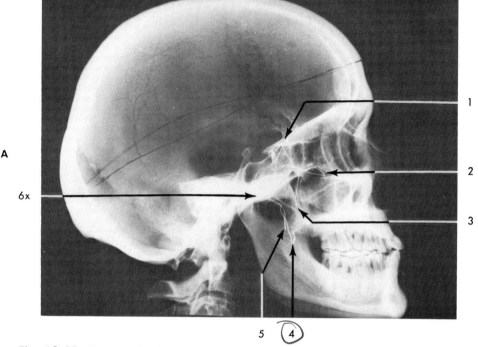

Fig. 13-23. Extraoral landmarks. **A,** Lateral view. **B,** Maxillary sinus view. **C,** Bregmamentum view.

1. Superior orbital fissure
2. Inferior orbital fissure
3. Pterygomaxillary fissure
4. Posterior border and hamular process of the medial pterygoid plate

5. Posterior border of the lateral pterygoid plate
6. Articular eminence

X. Approximate location—opaque outline of the landmark cannot be seen.

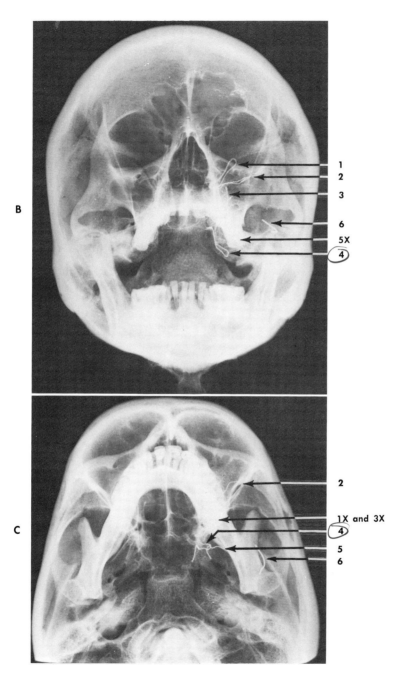

B

1
2
3
6
5X
4

C

2
1X and 3X
4
5
6

Fig. 13-23, cont'd. For legend see opposite page.

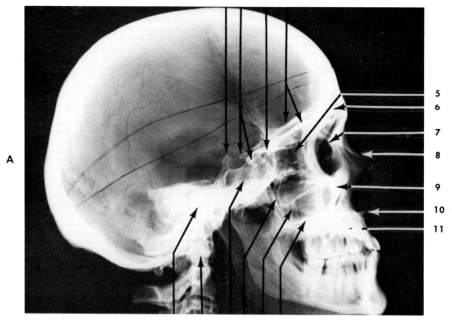

Fig. 13-24. Extraoral landmarks unidentified with opaque medium. The more common landmarks identified in Figs. 12-19 to 12-23 are reidentified. Some landmarks not included in prior illustrations are identified.

A, Lateral view:

1. Posterior clinoid processes and dorsum sellae
2. Anterior clinoid processes
3. Floor of the anterior cranial fossa in the midline
4. Roof of the orbit and floor of the anterior cranial fossa lateral to the midline
5. Ethmoid sinus
6. Frontal sinus
7. Orbit (medial wall)
8. Nasal bones

9. Zygoma
10. Anterior nasal spine
11. Roof of the palate (midline)
12. Floor of the nose and roof of the palate (midline)
13. Maxillary sinus
14. Pterygomaxillary fissure
15. Sphenoid sinus
16. Mastoid process of the temporal bone
17. Petrous portion of the temporal bone

B, Maxillary sinus view:

1. Frontal sinus
2. Orbit
3. Floor of the temporal fossa (temporal surface of the sphenoid and temporal bones)
4. Medial wall of the ethmoid sinus (both arrows); space between arrows, upper portion of the nasal airway
5. Zygoma
6. Maxillary sinus (above) and sphenoid sinus (below)

7. Zygomatic arch
8. Temporal fossa
9. Basilar portion of the occipital bone at the approximate area of union with the sphenoid bone
10. Odontoid process of the second cervical vertebra superimposed on the foramen magnum and midline of the mandible

C, Bregma-mentum view:

1. Medial wall of the ethmoid sinus
2. Orbit
3. Maxillary sinus
4. Temporal and infratemporal fossa
5. Ethmoid sinus
6. Sphenoid sinus
7. Foramen ovale

8. Foramen spinosum
9. Foramen lacerum
10. Basilar portion of the occipital bone at the approximate area of union with the sphenoid bone
11. Petrous portion of the temporal bone
12. Odontoid process

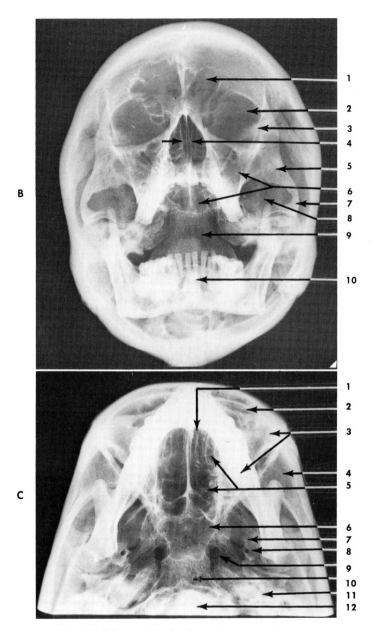

Fig. 13-24, cont'd. For legend see opposite page.

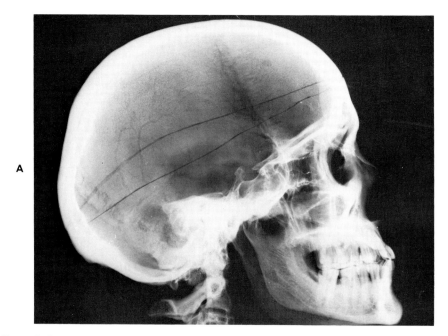

Fig. 13-25. Extraoral landmarks totally unidentified. These illustrations can be used to test understanding of extraoral anatomic landmarks. **A,** Lateral view. **B,** Maxillary sinus view. **C,** Bregma-mentum view.

B

C

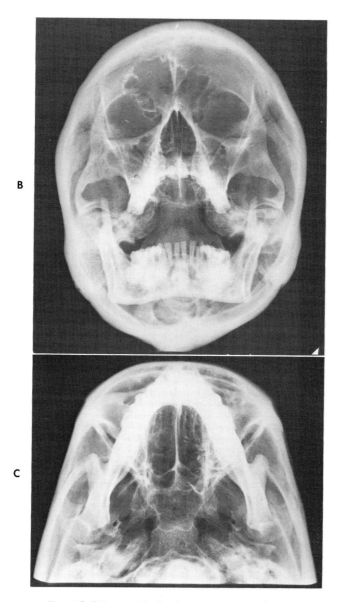

Fig. 13-25, cont'd. For legend see opposite page.

Fig. 13-26. A, Anatomic landmarks observed on a panoramic view of the mandible and maxilla. **B,** Position of skull in chin rest prior to exposure. Metal outlining various landmarks can be seen.

1. Orbit
2. Superior and inferior borders of the zygomatic arch (The wire on the superior border continues upward on the distal aspect of the frontal process of the zygoma. The wire on the inferior border passes downward along the inferior border of the zygomatic process of the maxilla [jugal ridge].)
3. External auditory meatus
4. Anterior border of the nasal cavity
5. Posterior and inferior aspect of the lateral ptery-goid plate; a heavy wire was used to determine if the structural outline could be seen on the op-posite side
6. Infraorbital foramen
7. Posterior and inferior border of the mandible (A heavy saw-toothed lead marker was used to de-termine if its outline could be seen on the op-posite side. As with landmark 4, it can be seen. Note that the direction of the saw teeth is the same as that seen on the right side. It can be concluded that anatomic landmarks, when ob-served on the contralateral side, will be blurred and, in relation to comparable structures on the side being examined, will be rotated 180°.)
8. Mandibular foramen (at apex of the wire marker) leading into the mandibular canal.
9. Wire outlining the posterior border of the ramus, condyle, sigmoid or mandibular notch, coronoid process, anterior border of the ramus, and ex-ternal oblique line
10. Mylohyoid ridge
11. Mental foramen
12. Wire outlining the plastic chin rest; the shadow of the chin rest can also be seen on the left side
13. Incisive foramen (Note that the same marker is seen on both the right and left sides. A wire extends from the foramen distally along the mid-line of the palate to landmark 14.)
14. Posterior aspect of the hard palate; note that the same marker is seen on the right side
15. Inferior border of the vomer (The angle at land-mark 14 is the termination of the hard palate. Note that this marker also is observed on the right side.)

This film was exposed with a Panorex. A similar film made with an Orthopantomograph or a Rotograph would not show the nonexposed center strip, and structures (for example, the incisive foramen) in the anterior midline would appear only once. However, the more distal midline structures would probably show, with some loss of definition, much as do land-marks 14 and 15.

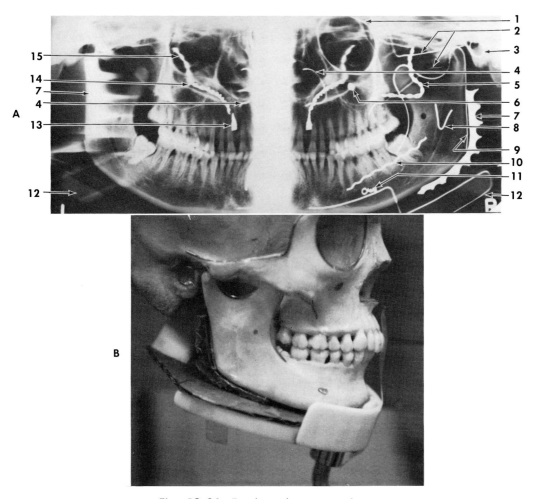

Fig. 13-26. For legend see opposite page.

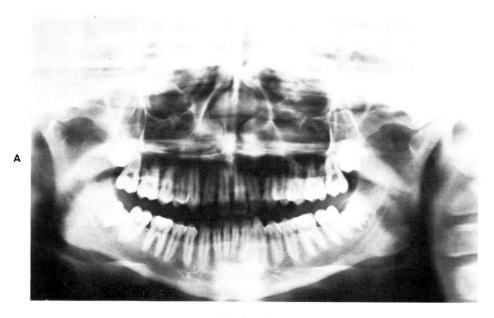

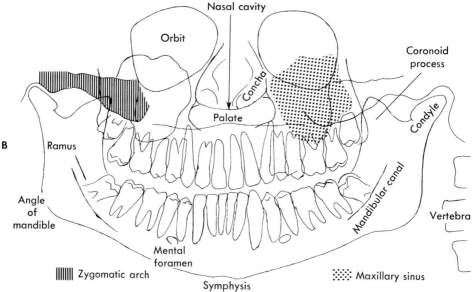

Fig. 13-27. Panoramic radiograph and tracing of the radiograph showing outlines of the major anatomic structures. (From Manson-Hing, L. R.: Panoramic dental radiography, courtesy of Charles C Thomas, Publisher, Springfield. Ill.)

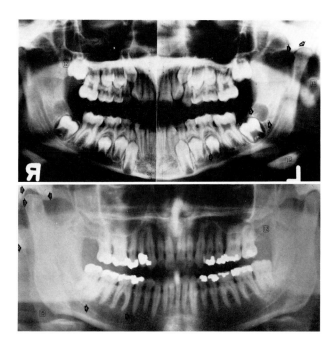

Fig. 13-28. Normal pantomographic anatomy of a child (Panorex) and an adult (Panelipse). (From Manson-Hing, L. R.: Paroramic dental radiography, courtesy of Charles C Thomas, Publisher, Springfield, Ill.)

1. Articular eminence
2. Glenoid fossa
3. Mandibular condyle
4. Mandibular canal
5. Third molar crypt
6. Enamel organ
7. Dentinal papillae
8. Mental foramen
9. Styloid process
10. Nasal septum
11. Conchae
12. Maxillary tuberosity
13. Ear lobe
14. Hyoid bone
15. Lateral head positioner
16. Chin rest

The second mode of approach is simply that of indicating on the three projections under discussion the anatomic landmarks observed on a particular film (Fig. 13-24). Only the more common landmarks identified in Figs. 13-19 to 13-23 are reidentified in Fig. 13-24. The combination of the two methods used simultaneously should provide the observer with a reasonably comprehensive understanding of skull osteology from a radiographic standpoint. Fig. 13-25 is the same as Fig. 13-24, but the landmarks are not identified. These illustrations can be used for self-examination.

The location of anatomic landmarks, as observed in a panoramic radiogram, is seen in Figs. 13-26, 13-27, and 13-28.

If a suitable skull is not available, the reader should make continual use of Chapter 12 as he learns to identify radiographic landmarks, particularly extraoral landmarks.

CHAPTER 14

Growth of the head and face

Radiographic technics of primary interest to dentistry are concerned with observations of structural alterations in the entire head. An understanding of the growth patterns of the head and face should be of academic interest to the general practitioner, the dental radiologist, and other specialists of dentistry. In addition to pure academic interest, a knowledge of growth patterns will assist one in understanding developmental abnormalities and certain types of pathologic changes. For example, some cysts found in the mandible and maxilla as well as palatal and lip clefts can be explained theoretically through an understanding of growth patterns. An appreciation of facial and skull developmental abnormalities is based on a knowledge of normal growth patterns.

The sequence of subjects that are discussed in this chapter include mechanisms of bone growth, basic factors influencing bone growth, embryology of the facial skeleton, growth patterns of the skull, growth patterns of the dentition, and anthropometric landmarks.

MECHANISMS OF BONE GROWTH

The development of bones is divided basically into membranous and endochondral types. The former type develops in connective tissue without being preformed in cartilage; the latter is preformed in cartilage. A third type exists; it is exemplified by the mandible and the clavicle. This third type develops as membranous bone, but during its formation cartilage is differentiated from connective tissue and plays an important part in growth. The long bones of the extremities and the vertebrae are examples of endochondral bone formation; such bones increase in size by interstitial growth of cartilage that is subsequently replaced by bone. The parietal and frontal bones and all bones of the upper face as well as the squamous portion of the temporal bone are among examples of the membranous type; membranous bone formation is by osteoblastic activity on the outer bone surfaces. Some texts differentiate bone formation into interstitial and appositional types. The former implies bone development through the replacement of cartilage; the latter suggests the growth of bone on its outer surface. Actually, all bone growth is by the apposition of one layer of bone on another through osteoblastic activity. Knowledge of the kind of tissue from which bones form evokes an appreciation of normal and abnormal growth.

Longitudinal growth centers of long bones are located near the surface of the epiphyses and between the epiphyses and the diaphysis or shaft. They are known respectively as articular and epiphyseal cartilages. Most growth takes place in the epiphyseal plates between the epiphysis and diaphysis.

Flat bones start developing from a center of ossification. Trabeculae radiate from the center of ossification and form a circular plate having rough, irregular borders. Growth is by apposition at the borders and on the outer and inner surfaces until a given bone approximates the edges of another bone. Continued growth of flat bones is the result of proliferation of sutural connective tissue and is followed by apposition of bone at the sutures and, in the case of the skull, an enlargement of the skull as a whole. Similarly, cartilage proliferates at the synchondroses, for example, in the area of junction between the sphenoid and occipital bones.

Cartilage develops both appositionally and interstitially. Interstitial growth is the result of mitotic division of cartilage cells within the cartilage, whereas appositional growth takes place on the surface of the cartilage as a result of chondroblastic activity in the perichondrium. Whereas longitudinal growth of cartilage occurs only interstitially, the transverse diameter of cartilaginous growth is increased through apposition.

Hyaline cartilage is found after birth primarily in three skull locations: (1) it forms part of the nasal skeleton; (2) it joins the occipital and sphenoid bone and the different parts of the occipital bone to each other; and (3) it forms part of the mandibular condyle. In the spheno-occipital synchondrosis, hyaline cartilage plays the same role for the anteroposterior extension of the cranial base as the epiphyseal cartilage plays for the longitudinal growth of the tubular or long bones. This cartilaginous plate grows interstitially, thereby lengthening the cranial base.

The cartilage in the head of the mandible, however, is unlike epiphyseal cartilage. It is covered on its free surface by fibrous tissue that bounds the articular space; this probably explains the appositional growth of condylar cartilage. The mechanism of cartilaginous growth in the mandible increases the overall length of the mandible and at the same time, the height of the mandibular ramus. The replacement of the cartilage is radically different from that in an epiphyseal center of ossification; the condylar cartilage is apparently resorbed and is then invaded by osteoblasts on its outer surface.

BASIC FACTORS INFLUENCING BONE GROWTH

Apart from the genetic aspects of bone growth (which largely control face and skull shape), there are some basic factors that can significantly alter bone growth or the appearance of the bone. Although bone growth is an extremely complex phenomenon, a general framework can be developed for the clinician. Bone seen at a particular time is due to a balance between bone formation and bone resorption. Any factor affecting this balance will alter bone growth and/or the appearance of the bone. Bone formation occurs through the development of a matrix by a soft tissue component and the subsequent mineralization of the matrix. Bone resorption (of the calcified elements) appears to occur in more or less a single step.

When a bone is radiolucent and shows less calcified material, the basic cause can be due to either a reduction in bone formation or an increase in bone resorption. The reduction in bone formation can further be subdivided into a defect in matrix formation and a reduction in matrix calcification. An overly radiopaque bone results from increased bone formation or decreased bone resorption. In any event, the changed appearance of the bone is the result of an imbalance between bone formation and bone resorption.

Radiolucent bone can occur from poor osteoid matrix formation, which in turn can occur from a disturbance of the osteoblasts. Such is the case in disuse atrophy, estrogen deficiency, and osteogenesis imperfecta. The matrix can be defective without a disturbance of osteoblasts. Examples of this process include androgen deficiency and nutritional deficiencies such as a lack of protein or ascorbic acid. Poor matrix mineralization also results in radiolucent bone. Such is the condition in avitaminosis D and conditions that result in hypercalciuria. Radiolucent bone caused by increased bone resorption occurs when concurrent bone formation is normal; an example of this process occurs in hyperparathyroidism.

Radiopaque bone showing more calcified material results when there is a decrease in bone resorption. This mechanism occurs in osteopetrosis. The production of radiopaque bone by an increase in matrix formation is questionable; however, tumors such as osteomas demonstrate this process on a localized basis.

Radiolucent and radiopaque areas within bones can occur at the same time; Paget's disease presents this type of picture. In addition, soft tissue lesions that subsequently produce calcified materials, for example, cementomas, also show both radiolucency and radiopacity.

EMBRYOLOGY OF THE FACIAL SKELETON

The face develops from several components of the embryo. These include the cephalic end of the embryonic gut, which initially is a blind tube; paired mandibular arches, which are the first of several brachial arches; the frontal prominence (the tissues over the forebrain), which flexes over the upper end of the gut; and a stomodeum or primitive oral cavity, which invaginates toward the gut from the outer surface of the embryo. The facial development starts approximately 3 weeks after conception.

The mandibular arches are located just below the area where the stomodeum invaginates. The arches develop toward the midline to form the embryonic mandible. Continuous with the more posterior end of each arch and from their upper border, a maxillary process develops, which accounts for a major part of the upper face.

From the region of the forebrain in the 3-week embryo a frontal process develops, which extends downward over the anterior opening of the primitive oral cavity, or stomodeum. On each side of the frontal process near its inferior border an invagination known as the olfactory pit appears; the openings of these pits are the primitive nares. The two pits are bounded superiorly and on each side by a rather heavy ridge, which, as each pit continues to invaginate, becomes the lateral nasal process and the medial nasal process. Since there are two olfactory pits, these processes are paired. The region between the two medial nasal processes continues to be known as the frontal process. The medial nasal processes grow toward each other with consequent narrowing of the area between them. The depressed center portion, now known as the triangular area of the frontal process, extends backward to form the lower part of the nasal septum; its upper part develops into the bridge of the nose. The medial nasal processes continue growing toward each other. They finally contact in the midline and become known as the globular process. The globular process forms the premaxilla, the portion of the face that will ultimately support the maxillary central and lateral teeth. The lateral nasal processes form much of the structure comprising the nose and ethmoidal region. The original olfactory pits eventually become the nasal cavity.

Coincidental with the downward extension of the medial nasal processes, the maxillary processes grow medially to join with the premaxilla. Each maxillary process develops a palatal process that extends horizontally to join ultimately with its counterpart to form the floor of the nose and the roof of the mouth. The maxillary processes also form the lateral wall and floor of the orbits. They ultimately fuse with the lateral nasal and medial nasal (globular) processes to form the lateral aspect of the upper lip and the posterior boundary of the nares. The lateral wall of the nasal cavity also arises from the maxillary process.

The roof of the nose, the ethmoidal air spaces, the inferior nasal concha, the lateral cartilage of the nose, and the ala of the nose are formed from the lateral nasal processes. The calvarium develops from the region of the cephalic parts of the embryo covering the forebrain, midbrain, and hindbrain. The eye develops from both the cavity in the forebrain and the surface invagination of the ectoderm. The facial components resulting from the various embryonic entities are shown diagrammatically in Fig. 14-1.

From a strictly dental viewpoint, the most important aspects of skull development relate to the embryonic growth patterns of the medial (globular), maxillary, lateral, and palatal processes. Harelips, cleft palates, and inclusion or fissural cysts occur in the areas where these entities join and finally fuse. The lateral process joins with the maxillary process and globular process in the region of the ala of the nose; this is the site of nasoalveolar cysts. The globular process,

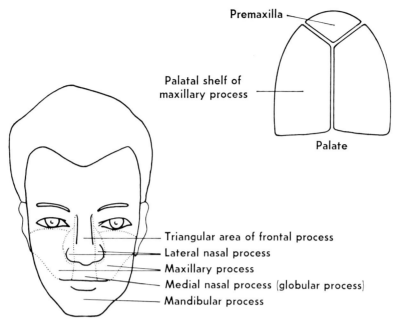

Fig. 14-1. Relationship of embryonic processes to facial development.

or premaxilla, joins with the maxillary process in the area between the cuspid and lateral teeth; this is the area where the globulomaxillary cyst and harelip occur. The median palatine cyst and the cleft palate appear where the palatal shelves of the maxillary process join in the midline to form the roof of the mouth and the floor of the nose. Incisal foramina and incisal canal cysts occur in the apex of the triangle formed by the premaxilla and the anterior borders of the palatal shelves of the maxillary process. Clefts and cysts in the globular process (between the paired medial nasal processes) in the center of the premaxilla are rare, as are clefts and cysts in the midline of the mandible.

GROWTH PATTERNS OF THE SKULL

Sicher has aptly stated:

> The complexity of the skull, in a phylogenetic, ontogenetic, and functional sense, is especially apparent if one tries to understand its growth. This is the reason it has taken so long to acquire a fairly clear picture of the intricate changes in the different parts of the skull during its development and growth. The single fact that the bony capsule of the brain is inseparably linked with the masticatory facial skeleton, so that these two parts of the skull are integrated into one anatomic and biologic unit, accounts for many complications. These complications arise because the growth of the capsule of the brain is entirely dependent upon that of the brain itself, whereas that of the masticatory skeleton is, to a great extent, dependent upon muscular influences, dentition, and the growth of the tongue. The two parts of the skull not only follow different paths of development, but also the timing of their growth rates is entirely divergent. The brain has, at the age of 12 years, almost completed its growth

by reaching about 90 per cent of its ultimate weight and volume. At this age, however, the dentition and therefore the jaws are only beginning their final phase of growth which will end eight or ten years later.[*]

Because of anatomic considerations as well as considerable variation in timing, it is advisable to discuss the development of the osseous structures of the head in two categories: the cranium and the facial skeleton.

Cranium

Lateral and posteroanterior development of the cranial base is caused largely by the proliferation of cartilage and its subsequent replacement with bone. This growth occurs principally between the sphenoid and ethmoid bones, between the sphenoid and occipital bones, and in the intraoccipital synchondroses. The spheno-occipital synchondrosis persists until about the age of 18 years, at which time it is replaced by bone. The other two areas disappear between birth and the fourth and fifth years. The rate of bone growth of the sphenoid and occipital bones at the spheno-occipital synchondrosis is not equal; the occipital bone grows more slowly than does the sphenoid bone. Thus the anterior portion of the skull base grows more rapidly than does the posterior part. This variation in growth rate is significant when pathologic conditions or genetic factors alter normal development.

Expansion of the cranial vault results mainly from appositional bone growth on the margins of bones in the sutural areas. Apposition of bone on the inner and outer surfaces of the flat bones occurs accompanied by some resorption. Although such growth does not account for major changes, it contributes to bone flattening and to the deepening of grooves and impressions on the inner cranial surface.

At birth, the borders of the bones forming the cranial vault are quite well approximated except at their rounded corners. These openings are called the fontanels. There are six—the frontal (bregma[†]), occipital (lambda[†]), sphenoid, and mastoid; the latter two are paired. All fontanels ordinarily close in the first 2 years of postnatal life. However, closure of the cranial sutures does not occur until the thirteenth or fourteenth year of life, and some sutures remain open for many more years. The difference in bone growth mechanism between the cranial base and the cranial vault associated with pathologic and genetic processes accounts for some peculiarities of skull shape.

Sutures, particularly the coronal, lambdoidal, and sagittal sutures, are not uncommonly misinterpreted as fractures when they are associated with a traumatic incident. Similarly, wormian bones are confused with bone fragments. These wormian, or sutural, bones are supernumerary bones that have developed from supernumerary centers of ossification in the suture sites.

---

[*]From Sicher, H., and DuBrul, E. L.: Oral anatomy, ed. 5, St. Louis, 1970, The C. V. Mosby Co., p. 88.
[†]Point of fontanel closure.

By the age of 12 years, the brain has grown to 90% of its volume. The rate of brain growth decreases materially after the third or fourth year. The bony capsule growth accompanies and is probably directly related to the growth of the inner soft tissue. Further changes in the skull result from functional demands placed on the bones by muscular stresses and the development of the facial skeleton. Development in the supraorbital region is a good example; the external occipital protuberance is another. The mechanical influence of the muscles gradually contributes to an alteration in skull shape and facial contour.

Facial skeleton

Upper facial skeleton. The growth of the facial skeleton is different from that of the calvarium and base of the skull. Much of the cranial growth has been completed during the first 2 years of life, and by the seventh year change is almost nonexistent. The facial skeleton grows considerably faster than the brain case after the first few years of life and continues its active growth until at least the eighteenth year. It ceases its growth much later.

During the growth period, the facial skeleton increases in size vertically and horizontally, and in an anteroposterior direction. The most important sites of growth for the maxillary complex are the following three bilateral sutures:

1. The frontomaxillary suture between the frontal process of the maxilla and the frontal bones.
2. The zygomaticomaxillary suture between the maxilla and the zygomatic bone as well as (but of lesser importance) the zygomaticotemporal suture between the zygomatic bone and the zygomatic process of the temporal bone.
3. The pterygopalatine suture between the pterygoid process of the sphenoid bone and the pyramidal process of the palatine bone.

It is significant that these four sutures are parallel with each other and course downward and posteriorly. Sicher points out that growth in these sutures has the effect of "shifting" the maxillary complex downward and anteriorly. This downward and anterior growth is accompanied by vertical and anteroposterior dimensional increases through growth of the maxilla. Growth at the alveolar border increases the vertical dimension, and palatal changes both broaden and increase the anteroposterior dimension of the facial skeleton.

Concurrently with the growth pattern just described, bone apposition and resorption that mold the face occur. Growth takes place at the site of all sutures in the facial skeleton. The lateral dimension of the maxilla is increased through growth in the median suture, and maxillary and interpterygoid lateral expansion results from the downward growth and divergence of the pterygoid processes. Increased height of the nasal cavity and an adjustment in the orbital height-to-width ratio is accomplished by apposition of bone on the orbital floor and resorption on the nasal floor. As the bone on the nasal floor is resorbed, the surface of the hard palate gains bone through apposition. All of this is attended by considerable growth of the alveolar process. It is clear that a definite growth interrelationship exists between all bones of the facial skeleton.

Mandible. Mandibular growth results largely from the proliferation of cartilage in the condylar head and the replacement of cartilage by bone. The cartilage in this area grows both interstitially and appositionally. The mandible develops as a membranous bone, and the two halves are still separated at the symphysis at birth; although separated by cartilage and connective tissue, little or no growth seems to occur in this region.

Growth of the condylar cartilage increases the vertical height of the ramus, and because the ramus is connected to the body by an oblique angle, it contributes to the overall length of the entire mandible. The actual length of the body, its cross-sectional dimensions, and those of the ramus are accomplished through appositional growth. The latter also provides for growth of the coronoid process. Concurrently with this growth process, there takes place resorption activity, especially along the anterior border of the ramus, that alters the anteroposterior dimension of the mandible and provides increased space for the alveolar ridge.

While the ramus is growing downward and forward, the alveolar ridges are growing upward by appositional growth. Thus the vertical height of the mandible is increased, and the relative position of the mandibular and maxillary alveolar processes is maintained. Teeth erupt as an integral part of this vertical growth process. The role played by tooth eruption in fostering normal mandibular and maxillary growth is still open to question. It appears unlikely, however, that the teeth play a dominant role. The alveolar processes must grow if the teeth are to erupt in a normal fashion; the latter appears to be dependent on the former.

Alterations in growth patterns do occur as a result of pathologic situations. Mandibular growth is the product of two different growth mechanisms. Interruption or acceleration of growth rarely concerns both mechanisms to an equal degree. Disorders in the growth of the mandible result in maxillary changes, particularly in the anterior part of the upper facial skeleton.

Paranasal sinuses. Air spaces that can be considered of dental importance include the frontal, maxillary, and sphenoid sinuses; ethmoid and mastoid air cells; and evaginations of the nasal cavity. The development and growth of these air-filled cavities can probably be understood best if their functional role is clarified.

These air-filled cavities theoretically can be thought of as contributing to the structural efficiency of the bone. Since heavy bony structure would unnecessarily add substantially to the bone weight, there develops a bone architecture that best meets the need of the living individual. These air spaces under discussion either are not present or are extremely small in the newborn and growing child. When the mechanical stresses on the facial skeleton are greatest, the sinuses are proportionately smaller than in a later stage, when the structures have developed fully and mechanical stresses tend to diminish. This is particularly true in older individuals, especially when they become edentulous, but it is true in all people as facial development begins to terminate and pillars that support the major mechanical stresses are developed.

The frontal sinus develops at the time that the supraorbital ridge is being formed. Prior to this time, the outer and inner plates of the anterior part of the skull are in close approximation. As the outer plate of the skull increases in size as a buttress for certain masticatory forces, the need for increased bone thickness becomes no greater. As a compensatory mechanism, a space known as the frontal sinus develops as a diverticulum of the most anterior cells of the ethmoid labyrinth. The maxillary sinus develops in much the same manner as an evagination from the middle nasal meatus and reaches its average size at puberty. In most individuals, the maxillary sinus continues to expand throughout life; it penetrates deeper into the alveolar process and expands into the zygomatic process of the maxilla. The development of the maxillary sinus is dependent on the fact that the facial skeleton does not need dense bone in the area of the maxillary sinus in order to support the stresses placed on it. As a result, the maxillary bone becomes pneumatized. A similar type of reaction occurs in the case of the other pneumatic cavities of the skull.

Skull alterations in older persons

Senile changes in the skull and jaws are largely related to muscular function and thus to the stresses placed on the various bony parts. Incidentally, differences in the adult male and female skeleton are similarly related to structural demands placed on osseous tissues. As the individual ages, ridges to which muscles are attached often become somewhat less broad and thick. The pneumatic cavities of the skull tend to enlarge because of reduced demands on the surrounding bone structure and the consequent resorption of bone directly surrounding the sinuses. The condylar angle of the mandible (the angle formed by the lower border of the mandible and a line that is a common tangent to the condylar head and the posterior border of the mandible) increases and thus tends to revert to a situation that existed before the adult mandible was fully developed. This is again due to masticatory demands and to some resorption of bone at the angle where the masseter and internal pterygoid muscles attach. This also results in a change in the gonial angle (the angle formed by the lower border of the mandible and the posterior border of the ramus directly above the gonion).

In the edentulous mouth, the height of the alveolar ridges decreases, and the result is that such structures as the mental foramen, the incisive foramen, the mylohyoid ridge, and so forth, approximate the crest of the alveolar ridge. The bone density at the lower border of the mandible and in such areas as the mylohyoid ridge and the mental ridges is reduced. The median alveolar suture found between the maxillary central teeth in the young person rarely is evident in the older individual. The size of the trabecular spaces in the older individual may increase because of the reduced masticatory stresses placed on the bone. On the other hand, particularly in the lower anterior portion of the mandible, the trabecular spaces are frequently reduced in size as compared to the young adult structure. These changes may have to do directly with bone metabolism rather than with functional stress since it is also common to observe reduced size of trabecular spaces following bone repair after infection has been eliminated. Last, the presence of nutrient vessels is frequently observed, particularly

Table 14-1. Chronology of the human dentition*

Tooth	Hard tissue formation begins	Amount enamel formed at birth	Enamel completed	Eruption	Root completed
Primary dentition					
Maxillary					
Central incisor	4 mo. in utero	Five sixths	1½ mo.	7½ mo.	1½ yr.
Lateral incisor	4½ mo. in utero	Two thirds	2½ mo.	9 mo.	2 yr.
Cuspid	5 mo. in utero	One third	9 mo.	18 mo.	3¼ yr.
First molar	5 mo. in utero	Cusps united	6 mo.	14 mo.	2½ yr.
Second molar	6 mo. in utero	Cusp tips still isolated	11 mo.	24 mo.	3 yr.
Mandibular					
Central incisor	4½ mo. in utero	Three fifths	2½ mo.	6 mo.	1½ yr.
Lateral incisor	4½ mo. in utero	Three fifths	3 mo.	7 mo.	1½ yr.
Cuspid	5 mo. in utero	One third	9 mo.	16 mo.	3¼ yr.
First molar	5 mo. in utero	Cusps united	5½ mo.	12 mo.	2¼ yr.
Second molar	6 mo. in utero	Cusp tips still isolated	10 mo.	20 mo.	3 yr.
Permanent dentition					
Maxillary					
Central incisor	3 - 4 mo.	—	4 -5 yr.	7- 8 yr.	10 yr.
Lateral incisor	10 -12 mo.	—	4 -5 yr.	8- 9 yr.	11 yr.
Cuspid	4 - 5 mo.	—	6 -7 yr.	11-12 yr.	13-15 yr.
First bicuspid	1½- 1¾ yr.	—	5 -6 yr.	10-11 yr.	12-13 yr.
Second bicuspid	2 - 2¼ yr.	—	6 -7 yr.	10-12 yr.	12-14 yr.
First molar	At birth	Sometimes a trace	2½-3 yr.	6- 7 yr.	9-10 yr.
Second molar	2½- 3 yr.	—	7 -8 yr.	12-13-yr.	14-16 yr.
Mandibular					
Central incisor	3 - 4 mo.	—	4 -5 yr.	6- 7 yr.	9 yr.
Lateral incisor	3 - 4 mo.	—	4 -5 yr.	7- 8 yr.	10 yr.
Cuspid	4 - 5 mo.	—	6 -7 yr.	9-10 yr.	12-14 yr.
First bicuspid	1¾- 2 yr.	—	5 -6 yr.	10-12 yr.	12-13 yr.
Second bicuspid	2¼- 2½ yr.	—	6 -7 yr.	11-12 yr.	13-14 yr.
First molar	At birth	Sometimes a trace	2½-3 yr.	6- 7 yr.	9-10 yr.
Second molar	2½- 3 yr.	—	7 -8 yr.	11-13 yr.	14-15 yr.

*From Finn, S. B.: Clinical pedodontics, ed 2, Philadelphia, 1962, W. B. Saunders Co.; after Logan, W. H. G., and Kronfeld, R.: Development of the human jaws and surrounding structures from birth to the age of fifteen years, J.A.D.A. 20:379, 1933 (slightly modified by McCall and Schour).

in the anterior portion of the mandible, in older persons. Nutrient vessels are relatively rare in young, vigorous people.

GROWTH PATTERNS OF THE DENTITION

The chronology of the human dentition is of practical importance to the dental diagnostician. Variations from normal in development, calcification, and eruption times should raise questions and provoke answers. It is not within the province of this text to provide the answers; other reference material must be used. It is desirable, however, to make available normal schedules. Two tables are given (Tables 14-1 and 14-2). Table 14-2 complements Table 14-1 in that it differentiates between the sexes; it also differs somewhat from Table 14-1. The data in Table 14-2 are said to be the more reliable; however, in the case of a specific patient, individual variability from the statistical norm may be greater than indicated in the tables.

ANTHROPOMETRIC LANDMARKS

Embryologic and postuterine factors that play a major role in the growth of the head and face have been reviewed in this chapter. One method of evaluating the normalcy of development is by means of cephalometric radiograms. The technic for making lateral cephalometric radiograms is discussed in Chapter 7, and a portion of Fig. 7-13 is reproduced in Fig. 14-2. Although considerable study

Table 14-2. Ages for completion of calcification of permanent teeth*

Teeth	Crown completed (Nolla)		Root completed (Nolla)		Root completed (Logan and Kronfeld; modified by Schour and Massler)
	Boys	Girls	Boys	Girls	
Mandibular					
1 1	3 yr. 8 mo.	3 yr. 6 mo.	10 yr.	8 yr. 6 mo.	9 yr.
2 2	4 yr. 4 mo.	4 yr.	10 yr. 6 mo.	9 yr. 8 mo.	10 yr.
3 3	6 yr.	5 yr. 8 mo.	13 yr. 6 mo.	12 yr.	12-14 yr.
4 4	7 yr.	6 yr. 6 mo.	14 yr.	12 yr. 6 mo.	12-13 yr.
5 5	7 yr. 8 mo.	7 yr. 2 mo.	15 yr.	14 yr. 6 mo.	13-14 yr.
6 6	4 yr.	3 yr. 10 mo.	11 yr. 6 mo.	10 yr.	9-10 yr.
7 7	8 yr. 2 mo.	7 yr.	16 yr. 6 mo.	15 yr. 6 mo.	14-15 yr.
Maxillary					
1 1	4½ yr.	4½ yr.	11 yr.	10 yr.	10 yr.
2 2	5½ yr.	5 yr. 2 mo.	12 yr.	11 yr.	11 yr.
3 3	6½ yr.	5 yr. 10 mo.	15 yr.	12½ to 13 yr.	13-15 yr.
4 4	7 yr. 4 mo.	6 yr. 4 mo.	14½ yr.	12 yr. 9 mo.	12-13 yr.
5 5	8 yr. 5 mo.	7 yr. 3 mo.	15½ yr.	14 yr.	13-14 yr.
6 6	4½ yr.	4 yr. 2 mo.	11½ yr.	9½ yr.	9-10 yr.
7 7	8 yr. 2 mo.	7 yr. 6 mo.	16½ yr.	15 yr. 6 mo.	14-16 yr.

*From Nolla, C. M.: Development of the permanent teeth, J. Dent. Child. **27**:254, 1960.

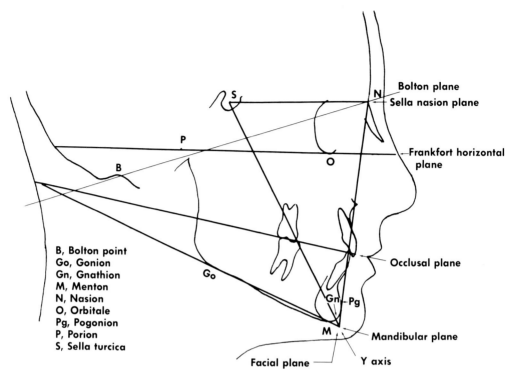

B, Bolton point
Go, Gonion
Gn, Gnathion
M, Menton
N, Nasion
O, Orbitale
Pg, Pogonion
P, Porion
S, Sella turcica

Fig. 14-2. Anthropometric landmarks of the face and skull.

has been made of variations in the posteroanterior dimension, there is a dearth of reliable radiographic information relating to lateral growth of the skull and face.

The purpose of Fig. 14-2 is to acquaint the reader with the more common anthropometric landmarks used in cephalometry. No attempt is made to discuss the normal relationship between several planes or to comment about the variations from normal. The dental practitioner should be conversant with the planes and landmarks and, if he plans to use this type of material instead of referring the patient to a specialist, should utilize other texts and periodicals to qualify himself to evaluate cephalometric radiograms.

CHAPTER 15

Common diseases of teeth and supporting structures

A very large percentage of all radiographic interpretation done in the dental office is concerned with an understanding of the normal intraoral radiographic landmarks and of variations from normal that manifest the presence of dental caries, the probable existence of some type of apical change, and alterations in the supporting structures of the teeth. Even though caries, apical changes, and periodontal disease may not be as dramatic as some other radiographic manifestations, the frequency of their occurrence requires a thorough understanding of these conditions. In addition, other conditions are frequently observed. Some of these are discussed in Chapter 16; the following are included in this chapter: tooth resorption; hypoplastic defects; pulp calcifications; tooth fractures; erosion, abrasion, and attrition; pericoronitis; and dry sockets and pulpitis.

DENTAL CARIES

Moderately advanced caries on any tooth surface can be demonstrated on a properly angulated, exposed, and processed intraoral film. Caries on some surfaces of a tooth is observed more readily radiographically than on other surfaces and may become visible at an earlier stage in the decay process. The appearance of dental caries is described in the following order: interproximal, occlusal, buccal and lingual, and cemental. Pulp exposure and factors affecting caries interpretation are discussed separately.

Interproximal caries

The intraoral radiographic film, notably the bite-wing film or the periapical radiogram made with the paralleling technic, is extremely useful in detecting interproximal carious lesions, particularly in the early stages. The first evidence of the interproximal carious lesion consists of an extremely small notching on the enamel surface below the interproximal contact point. It is pertinent to emphasize that interproximal caries ordinarily commences in the small space located between the free gingival margin and the point of contact with the adjacent tooth. As the carious lesion in the enamel increases in size, it continues to demonstrate a more or less triangular pattern with its base toward the outer surface of the tooth and with a somewhat flattened apex toward the dentoenamel junction. The carious lesion, after reaching the dentoenamel junction, tends to spread in it. From this second base, the carious process proceeds toward the pulp, roughly along the dentinal tubules, and forms another triangular radiolucency. The tendency for dentinal caries to be restricted by the paths of the tubules is not as great as in the enamel; large lesions in the dentin give an appearance of more or less diffusing through the dentin as they expand toward the pulp. When the undermined enamel fractures, the entire carious lesion radiographically acquires a kind of U shape.

Studies have shown that, when radiograms are used in addition to clinical observations, the detection of interproximal caries increases materially. The percent of increase is difficult to determine, but in one study confined to posterior proximal cavities, it was found that the increase in cavity detection was as high as 215%.* The same study (on 100 naval reserve personnel) showed that the use of bite-wing films increased caries detection in the entire mouth by 78% over the use of a mirror and explorer alone. The typical radiographic appearance of interproximal decay is illustrated and described in Fig. 15-1.

Occlusal caries

Occlusal caries in the bicuspid and molar teeth is ordinarily observed radiographically only after the decay process has penetrated through the enamel fissures to the dentoenamel junction. The first radiographic sign is a thin dark line between the enamel and the dentin. As decay progresses, this slightly dark region expands pulpally with no readily discernible margin between the carious and noncarious dentin. Occasionally, occlusal caries is confused with buccal or lingual decay. This diffuse quality permits differentiation from the buccal or lingual caries since the margins of the latter ordinarily are well defined; the shape and position of occlusal caries also differs from buccal or lingual caries. Definitive differentiation may have to be done clinically.

Occlusal caries follows the enamel rods, as in interproximal caries. The shape of the caries in the fissures is triangular, but occlusal caries differs from interproximal enamel caries in that the base or widest portion of the former is toward the dentoenamel junction and the apex of the triangle is toward the occlusal surface of the tooth. It is for this reason that occlusal caries occasionally avoids clinical detection until sufficient enamel in the region of the fissures has been undermined and fractured. Thus, the radiogram occasionally gives the first indication of occlusal caries. The **diligent use of a mirror and explorer will ordinarily detect occlusal caries before it becomes observable radiographically.** Fis-

---

*Dunning, J. M., and Ferguson, G. W: Effect of bite-wing roentgenograms on navy dental examination findings, U.S. Naval Med. Bull. **46:**83, 1946.

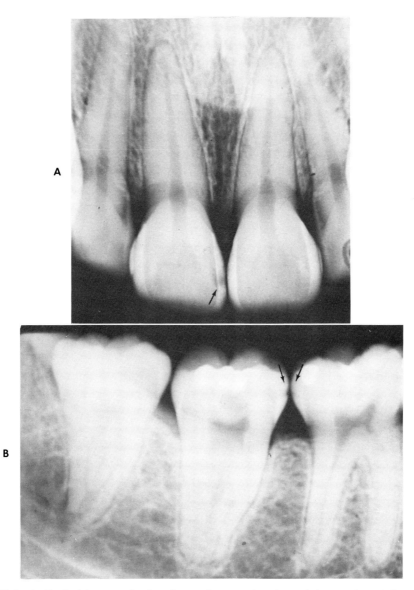

Fig. 15-1. A, Typical interproximal caries on the mesial surface of the maxillary left central incisor. Note the spread of caries at the dentoenamel junction. **B,** Interproximal caries on the distal surface of the mandibular first molar and on the mesial surface of the second molar. The dentin of the second molar is shown to be involved even though the caries does not appear to have penetrated the enamel. The radiolucent area in the center of the crown is buccal caries.

sural caries ordinarily is obscured radiographically because of the superimposition of buccal, lingual (or palatal), and occlusal enamel on a relatively small area of decay. In Fig. 15-2 is demonstrated an initial and continuing occlusal carious lesion as it is seen radiographically.

Buccal and lingual caries

Buccal and lingual, or palatal, caries ordinarily occur in the pits and grooves or in the region of the free margin of the gingiva. They penetrate toward the dentoenamel junction in the same manner as do the interproximal and occlusal caries; the enamel caries tends to follow the lines of the enamel rods. The x-rays entering the enamel defect on the buccal or lingual surface penetrate approximately parallel with the enamel rods. This is like looking into a hole. The periphery of the hole produces a relatively sharp separation of the lost and intact enamel. It is for this reason that radiographically caries on the buccal or lingual surfaces of the tooth is ordinarily well demarcated from the surrounding sound enamel. Even after the decay process has penetrated to the dentoenamel junction and has spread in this area, the undermined enamel tends to retain its integrity and provides a fairly definite periphery to the lesion. This usually clear-cut outline assists in differentiating such lesions from occlusal caries; the periphery of the latter is diffuse. Occasionally, diffuse decalcification on the buccal or lingual surfaces occurs; such lesions tend to produce less sharp radiographic images. The appearances of several different buccal and/or lingual caries are shown in Fig. 15-3.

Fig. 15-3 shows that the shape of the various lesions is either round, oval, or more or less semilunar. These shapes are largely dependent on the location of the lesion and the degree of extension. Carious lesions developing in the buccal and palatal pits are ordinarily round (Fig. 15-1). Lesions developing at the free margin of the gingiva may be round in the initial stages, but as they increase in size, they become elliptical and/or semilunar.

The location of carious lesions (that is, the differentiation of buccal from lingual, or palatal, lesions) can be done radiographically. However, this is only of academic interest. The radiographic film serves its purpose by directing the clinician's attention to the lesion; its actual location and extent can be determined through clinical observations. For this reason, no attempt is made to differentiate buccal from lingual lesions radiographically.

Because of the superimposition of the carious lesion onto the remaining dentin and the pulp, it is not possible to determine caries depth. Large buccal lesions often suggest pulp exposure when in reality the lesion may be relatively superficial.

Cemental caries

Cemental caries develops in an area between the enamel border and the free margin of the gingiva. It does not occur in areas covered by a well-attached

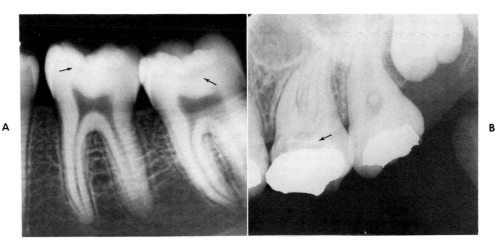

Fig. 15-2. Occlusal caries. **A,** Diffuse radiolucency can be seen in the center of the second molar just under the enamel cap. A similar but less extensive radiolucency can be observed in an identical position in the first molar. **B,** Hypercalcified or sclerosed layer is sometimes seen in the dentin below the carious lesion.

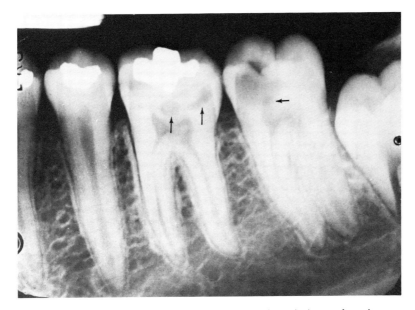

Fig. 15-3. Buccal and/or lingual caries. Several carious lesions of various types are illustrated. Buccal or lingual caries can be observed in the first molar in the center of the tooth and distal to the tooth center below the opaque metallic restoration. Occlusal caries exists in the second molar, and a buccal or lingual lesion can be seen through it. Inter-proximal caries is seen on the distal aspect of the second bicuspid and on the mesial aspect of the first molar; in the latter case, the caries has extended well into the dentin. A relatively slight amount of enamel destruction is also located interproximally between the first and second molars.

gingiva; it occasionally does invade under the thin gingival margin of enamel. Histopathologically, decay in the cementum simply invades without any particular pattern. The effect is a kind of scooping-out process that may have a broad or a narrow base, depending largely on the amount of root surface exposed. Radiographically, this is usually described as a saucer-shaped lesion of varying depth. The periphery is diffuse. This fact, accompanied by its location, differentiates the cemental carious lesion from the buccal, lingual, or interproximal lesion. Cemental caries occurs less frequently than do the other types previously discussed. Such lesions are ordinarily not missed by the clinician, because interproximally they stand out rather clearly on the radiogram and are easily detected clinically on the buccal and lingual surfaces. A frequent error is of great importance in the radiographic detection of cemental carious lesions and/or carious lesions under the interproximal step of metallic restorations. This error is that of confusing such carious lesions with cervical burnout. A typical carious lesion of the cementum is illustrated in Fig. 15-4. Cervical burnout is also discussed on p. 311.

Pulp exposure

Teeth frequently are removed or treated endodontically because radiographic evidence suggests carious exposure of the pulp. Radiographic evidence suggesting pulpal exposure, with or without apical change, should not be used as the only definitive criterion for either tooth removal or endodontic therapy. It is possible, through angulation changes, to create an appearance radiographically that

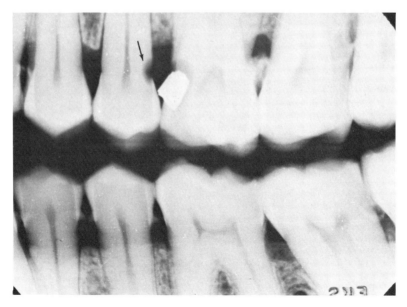

Fig. 15-4. Cemental caries. A typical carious lesion of the cementum can be observed on the distal aspect of the maxillary second bicuspid.

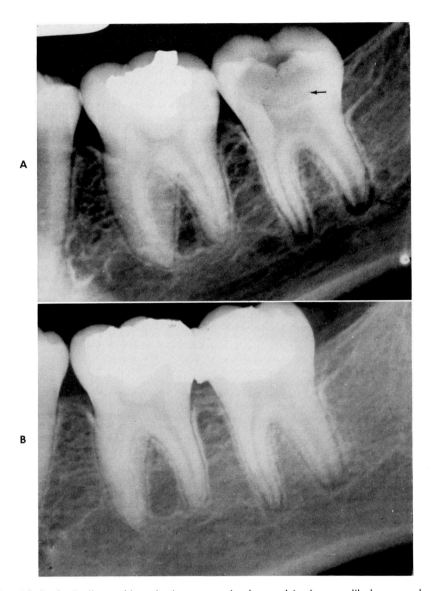

Fig. 15-5. A, Radiographic pulpal exposure is observed in the mandibular second molar, and apically there is radiographic evidence of a thickened periodontal space. Careful excavation of this tooth failed to produce clinical exposure. **B,** Same molar was restored using a calcium hydroxide subbase followed by a zinc phosphate base and a zinc oxide—eugenol treatment restoration. The tooth retained its vitality. The apical thickening is the end product of root formation.

simulates pulpal exposure. It is also possible to observe a normal widening of the periodontal space at the apex of the same tooth.

Although most instances of radiographic pulpal exposure will be substantiated clinically, it is important for the dentist to verify clinically the presence of pulpal exposure. Careful restorative procedures can result in the retention of many teeth condemned solely on the basis of radiographic evidence of pulpal exposure. The data given in Fig. 15-5 should assist in substantiating these remarks.

Factors affecting caries interpretation

Throughout this text, stress has been placed on the need for excellence in radiographic technics. A number of factors affect the ability of the operator to detect carious lesions accurately. These potential shortcomings are discussed rather fully in this section; however, they relate to radiographic interpretation in general. It is hoped that these remarks will serve to emphasize the critical need for technical excellence on the part of the individual producing the films.

Contrast scale. The contrast scale observed in the radiogram can be varied clinically. The principal factors involved include kilovoltage, filtration, film exposure, and darkroom processing.

Much has been written in recent years concerning the use of kilovoltage variation in dental radiography. Modern dental x-ray machines have a range of approximately 50 to 100 kVp. Changes in kilovoltage control the penetrability of the x-rays and alter radiographic contrast. The desirable degree of contrast varies and depends on the structures being observed. The detection of carious lesions appears to be easier when kilovoltages in the range of approximately 65 to 70 kVp are used. Kilovoltages lower than this necessitate excessive exposure in order for the rays to penetrate the heavy enamel; kilovoltages above this level result in films that have a broad scale of contrast and hence tend to impair the operator's ability to observe the carious lesion. It is recommended that bite-wing films taken for the detection of interproximal caries be exposed at 65 to 70 kVp. It may be advantageous to expose periapical and periodontal films at higher kilovoltages. There is evidence suggesting that the use of higher kilovoltages combined with relatively dark films and specialized viewing technics produces optimal results.

Excessive filtration overly hardens the x-ray beam. Insofar as caries interpretation is concerned, it has approximately the same effect on caries interpretation as does high kilovoltage.

The interpretation of dental caries is probably best done on films that have been rather heavily exposed and thus are quite dark. Such procedures tend to produce a dark carious area surrounded by a rather light enamel through which the x-rays found difficulty in penetrating. Dark films, which may be highly satisfactory for the interpretation of caries, are not ordinarily satisfactory for the interpretation of other disease processes.

Film processing will affect the contrast observed on the radiogram. High solution temperatures result in high contrast; cold solutions broaden the scale of contrast and give a gray-looking film. Underdeveloped films result in a light image; this underdevelopment can result from weak solutions or insufficient developing time. For sufficient contrast to be obtained for caries interpretation, film processing must be rigidly controlled.

Inaccuracy of caries size. The size of the carious lesion as seen radiographically is usually not the same as is seen microscopically or after clinical excavation of the decay. The size usually appears smaller on the radiogram than actually exists. Under some circumstances the lesion may appear to extend into areas of the crown that in reality are not carious; in these instances the carious lesion is exaggerated.

Minimization of caries. The minimization of caries should be considered from two aspects: (1) the incipient carious lesion and (2) the small to moderately large lesion. The incipient carious lesion cannot be seen radiographically until there has been a sufficient degree of enamel decalcification to permit an observable radiographic density difference between the decay and the enamel. For example, slight etches found on the mesial surface of a first molar after the deciduous second molar has been removed are often not observable radiographically. It is also important to mention that overexposure of the peripheral surface, particularly when low kilovoltages are used, tends to burn out the enamel peripheral surface and thus obliterate the decayed area. In Fig. 15-6 are shown two

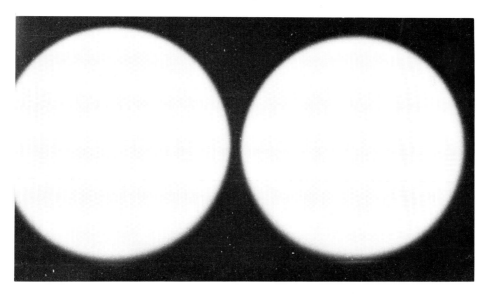

Fig. 15-6. Peripheral burnout. The two ivory spheres, which clinically were in *direct contact,* demonstrate so-called burnout of the spheres' peripheries. This was accomplished using a relatively light exposure; heavier exposure produces greater separation of the spheres. It is useful to note that an intense light would assist in visualizing the burned-out surfaces.

contacting ivory spheres that received a light exposure. It is obvious that a simulated carious lesion in the burned-out periphery of the sphere could not be observed radiographically. This phenomenon also can be illustrated clinically. Teeth in proximal contact are shown in Fig. 15-7. The space between the two bicuspid teeth has been artificially widened through the use of increasing amounts of exposure. It is also pertinent that incipient occlusal, buccal, and lingual carious lesions are not ordinarily observed radiographically, because they are superimposed on a large amount of tooth structure.

As the small to moderately large carious lesion progresses, its depth is minimized radiographically. This is true for two reasons: (1) radiographic evidence of caries will not be observed until there is sufficient decalcification to provide

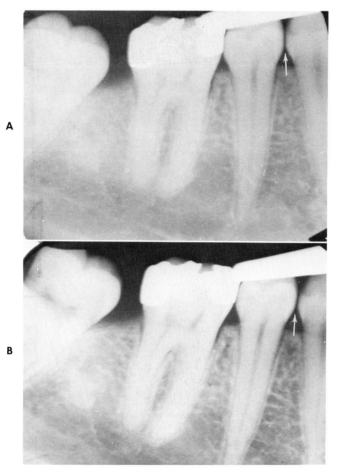

Fig. 15-7. Peripheral burnout. The interproximal contact between the mandibular bicuspids was sufficiently tight to necessitate forcing of dental floss through the interproximal space. A space was created radiographically in both **A** and **B**. The space in **B** is slightly wider because of increased exposure.

a difference in density between normal and carious structures. It is well known that the carious process precedes massive decalcification. (2) The ratio of sound tooth structure through which the x-rays must penetrate to the size of the lesion will vary in different areas of the tooth. In interproximal caries, the greatest ratio of sound tooth structure to decay exists in the enamel just peripheral to the den- toenamel junction. The carious area is relatively narrow, whereas the thickness of enamel through which the rays must penetrate, particularly in the molar teeth, is great. As a result, the heavy overlying sound enamel often attenuates the x-ray beam to the extent that little radiation reaches the film; since the film remains relatively unexposed at this point, little or no caries can be observed. Once the interproximal carious lesion has reached the dentoenamel junction, it can usually be observed quite readily in the radiogram. However, the observable extent of the lesion continues to be less than the *actual* extent of the process. This phe- nomenon is diagrammatically shown in Fig. 15-8.

The occlusal carious lesion ordinarily is first observed radiographically after it has reached the dentoenamel junction (Fig. 15-2). Like the interproximal lesion, its size in the dentin is minimized.

Buccal and lingual carious lesions will be observed radiographically as soon as the amount of decalcification produces a significant difference in density be- tween normal and carious tooth structures.

Exaggeration of caries. The carious lesion may appear enlarged as a result of a burnout of thin normal tooth structure existing between a large carious lesion and the pulp or the outer surface of the tooth. In addition, the large

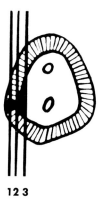

1 2 3

Fig. 15-8. Diagram of a bicuspid tooth illustrating the ratio of enamel to caries through which x-ray photons must penetrate. Photon 1 is seen to be penetrating a minimum amount of enamel and a maximum amount of caries. Photon 2 is penetrating a maximum amount of enamel and a minimum amount of caries. Photon 3 penetrates buccal and lingual enamel plus dentin or carious dentin. The attenuation of photons in region 2 will obviously be greater than that of those in region 1 or 3. Thus the radiograph frequently shows little or no radiolucency in the area just peripheral to the dentoenamel junction.

carious lesion may be superimposed on the pulp chamber and give the illusion of an increase in the size of the carious lesion (Fig. 15-5).

Angulation. Faulty angulation, both horizontal and vertical, frequently interferes with the detection of the interproximal carious lesion, particularly the small defect. Once the carious process has reached the stage at which it is observable clinically, angulation errors do not impair the observance of the lesion. However, the radiographic film is most useful in the detection of the early lesion, and it is for this reason that angulation must be accurate.

If the paralleling technic is used, the vertical angulation is optimal; the rays are directed at right angles to the tooth and the film, both of which are parallel with one another. The carious lesion is superimposed on a minimum amount of sound tooth structure; also, the x-ray beam is directed through the greater dimension of the carious lesion since the interproximal lesion spreads more buccolingually than in a vertical direction. When the bisecting technic is used, the central ray is directed through the area of the carious lesion in such a manner that the small lesion is superimposed on a great amount of sound tooth structure; the lesion is frequently obliterated. In addition, the x-ray beam crosses the carious lesion in a relatively narrow dimension. The effect of vertical angulation is illustrated in Fig. 15-9. When an angle-bisecting technic is used, bitewing films are imperative. The bite-wing film procedures employ the principles of the paralleling technic.

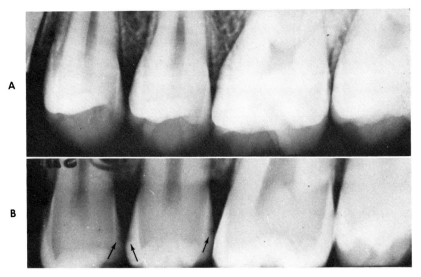

Fig. 15-9. Effect of vertical angulation on caries detection. **A,** Radiogram taken using the bisecting technic. **B,** Radiogram taken using the paralleling technic. The same results could be obtained on a bite-wing film. Note that carious lesions can be observed in the lower film interproximately between the biscuspids and on the distal surface of second bicuspid These lesions are not observable in **A.**

Faulty horizontal angulation can be defined as failure to project the x-rays directly through the interproximal space or spaces of the teeth under observation. This procedure results in superimposition of one adjacent tooth on another. Such faulty angulation tends to hide the small interproximal carious lesion in the dense, superimposed enamel. Such superimposition is illustrated in Fig. 15-10.

Faulty angulation has a greater influence over interproximal caries detection than over occlusal, buccal, or lingual caries detection. Excessive vertical angulation occasionally results in the detection of occlusal caries that would not be observed if optimal technic were used. When the x-rays strike the occlusal surface at an increased angle, the outline of the occlusal fissures becomes increasingly well defined.

Restorative materials. Restorative materials of relatively high atomic weights, notably the metals, appear radiopaque when observed on the x-ray film and hence are not confused with dental caries. Conversely, restorative materials such as the silicates and particularly the plastics tend to be radiolucent and to simulate dental caries.

The radiographic differentiation between silicate and plastic restorations is not a critical matter, since clinical observation will provide the desired answer.

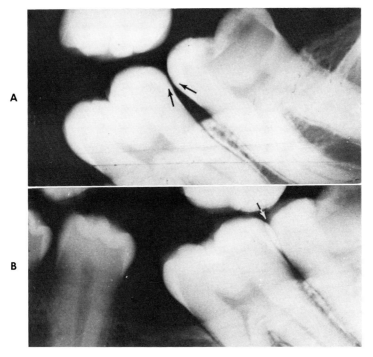

Fig. 15-10. Effect of horizontal angulation on caries detection. **A,** Interproximal caries between the two mandibular molars. **B,** Same two teeth, but the interproximal surfaces are overlapped through faulty angulation, and the carious lesions are obliterated.

The fact that these materials require the use of a suitable radiopaque base assists the clinician in differentiating them from caries. Both zinc oxide–eugenol and zinc phosphate cements appear radiopaque. In addition, the typical Class III cavity preparation into which the silicate and plastic restorative materials are ordinarily placed shows a U-shaped appearance quite different in outline from the beginning carious lesion.

It is important to realize that calcium hydroxide also may be radiolucent. The amount of calcium in relation to the radiolucent carrier or binding material is relatively small. However, some commercially available preparations containing calcium hydroxide are quite radiopaque. Calcium hydroxide is ordinarily used as a subbase between an exposure or a near exposure and conventional restorative base materials. Since it cannot be observed clinically, the operator would be aided if the radiographic film could assist him in differentiating caries under restorations from calcium hydroxide. Unfortunately, such a differentiation cannot be made if the calcium hydroxide is radiolucent, but there are a few clues that may be helpful. When properly placed, calcium hydroxide appears radiographically as a thin radiolucent line. If the radiographic appearance is much wider than approximately the thickness of a pencil line, the operator should be suspicious that he is dealing with caries rather than with calcium hydroxide. In addition, it will be helpful for the operator to observe the sharpness or unsharpness of the cavity preparation. The border of the carious lesion in dentin is ordinarily poorly defined. If this border is sharply demarcated, it is likely

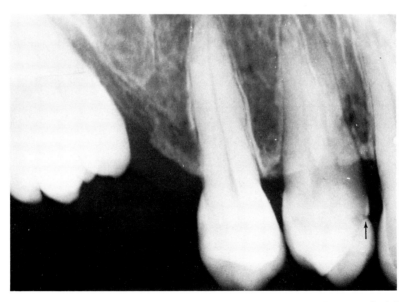

Fig. 15-11. Mesial surface of the first bicuspid illustrates a developmental defect that simulates caries. Note that the proximal surface of the tooth tends to curve inward. This is not a characteristic of the normal tooth with a typical carious lesion.

that the carious material has been removed and that the dark line under the restoration represents a layer of calcium hydroxide. Restorative materials are illustrated in Chapter 13.

Developmental pits. Developmental defects, particularly isolated hypoplastic areas, can simulate caries radiographically. In the case of a hypoplastic pit, the enamel surface tends to curve inward into the defect. If a carious lesion is present, the contour of the enamel is normal but its periphery is interrupted by the notch of caries. These characteristics are useful in differentiating interproximal caries from a hypoplastic pit on the proximal surface. Pits on the buccal or lingual surface simulate caries but are readily identified on clinical examination. An interproximal developmental pit that simulates caries is illustrated in Fig. 15-11.

Cervical burnout. The neck of the tooth, the area between the crown and that portion of the root covered by supporting bone, absorbs less of the x-rays than do the areas above and below it. This is due to the presence of the enamel and supporting alveolar bone in the latter areas. As a result, radiograms often show either a radiolucent band running across the tooth (Fig. 15-12) or a triangular radiolucency in the same region on the mesial and/or distal surface.

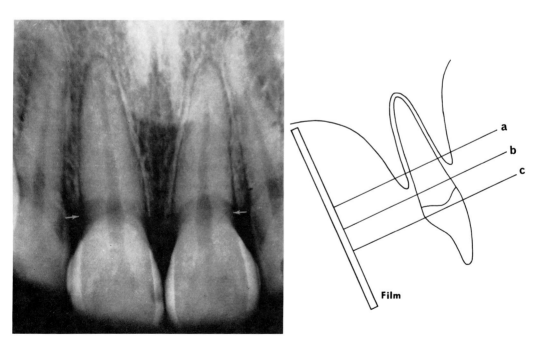

Fig. 15-12. Cervical burnout. A radiolucency can be observed, particularly in the necks of the maxillary central incisors, running across the entire width of the tooth. Such burnout is the result of a decrease in total structural thickness and/or a change in the hard tissue composition. The accompanying diagram illustrates this concept. Lines *a* and *c* penetrate more or more dense tissue than does line *b*.

In addition to density differences resulting from the enamel and the supportive bone, the appearance of cervical burnout is caused by root configuration and the shape of the cementoenamel contour. These principles are illustrated in Fig. 15-13. Cervical burnout should not be confused with cemental caries or with caries under the proximal step of Class II restorations. The practitioner must remember that cemental caries will not occur unless the free margin of the gingiva has receded from its normal position. Areas of cervical burnout are most often observed when no alveolar bone has been lost, because these radiolucencies depend partially on the presence of the alveolar bone to provide the necessary contrast. It is essential that clinical exploration verify the presence of cemental caries.

Optical illusion. When the interproximal surfaces of two teeth overlap, the overlapped radiopaque enamel is outlined by what appears to be a radiolucent line. This is actually an optical illusion. Optical illusions are discussed in Chapter

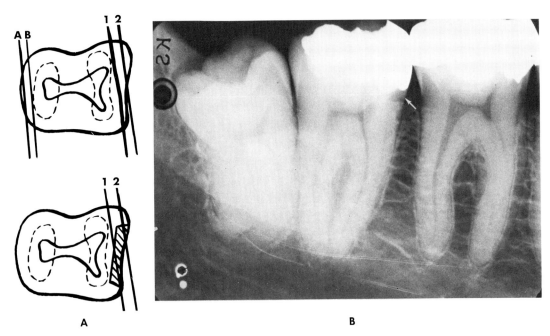

A   B

Fig. 15-13. A, Upper figure illustrates the reasons for cervical burnout. In the top figure, x-ray photons A and 2 have considerably less structural thickness through which to pass than do photos B and 1. The lower figure illustrates the same phenomenon except that the diagonal lines are added to represent the proximal step of a metallic restoration. The addition of this radiopaque material results in a sharp radiographic contrast between the opaque restoration, the moderately light portion of the tooth represented by photon 1, and the comparatively dark portion of the tooth represented by photon 2. **B,** Mesial surface of the mandibular second molar below the opaque restoration illustrates this type of burnout. Burnout can also be observed on the mesial and distal surfaces of the first molar, particularly on the mesial surface.

11 (Fig. 11-4). This phenomenon of optical illusion is of significance clinically because the apparent radiolucency surrounding the overlapped interproximal enamel tends to mask small lesions. Somewhat similarly, the apparent radiolucent line differentiating occlusal enamel from dentin sometimes is confused with a spread of caries at the dentoenamel junction.

APICAL LESIONS

The radiographic film serves an extremely important need in detecting disease processes that affect the tooth root and surrounding bone. In the absence of clinical symptoms, pathologic changes in bone are ordinarily not detected except through radiographic means. The dental practitioner must understand fully the significance of changes occurring at the root end. It is equally essential that the practitioner recognize the limitations of radiographic information.

Apical changes considered in this section are those common to general practice. They include periapical radiolucencies, early radiographic periapical signs, root apex changes, and bone changes associated with apical alterations. No emphasis is placed on changes occurring on the lateral surface of the tooth root because of the presence of accessory root canals. Suffice it to say that changes occurring apically can also occur on the lateral surface of the root. Radiographic findings not commonly observed in a general dental practice are discussed in Chapters 16 and 17.

Periapical radiolucencies

The average practitioner of dentistry usually thinks of an apical lesion as being either an abscess, a granuloma, or a cyst. He may envision some rather specific radiographic characteristics for each of these lesions, and he may attach significance to the radiographic appearance. The practitioner often bases his treatment on this appearance; he usually feels the need for enucleating cysts but feels justified in permitting abscesses and granulomas to remain in situ.

Investigative work has clearly established that the abscess, granuloma, and cyst cannot be differentiated on a radiographic basis. The apical lesion measuring approximately a half inch or less in diameter, which was formerly thought of as either a granuloma, abscess, or cyst, must simply be considered evidence of bone change in the region of the root apex. One modification to this statement exists: if a lesion has the usually accepted radiographic characteristics of a cyst, it is likely to be a cyst.

Radiographic signs. The apical lesion will show an interrupted lamina dura. The peripheral appearance of the lesion can vary greatly. It may be indistinct and tend to blend into the surrounding bone; a definite demarcation may exist between the lesion and the bone; or the lesion may exhibit a distinct bone lamina encircling the radiolucency. The shape of apical lesions is basically spherical; however, they may be irregular in outline or may show a smooth periphery. The immediately surrounding bone may appear normal; it may give the appearance

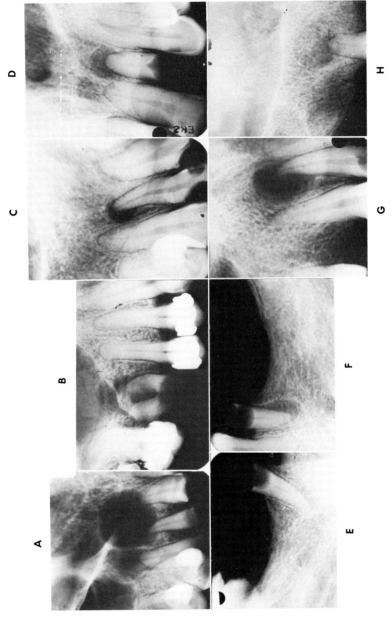

Fig. 15-14. From among 101 cases, these eight examples illustrate the diagnostician's inability to interpret apical lesions accurately on a radiographic basis. Each of the films was interpreted clinically and then evaluated histologically, with the following results: **A,** Interpretation, cyst; microscopic evaluation, cyst. **B,** Interpretation, granuloma; microscopic evaluation, cyst. **C,** Interpretation, cyst; microscopic evaluation, granuloma. **D,** Interpretation, granuloma; microscopic evaluation, cyst. **E,** Interpretation, granuloma; microscopic evaluation, cyst. **F,** Interpretation, granuloma; microscopic evaluation, granuloma. **G,** Interpretation, cyst; microscopic evaluation, cyst. **H,** Interpretation, granuloma; microscopic evaluation, granuloma.

of porosity; or it may present evidence of sclerosis or condensing osteitis—increased bone opacity with a reduction in the size of the trabecular spaces. The center of the lesion can vary from almost total blackness to a shade of gray that is approximately the same as the surrounding bone.

Common pathologic conditions. The above radiographic signs have been given meaning by some diagnosticians based largely on intuitive analysis rather than on research data. An ill-defined periphery suggests invasion of the surrounding bone. Conversely, a well-defined periphery indicates that the lesion is more self-contained and that its enlargement is by expansion rather than by invasion. The presence of a lamina dura–like periphery is suggestive of a very slow growing lesion. An irregular shape, in contradistinction to a rounded form, suggests invasion rather than expansion. The surrounding bone that shows no change suggests a static lesion. Porosity indicates bone breakdown suggestive of an invasive process. Sclerosis shows resistance to the pathologic process. Dark, well-outlined, spherical lesions are thought of as being cystic; lesions that tend to blend more closely with the surrounding bone often are considered to be abscesses or granulomas.

The significance of these signs is questionable. The varied appearances of the abscess, granuloma, and cyst are shown in Fig. 15-14; each has been confirmed histologically. It is obvious that apical lesions can easily be misinterpreted if one tries to differentiate the abscess, granuloma, and cyst from radiographic data.

Less common pathologic conditions. Any condition that reduces the density of the bone in the area of the tooth apex can give the appearance of a periapical radiolucency. There are many conditions that could be discussed under this category—for example, fibro-osseous lesions, neoplastic changes, and various infections.

The most frequently observed lesion in this category is the cementoblastoma, the first stage of cementoma formation. This lesion occurs most frequently in the lower anterior region. A typical cementoblastoma is shown in Fig. 15-15.

Superimposition. It must be remembered that anatomic entities such as the mental and incisive foramina, as well as pathologic cavities separated from the tooth apex, can be superimposed on the tooth apex. Such superimpositions may simulate apical pathology. This situation is shown in Fig. 15-16.

Early radiographic periapical signs

The abscess, granuloma, and cyst have been discussed first because they offer points of greatest controversy and because they are the lesions most frequently observed by the dental practitioner. However, there are some radiographic signs that, in point of time, precede the formation of periapical radiolucencies. Other appearances, though normal in nature, resemble early periapical signs. Under certain circumstances, pathologic change is not observable radiographically. Early radiographic periapical signs are categorized and discussed as follows: (1)

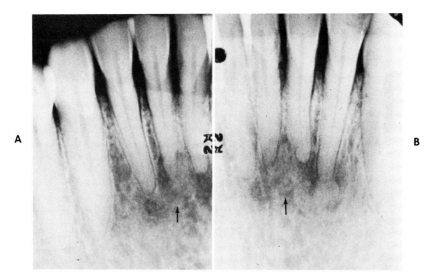

Fig. 15-15. Cementoblastoma. Technically, the cementoblastoma should have no areas of calcification within the lesion. If calcified areas exist, the lesion is a Stage 1 cementoma. **B** shows one definitely calcified area at the apex of the lateral tooth; in all other respects the appearance is that of a typical cementoblastoma.

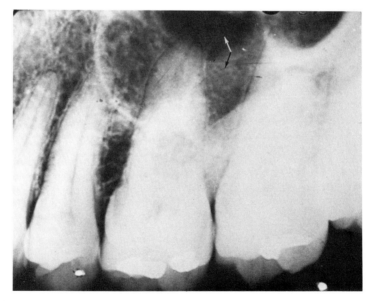

Fig. 15-16. Superimposition of a portion of the maxillary sinus on the apex of the palatal root of the first molar suggests the possibility of apical disease. A close observation of the apical area indicates the continuity of the periodontal space. The dark area (upper arrow) is simply a portion of the sinus that has greater horizontal depth than does the area below (lower arrow).

no change in osseous configuration, (2) periodontal space thickening, and (3) interruption in the continuity of the lamina dura.

No change in osseous configuration. It must be recognized that the radiographic film is an adjunct to oral diagnosis, and clinical findings are important. The most obvious example of this is the absence of radiographic alterations in the presence of acute clinical symptoms. Unless the acute symptoms have resulted from a flare-up of a prior chronic lesion, destruction of the hard tissues will not ordinarily have proceeded sufficiently within a matter of a few days to be observable radiographically. Thus acute conditions such as an acute abscess or the beginning stages of osteomyelitis will not demonstrate radiographic change.

It is important to emphasize that curved roots turning toward either the buccal or lingual aspect ordinarily do not show the root end in the conventional periapical film. The apparent root end is merely the curved root surface; the apex is superimposed on the root. It becomes obvious that slight changes at the apex of such a root cannot be observed radiographically. This type of root curvature is shown in Fig. 15-17.

Pulp disease detected clinically is ordinarily expected to show some periapical change. Apical changes that might be anticipated as a result of pulp exposure may not be recognized either clinically or radiographically if the apical foramen

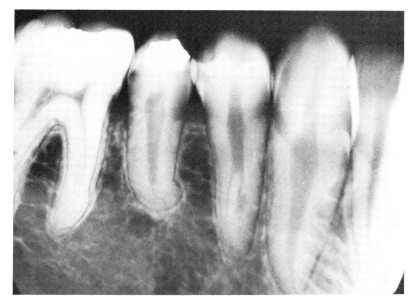

Fig. 15-17. Root curvature of the mandibular second biscuspid results in the root end, as seen radiographically, being different from the apical end; the latter is literally buried behind root structure. Under these circumstances, beginning apical disease would be difficult, if not impossible, to observe. The radiolucency directly below the blunted root is likely to be the mental foramen, or it may be normal trabecular structure.

becomes sealed through the production of cementum or dentin. Apical closures are ordinarily associated with diminution in size of the pulp canal.

Periodontal space thickening. Periodontal space thickening can occur from both pathologic conditions and nonpathologic circumstances.

Pathologic periodontal space thickening. Pathologic thickening of the periodontal space can occur as a result of tooth extrusion, root resorption, or resorption of the lamina dura. Clinical manifestations of acute initial pericementitis are usually not accompanied by radiographic evidence of periodontal space thickening. The lack of significant decalcification accounts for the absence of radiographic signs.

A thickening of the periodontal space because of tooth extrusion ordinarily is associated with the initial symptoms of osteomyelitis or with trauma; it is not usually associated with common types of periapical pathology. Thickening of the periodontal space can also occur as a result of root resorption associated with periapical change; root resorption is discussed separately in this chapter. The most common cause of pathologic periodontal space thickening is the progressive destruction of the lamina dura because of infection; such thickening is illustrated in Fig. 15-18.

Nonpathologic periodontal space thickening. It is important for the dentist to recognize that the periodontal space surrounding the tooth root, particularly

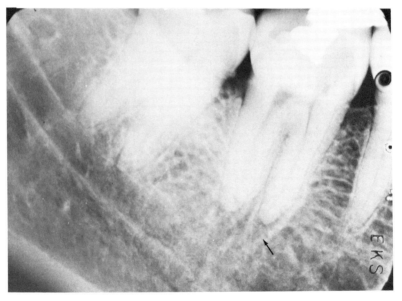

Fig. 15-18. Thickening of the periodontal space at the root ends of the mandibular first molar. A large occlusal carious lesion can be observed; the tooth was clinically determined to be nonvital.

the area at the tooth apex, is frequently widened from causes other than those of a pathologic nature. It is also important to emphasize that the normal periodontal space in different individuals varies and occasionally may be wider than expected. However, in these instances, the entire space rather than the area just at the apex of the tooth is ordinarily thickened.

Probably the most frequent cause of a wide periodontal space is the terminal stage of root formation. The radiographic appearance of the forming root is well known. Somewhat less well understood is the fact that a wide periodontal space at the root end may persist for approximately 6 months after the completion of root development. When evidence of periodontal space thickening is associated with the presence of extensive caries that appears radiographically to involve the pulp, a tendency exists to condemn the tooth. A mandibular second molar with extensive caries that appears to involve the pulp is shown in Fig. 15-5; the tooth apex demonstrates thickening of the periodontal space. There was no pulp exposure. The tooth was restored uneventfully. The purpose of this illustration is to emphasize a possible error when a diagnosis of pulpal exposure is made solely on radiographic evidence and is not substantiated clinically through exploration with an explorer or a bur.

The superimposition of a tooth apex on a radiolucent area such as the nasal fossa, the maxillary sinus, the mental foramen, or the submandibular fossa, or on

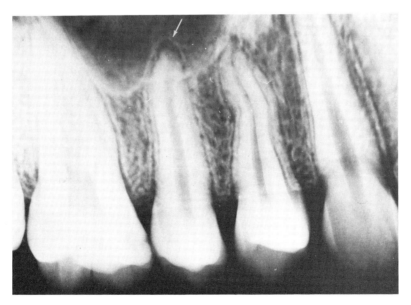

Fig. 15-19. Widening of the periodontal space can result from tooth trauma or from superimposition of the apex on a radiolucent area. In this illustration the tooth apex is superimposed on the maxillary sinus. Traumatic occlusion was also a factor. Such thickening should not be considered pathologic.

any other indentation or cavity in the bone will often result in an appearance of periodontal space thickening. This can be explained on the basis of localized film overexposure or burnout. As a result of superimposing an anatomic landmark of minimum density on the apex, the rays passing through the apical area are attenuated less than they normally would be if the structures were more dense. Because of this, the peripheral surface of the root end as well as the inner surface of the lamina dura are burned out in a manner not unlike that described earlier in this chapter in the discussion of cemental caries and the incipient interproximal carious lesion. This condition is demonstrated in Fig. 15-19. Overly heavy exposure of the entire film produces the same result. It is important to reemphasize that such widening of the periodontal space must not be interpreted as a pathologic periapical change.

Trauma to a tooth results in a thickening of the periodontal space. If the individual is capable physiologically of withstanding this trauma, the periodontal space will return to its normal appearance after the elimination of the trauma. Orthodontic tooth movement is a frequent cause of periodontal space thickening. The degree of space thickening associated with orthodontic treatment is some-

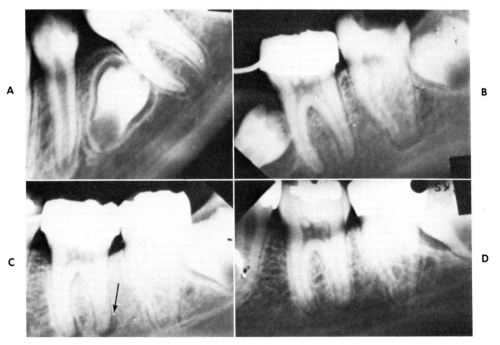

Fig. 15-20. Trauma in the form of orthodontic treatment frequently results in thickening of the periodontal space. This illustration shows sequential films wherein considerable orthodontic stress was placed on the mandibular first molar. **A,** Preorthodontic treatment film. **B,** Same general area soon after the start of treatment. **C,** Periodontal space thickening in a tooth that was clinically completely normal. **D,** Same tooth in normal position some time later.

times alarming to the beginning practitioner (Fig. 15-20). Transient trauma resulting from a blow or a slight, persistent trauma, such as that resulting from occlusal imbalance, may create varying degrees of periodontal space thickening. Any of these circumstances in the presence of massive caries or obscure clinical symptoms could influence the practitioner to make a hasty decision and to institute endodontic or exodontic measures.

Interruption in the continuity of the lamina dura. The lamina dura at the tooth apex may be destroyed as part of the development of an apical radiolucency. In slowly expansive lesions the lamina dura is often pushed back away from the tooth apex. It tends to surround such lesions and to remain continuous with the lamina dura on the lateral surface of the tooth root.

Superimposition of the lamina dura on an anatomic entity of minimum density or an excessively heavy total film exposure can produce an apparent break in the lamina dura. This situation is illustrated in Fig. 15-21. Root apices that extend into the maxillary sinus often demonstrate a lack of lamina dura. This may be due to the actual nonexistence of a bony lamina.

Root end changes

Root end changes associated with apical lesions are restricted to hypercementosis and root resorption.

Hypercementosis. Hypercementosis is a rather frequently observed condition; it probably occurs as a result of several etiologic factors. Typical hypercemento-

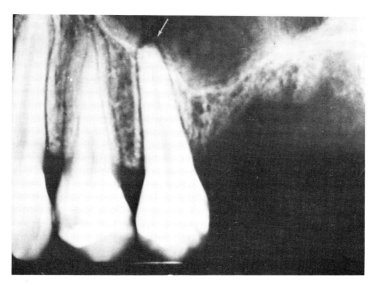

Fig. 15-21. Periodontal space thickening and loss of lamina dura are illustrated at the apex of the second biscuspid. This condition is partially due to superimposition on the maxillary sinus (see Fig. 15-19); it also resulted from tooth trauma caused by the stress placed on this tooth as a partial denture abutment. The tooth vitality was normal.

sis is illustrated in Fig. 15-22. It is ordinarily described as clubbing of the root end. The lamina dura and periodontal space are generally intact, and sometimes the outline of the original tooth can be observed within the mass. Hypercementosed teeth are often vital, but a pathologic condition can be superimposed.

Root resorption. Apical root resorption occurs in two forms, smooth and rough.

Smooth root resorption. Smooth root resorption at the apex of the tooth is frequently associated with a history of transient trauma or orthodontic therapy. The root appears shortened and blunted, but its surface is relatively smooth, and it is clearly surrounded by a distinct periodontal space and lamina dura. The tooth is ordinarily vital, although the pulp canal may be partially or totally obliterated. Fig. 15-23, *A*, illustrates smooth apical root resorption.

Rough root resorption. Rough apical root resorption (Fig. 15-23, *B*) is characterized by a roughened surface of the root periphery; it is often associated with infection. The periodontal space is ordinarily widened and may be nonexistent. The lamina dura is usually absent. A distinct apical lesion may be present. Root resorption can occur within the canal and/or on the external root surface. The presence and extent of apical root resorption are of special significance when endodontic therapy is contemplated.

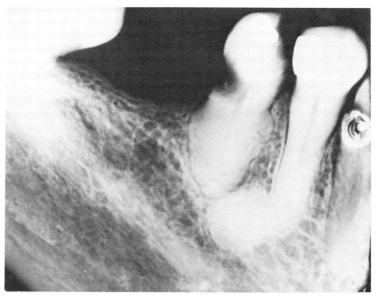

Fig. 15-22. Typical hypercementosed clubbing of the second bicuspid root. The periodontal space is intact and the tooth is vital in spite of the fact that carious exposure of the pulp exists (the carious exposure was determined clinically). The first biscuspid demonstrates a cementoma and possibly some hypercementosis.

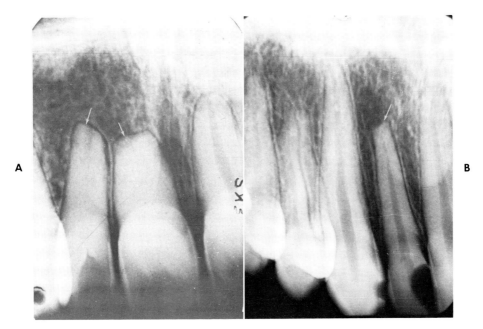

Fig. 15-23. Apical root resorption. **A,** Smooth root resorption is shown on the maxillary central and lateral teeth. Patient had a history of trauma several years previously. **B,** Rough root resorption is illustrated on the lateral tooth. Patient demonstrated a clinically nonvital tooth.

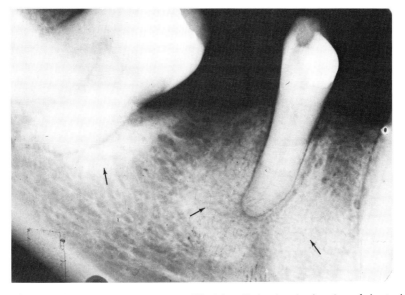

Fig. 15-24. Condensing osteitis, as exemplified by diminution in the size of the trabecular pattern, is illustrated in the area of the mandibular bicuspid root as well as mesial to the first molar root.

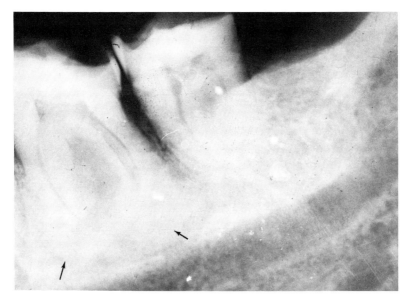

Fig. 15-25. True ankylosis of tooth to bone is a fairly rare occurrence. In this instance, there was complete fusion of these teeth, particularly the one on the left, to bone. Evidence of this was established through surgical removal.

Bone changes associated with apical alterations. Radiolucent bone changes directly related to apical alterations have been discussed. Radiopaque changes include condensing osteitis and ankylosis.

Condensing osteitis. Bone sclerosis, condensing osteitis or sclerosing osteitis, is believed to develop as a result of stress, trauma, or infection. It is generally characterized radiographically by reduction in the size of both the trabecular spaces and trabeculae, an increase in their number, and an increase in the opacity of the involved bone. The extent of the area involved varies greatly. This condition is illustrated in Fig. 15-24.

Ankylosis. Bone and tooth roots occasionally become fused. Such a union is called ankylosis. Root resorption, particularly that of an idiopathic nature, often is accompanied by a bony replacement of tooth structure (Fig. 15-34). This type of fibrous union is sometimes described as a pseudoankylosis. Quite infrequently, strong bonding occurs between root and bone; under these circumstances it is impossible to observe separation between tooth and bone radiographically. Ankylosis is illustrated in Fig. 15-25.

PERIODONTAL DISEASE

The use of periapical and bite-wing films is probably less important in the diagnosis of periodontal disease than it is in the detection of dental caries and apical lesions. This is true because the radiogram cannot show soft tissue changes. However, the radiogram can be of considerable value when used as an adjunct to clinical findings and laboratory tests. The radiographic film can be of assistance in observing the presence of incipient periodontal disease and in locating the areas of bone loss. Radiographic film can help evaluate the amount of bone remaining, the direction of bone loss, and the relative activity of the destructive process. The radiogram assists the practitioner in establishing a prognosis and in evaluating the healing process. In addition, the radiographic film is of value in locating irritants such as calculus, overhanging restorations, rough carious margins, and so forth. There is now some research evidence that the radiogram, by showing variations in the trabecular pattern of bone and the existence of nutrient vessels, can suggest the possibility of systemic complications that may relate to periodontal disease. Studies of this nature are limited; this is an area of investigation and probable clinical significance that has been ignored by the profession. Because variations in bone pattern and the existence of nutrient vessels are not, of themselves disease entities or clinically definitive conditions, they are discussed in Chapter 17 rather than in this chapter. The reader's attention is directed to pp. 427 and 448 and to Figs. 17-32 and 17-33.

Commonly used radiographic technics do not permit evaluation of soft structures. However, the depth of pockets can be determined radiographically by the use of opaque media such as metal probes, gutta-percha points, and radiopaque pastes. These technics ordinarily are not used because the same information can be secured clinically. For this reason, the use of opaque media in the diagnosis of periodontal disease is not discussed.

Incipient periodontal disease

Incipient periodontal disease can be recognized both clinically and radiographically. The high prevalence of moderate to advanced periodontal disease suggests that the incipient stage of the disease process is not being recognized and/or treated.

Radiographic evidence of incipient periodontal disease takes the form of three signs: triangulation, irregularities in the crest of the interproximal bone, and alteration in the alveolar bone. Each may be observed singly, but they are ordinarily found in combination.

Triangulation. Triangulation is the term given to a widening of the periodontal space at the crest of the interproximal bone. The sides of the triangle are formed by the lamina dura and the root surface; the base is toward the tooth crown. In the incipient stages, triangulation is small to the point of being hardly noticeable. Triangulation is illustrated in Fig. 15-26. The presence of such a triangular space is a sign of possible bone degeneration. Such a sign necessitates a search for possible etiologic factors.

Crestal irregularities. Ordinarily, the lamina dura extends to a point approximately 1 to 1.5 mm. from the cementoenamel junction. The bone crest running from the lamina dura of one tooth to that of the adjacent tooth ordinarily appears rather flat and should be parallel with a line drawn from the dentoenamel junction of one tooth to that of the adjacent tooth. The normal alveolar crest may

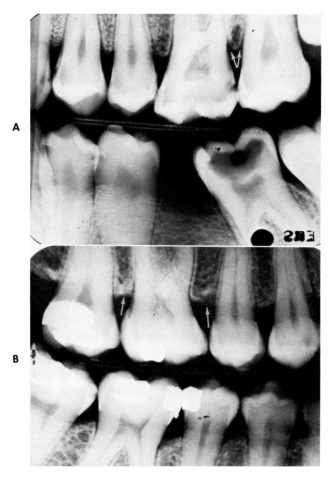

Fig. 15-26. Intraoral radiograms can assist the diagnostician in detecting periodontal disease. Triangulation can be observed in several areas but is best illustrated in **A** between the maxillary first and second molars. Irregularity and destruction of the crest of the alveolar bone is classically illustrated in **B** interproximally between the maxillary second bicuspid and first molar. The bony crest between the maxillary first and second molars in the lower film illustrates increased condensation. Since bone reacts to stress, the clinician should interpret such radiographic manifestations as indicative of the presence of etiologic factors that stimulate bone reaction.

have an opacity not unlike that of the lamina dura; it may appear slightly more opaque, or it may show decreased density. The difference can be explained on the basis of a variation in contour of the cementoenamel junction, the accompanying variation of the alveolar crest, and the relationship of the x-rays to the plane of crestal bone.

It is important to emphasize that angulation, exposure technics, and developing procedures must be ideal if radiographic results are to be truly informative. Angulation changes can grossly distort the appearance of the intercrestal bone; overexposure can burn out bone and give it an etched appearance; faulty developing technics, particularly the use of excessively warm solutions, can result in films of high contrast, which tends to obliterate fine bone trabeculae. Although the use of kilovoltages in the range of 65 to 70 kVp was advocated for the detection of caries, technics using higher kilovoltages in the vicinity of 90 kVp are probably more satisfactory for the interpretation of periodontal disease. Similarly, relatively light films rather than dark films are to be desired.* The paralleling technic is advocated. If the bisecting procedure is used, bite-wing films are mandatory.

Although the characteristics of the bone crest may vary, the bone surface should not be etched. Lack of a smooth bone surface across the interdental crest suggests the possibility of bone resorption. Crestal irregularity is illustrated in Fig. 15-26.

Alveolar bone change. Radiographic findings that show bone sclerosis between the lamina dura of two adjacent teeth in the area of an alveolar crest of normal height suggest an incipient periodontal disease process. In the past, bone condensation has not been regarded as a sign of periodontal disease; rather, it has been looked upon favorably. The following questions must be raised: Why is increased bone deposition needed? Bone responds to stress; is this condensation a stress response? If this is a stress response and if the individual's resistance should decrease, would the bone continue to resist the irritant? The type of bone change that is being discussed is illustrated in Fig. 15-26.

In our opinion, the presence of such a sign is an indication that incipient periodontal disease may exist. However, the presence of such a sign after the treatment of a known periodontal condition suggests that the body is responding favorably and should not be viewed in the same light as when it is found with little or no other evidence of a disease process.

Advanced periodontal disease

Advanced periodontal disease includes all stages that follow incipient periodontal changes. Only changes in osseous structure will be discussed. The periodontal pocket exists between soft tissue and tooth structure. Soft tissue cannot be evaluated from routine dental radiograms. The use of opaque media in diagnosing soft tissue changes can be helpful, but ordinary clinical means are simpler. Although pocket formation and bone loss are generally associated, the presence of bone loss radiographically should never be described as pocket formation. Bone loss can occur without pocket formation, or the degree of bone loss may be out of proportion to the depth of the periodontal pocket as measured clinically.

Complete mouth radiographic surveys are of assistance to the dental practitioner in determining the location of bone loss, the amount of bone loss, the direction of bone loss, and the activity of the destructive process. Some of this

---

*Relatively dark films can be very satisfactory if a high-intensity viewing light is available.

information can be obtained through clinical means, but neither radiographic nor clinical findings alone enable the practitioner to make accurate judgments; he must use all potential sources of information.

Location of bone loss. Periodontal bone loss may be restricted to one or a few areas, or it may be generalized throughout the dentition. Radiographic evidence assists in locating areas of bone loss. When periodontal bone loss is evenly distributed throughout the mouth, it is spoken of as generalized. In the past, this occasionally has been referred to as horizontal bone loss. This terminology is not recommended, since the term *horizontal bone loss* is also used to denote the direction of bone loss. When bone loss occurs in isolated areas, it is usually described as localized.

Evaluation of bone loss location is made primarily by examining the interproximal spaces. Bone loss occurs on all surfaces of the tooth root, but the thickness of the tooth tends to obscure the images of the buccal and lingual bones. However, methods will be described that can be helpful in evaluating bone loss on these surfaces.

Amount of bone loss. Under normal circumstances, the alveolar bone level is located 1 to 1.5 mm. from the cementoenamel junction. Bone loss is evaluated by estimating the amount of bone remaining. A measurement made from the

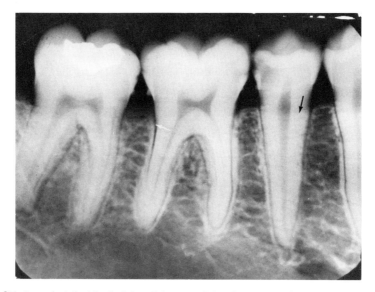

Fig. 15-27. Bone height (the height of the remaining bone) is ordinarily determined by one of two methods or a combination of the two methods: (1) Follow the line of the lamina dura on the distal of the first molar to the point where the lamina dura loses its opacity (white arrow); this is the true bone height. The bone above this level has been cast coronally by excessive angulation. (2) Starting at the tooth apex, note that the trabecular bone pattern on the bicuspid roots can be observed as the eye scans coronally to the level of the black arrow. Above the arrow the root appears denuded of bone. This is true bone height.

crest of the remaining bone to the cementoenamel junction minus approximately 1 mm. gives an indication of bone loss.

The bone height is determined by using two different procedures alone or in a combined fashion.

1. One observes the line of the lamina dura on the mesial or distal surface, starting at the apex of the tooth and continuing to a point where the lamina dura abruptly decreases in opacity. The periodontal space may continue toward the crown of the tooth beyond the point where the lamina dura loses this opacity. This is illustrated in Fig. 15-27. Ordinarily, the difference from the point of initial loss of lamina dura opacity to the maximum height of the bone is approximately equal to the distance between the buccal and the lingual or palatal cusp tips. This difference in bone (and cusp) levels is ordinarily caused by vertical angulation that has cast the buccal bone more coronally than the lingual or palatal bone. This is diagrammatically illustrated in Fig. 11-1. In most cases, if the distance between the point of maximum lamina dura opacity and the observable maximum bone height is greater than the distance between the cusp tips, the buccal bone height is probably higher than that of the lingual bone. Conversely, if the opacity of the lamina dura continues coronally to a level such that the distance between the point of maximum lamina dura opacity and maximum bone height is less than the distance between the cusp tips, the lingual bone level probably is higher than that of the buccal bone.

The foregoing generalizations are usually accurate because the clinical levels of buccal and lingual (or palatal) bone ordinarily are approximately the same. If considerable differences occur between buccal and lingual bone levels or if the x-rays are directed at a right angle to both the long axis of the tooth and the film plane (as in the paralleling technic or in the use of bite-wing films), it often becomes difficult to differentiate buccal from lingual bone levels. When the paralleling technic or bite-wing films are used, bone levels are superimposed if the buccal and lingual bone heights are equal. If the radiograms show the tooth cusp tips to be superimposed (or if in the anterior segment of the mouth, the teeth are of normal length) but the bone levels to be separated, the buccal and lingual bone heights are unequal; but to state with accuracy which bone level has undergone greatest destruction is difficult if not impossible.

2. There is a second procedure for evaluating bone height. Depending on circumstances, this method can be used alone or in conjunction with the previously described approach. At times, this procedure will prove difficult to use effectively.

Starting at the apex of the tooth, one examines the trabecular pattern of bone, which is superimposed on the tooth root. This trabecular pattern will terminate at some level on the tooth root and give the appearance of a line running across the root surface. That portion of the root between the line and the enamel will look bare or denuded. The bone line just described (running across the root surface) may be difficult to discern but ordinarily can be seen if viewed carefully.

This line usually represents the lingual bone level and will join the points on the lamina dura described in the preceding paragraphs as the terminal point of maximum lamina dura opacity.

Occasionally, a second trabecular line can be seen running across the root of the tooth from the points of maximum bone height (that is, the buccal bone level). This line usually cannot be observed, because the distance from the buccal bone to the film is relatively great, and because the slight thickness of the buccal bone is lost in the mass of root substance. In Fig. 15-27 is illustrated trabecular bone superimposed on root substance.

Considerable care must be taken so that the vertical angulation used in taking periapical films does not result in one's underestimating the amount of bone loss. This concept is illustrated and described in Fig. 15-28.

The amount of bone loss observed radiographically should not be used as the sole determining factor in deciding whether a tooth can be retained and

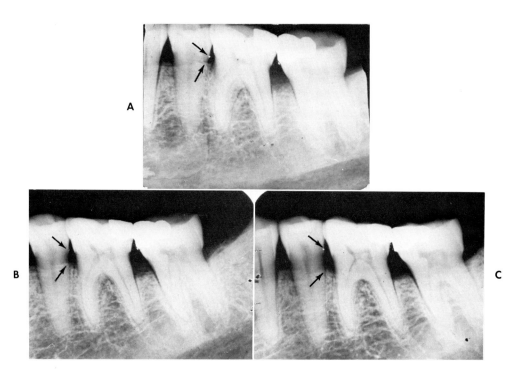

Fig. 15-28. Three views of the same teeth. In all three films, a white dot appears at the cementoenamel junction on the distal aspect of the mandibular second bicuspid. The distance between the dot and the bone crest varies in each film. Note also that the distance between the lingual and buccal cusps of the molar teeth also varies considerably. In **A** excessive vertical angulation caused the shadow of the bone to be cast coronally so that the bone height approximated normal. In **B** the angulation is decreased, and in **C** the rays were directed at right angles to both the tooth and the film. Under the latter circumstance, the true relationship between the bone height and the cementoenamel junction is portrayed.

treated or whether it should be removed. This fact is stressed because of the tendency to use such radiographic criteria, for example, bifurcation involvement, as an indication for tooth removal. Treatment should be determined by using radiographic evidence as adjunctive information; the final decision must be made on the basis of more complete evidence.

Direction of bone loss. As mentioned earlier, intercrestal bone should be parallel with a line drawn from the cementoenamel junction of one tooth to that of the contacting tooth. These lines are not always parallel with the occlusal plane; this is particularly true when teeth erupt or tilt. The direction of bone loss is determined by using the cementoenamel junction line as a plane of reference.

Bone loss can occur on a plane that is parallel with a line drawn from the cementoenamel junction of one tooth to that of an adjacent tooth; such loss is spoken of as *horizontal bone loss.* When there is greater bone loss on the proximal surface of one tooth than on the adjacent tooth, the bone level is not parallel with

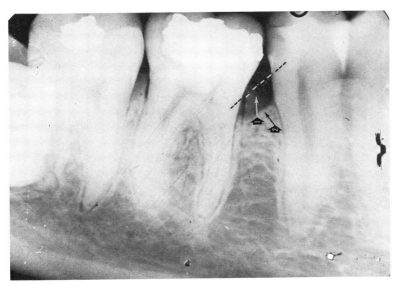

Fig. 15-29. Bone loss direction. Bone loss direction is measured by comparing the bone level with a line drawn between the cementoenamel junction of one tooth and that of the adjacent tooth. The dotted line between the mandibular second bicuspid and first molar joins the cementoenamel junctions. The buccal bone, *1,* which appears to run horizontally, actually has a vertical direction, whereas the lingual bone, *2,* is at a level parallel with the dotted line. Thus, the lingual bone has been lost in a horizontal direction, whereas the buccal bone on the bicuspid has been lost in a vertical direction. Note that the buccal bone is cast above the level of the cementoenamel junction on the molar tooth. This is due to excessive vertical angulation. The carious process on the distal aspect of the second bicuspid and the poorly contoured restoration on the mesial aspect of the first molar are likely contributing to food impaction, which in turn becomes a local etiologic factor in periodontal disease.

a line joining the cementoenamel junctions; such destruction is called *vertical bone loss*. Vertical and horizontal bone loss are illustrated in Fig. 15-29. The value of these terms is largely related to their use in communicating and in record keeping.

There is no definitive relationship between local and systemic conditions and bone loss direction. Clinical observations suggest that vertical bone loss is usually localized rather than generalized and is more often primarily related to local etiologic factors such as trauma, calculus, overhanging fillings, and food impaction. Horizontal bone loss may be localized or generalized. Generalized bone loss suggests a systemic etiologic factor.

Activity of the destructive process. Intraoral radiographic film can assist the practitioner in evaluating the activity of the destructive process. Activity is best measured by comparing radiograms taken over regular intervals of time. When only the current films are available, a subjective estimate of activity is still possible. When the intercrestal bone is rough and irregular and the bone below the crest is devoid of any suggestion of bone condensation, it is likely that the process is active. Conversely, if, in the presence of bone loss, sclerosing osteitis and a smooth surface to the crest of the interproximal bone are present, it is likely that the process is either static or only slowly destructive. It must be remembered that the shape of the interdental crest and x-ray beam angulation as well as exposure and developing factors have a direct effect on the radiographic appearance of bone. An active destructive process is illustrated in Fig. 15-30; relative inactivity is suggested in Fig. 15-29.

Detection of local irritating factors

Radiograms assist the practitioner in identifying some local etiologic factors. These include calculus deposits, overhanging restorations, faulty restorative margins, and carious lesions. These local factors must be eliminated if treatment is to be successful. After the elimination of these local factors, radiographic reexamination of the area is usually indicated to be certain that all operations have been performed adequately. The presence of local irritating factors is shown in Figs. 15-29 to 15-31.

Prognosis

The prognosis of any periodontal condition is made after all available information has been secured. Radiographic evidence is part of such diagnostic data and is used in evaluating the prognosis. The chances for returning the periodontal structures to a healthy state are reasonably good if the destructive process is not generalized, if only a limited amount of bone has been lost, if the destructive activity is minimal, and if correctable etiologic factors can be identified.

It must be reemphasized that radiographic films play no role in determining etiology other than that of detecting the presence of certain types of local irritation.

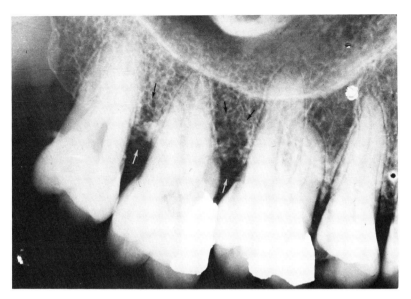

Fig. 15-30. Radiogram exemplifying the appearance of an actively destructive process. This is particularly true in the crestal areas between the maxillary molars. Clinically, this patient was suffering from acute Vincent's infection. This illustration should be compared with Fig. 15-29, which, particularly on the lingual bone level between the second bicuspid and first molar, illustrates a much more chronic process. Poorly contoured mesial proximal restorations on the first and second molars and the extrusion of the second molar probably contribute to the periodontal condition as local etiologic factors.

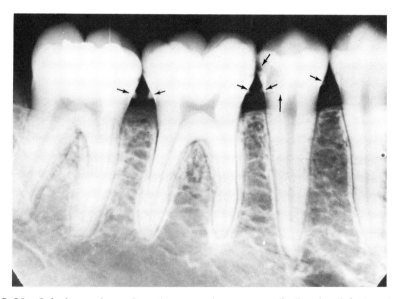

Fig. 15-31. Calculus and rough carious margins are contributing local factors to periodontal disease processes. Typical, rather extensive calculus deposits can be seen interproximally on the posterior teeth. These are located just above the cementoenamel junction in what is no doubt the gingival crevice. The shadow of the calculus ring is discernible on the crown of the second bicuspid tooth.

Treatment evaluation

Serial radiograms can be of considerable value in determining the success of treatment. Serial radiograms must be standardized; film placement, angulation, exposure, and film-processing factors must be kept constant. It is not generally expected that the bone height will increase in successfully treated conditions; however, it is anticipated that the radiographic features will change from those indicating an actively destructive process to those suggesting a static condition. The appearance of new bone interproximally in the diseased areas suggests satisfactory progress, as does the occurrence of a radiopaque lamina across the interproximal bone crest.

OTHER COMMON DISEASES OF THE TEETH AND SUPPORTING STRUCTURES

As mentioned in the introduction to this chapter, a number of common conditions are frequently seen by the dental practitioner. These include tooth resorption, hypoplastic defects, pulp calcifications, tooth fracture, erosion, abrasion, attrition, pericoronitis, dry sockets, and pulpitis. Other conditions that can be considered relatively common, for example, supernumerary and missing teeth, are considered along with less common diseases in Chapter 16.

Tooth resorption

Tooth resorption from the standpoint of etiology is subdivided into physiologic, idiopathic, and pathologic resorption. The resorbed surface may appear

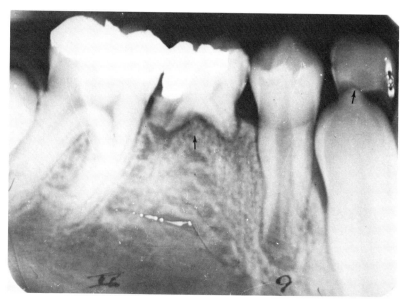

Fig. 15-32. Physiologic root resorption takes place in deciduous teeth. This illustration demonstrates root resorption of deciduous teeth in both the presence and absence of permanent replacements.

rough or smooth. Any portion of the tooth may be resorbed as long as such surfaces are associated with other living tissue. Thus tooth resorption can occur on the pulpal or external surfaces of the tooth. The enamel surfaces are resorbed only when the tooth is embedded.

Physiologic root resorption. Resorption of the roots of deciduous teeth normally precedes their exfoliation; it is a natural phenomenon. This condition is shown in Fig. 15-32. Resorption can occur with or without the presence of a permanent successor. Resorption often does not occur if the permanent successor is absent.

Idiopathic tooth resorption. Resorption of tooth surfaces, either internal or external, can occur from unknown causes. If the resorption occurs within the pulp, it is spoken of as internal idiopathic root resorption and is characterized by a localized increase in the size of the pulp. The radiographic shape of the resorbed area varies with its location and with the relationship of the x-ray beam to the involved tooth. Internal tooth resorption may continue until a spontaneous fracture of the tooth occurs. Internal root resorption is illustrated in Fig. 15-33.

External idiopathic tooth resorption can occur on any surface of the tooth. Tooth crowns are involved less often because they are not ordinarily surrounded by viable tissue. The resorption process in the root tends either to hollow out the root surface in a fairly smooth fashion or to resorb the root by creating a rough, irregular surface. The process is always covered by bone, and the root loss is ordinarily followed by filling-in of the excavated space by bone. Although there is little objective evidence available, it is generally believed that the process continues until the root spontaneously fractures or the crown exfoliates. Any portion of the root that is retained will be resorbed eventually. Idiopathic external root resorption is shown in Fig. 15-34 as follows: *A*, root resorption on the distal surface of the lateral incisor root; *B*, root resorption in the region of the root cervix; and *C*, root resorption on a tooth that had been crowned for a period of approximately 8 years prior to the date of spontaneous fracture. Although smooth external root resorption is usually associated with trauma, it is occasionally seen in patients who have a noncontributory history.

Pathologic tooth resorption. Pathologic tooth resorption usually is caused by pressure, infection, neoplasms, or trauma. Resorption can occur through pressure applied to another tooth. The resorbed area usually has a fairly smooth appearance (Fig. 15-35).

Portions of teeth surrounded by pus may be resorbed or absorbed. The smooth continuity of the root surface is broken. In Fig. 15-36 is demonstrated a long-standing area of infection associated with loss of tooth structure at the tooth apex. Infections of short duration do not produce tooth resorption.

Neoplasms of an expansive nature—for example, odontomas and slowly growing ameloblastomas—tend to produce tooth resorption not unlike that caused by pressure. Neoplasms of an aggressively infiltrating nature tend to produce a rough, external type of resorption. When neoplasms are extremely aggressive,

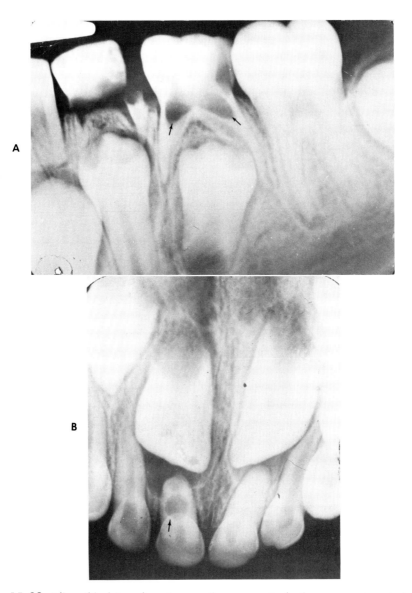

Fig. 15-33. Idiopathic internal root resorption occurs in both permanent and deciduous teeth. **A,** Idiopathic root resorption in the second deciduous mandibular molar. It is quite likely that the same phenomenon took place in the first deciduous molar and resulted in fracture rather than resorption of the deciduous molar roots. **B,** Note a circular area of resorption in or on (external or internal, but probably the latter) the root of the left deciduous central tooth.

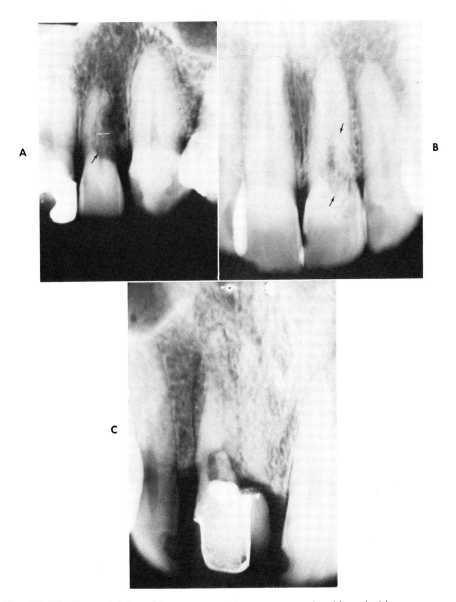

Fig. 15-34. External idiopathic root resorption can occur in either deciduous or permanent teeth. **A,** Resorption on the distal surface of the lateral root. The resorbed area ordinarily becomes replaced by bone. **B,** Resorption on the distal surface of the right central. The outline of the tooth is not clearly identifiable. **C,** Resorption process as it continues from the stage shown in **B** (though not of the same patient). The tooth root has almost completely resorbed. The apparent outline of the tooth root is an artifact that was drawn in by the practitioner who submitted this film for an opinion. The elapsed time interval between the stage represented by **B** and that represented by **C** was in the case of **C** approximately 8 years.

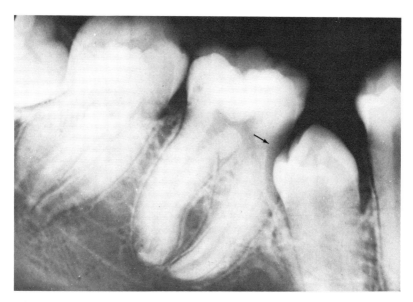

Fig. 15-35. Radiogram giving appearance of tooth resorption on the mesial surface of the mandibular first molar due to the presence of the erupting second bicuspid. In this case the molar tooth was actually resorbed, but radiographic pseudoresorption can be produced, particularly if the film is of high or short-scale contrast.

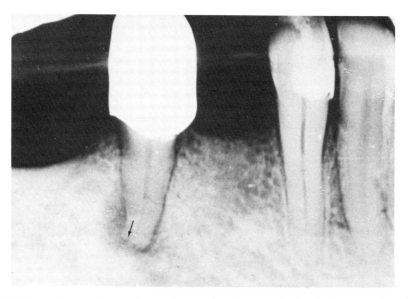

Fig. 15-36. Root resorption of the tooth apex is a frequent finding in long-standing chronic infections. Note also the rather considerable amount of condensing osteitis in the bone peripheral to the radiolucent area surrounding the tooth root. A similar type of pathologic root resorption can be observed in Fig. 15-23, *B*, without the condensing osteitis.

there is little time for tooth resorption to take place; teeth surrounded by such lesions will show little or no tooth resorption.

Trauma can produce tooth resorption. Teeth that have been replanted tend to have resorbed roots. The resorbed surfaces are usually rough and irregular. This characteristic is in contradistinction to the smooth type of resorption that sometimes is observed when there is a history of transient trauma or orthodontic treatment. This smooth type of resorption is usually localized in the apical region; the root apex is blunted, the lamina dura and the periodontal space are intact, and the tooth demonstrates normal vitality. Tooth resorption caused by transient trauma is shown in Fig. 15-23, A, and tooth resorption in a replanted tooth, in Fig. 15-37.

Hypoplastic defects

Hypoplastic defects alter the shape of the tooth and can be observed radiographically. Hypoplastic alterations in tooth root and crown result from many causes and take numerous forms. The most commonly observed changes are those resulting in a localized loss of enamel. This loss can take the form of a single pit defect or a series of pits encircling the tooth horizontally. The pits may coalesce to form a groove. The width of the band or groove can vary from an almost imperceptible line to a wide band covering an appreciable part of the tooth crown. The most commonly observed hypoplastic defects are illustrated in Fig. 15-38. Note that single hypoplastic defects resemble carious lesions; this is particularly true when the defects occur on the interproximal surface (Fig. 15-11).

Pulp calcifications

Pulp calcifications include pulp stones, secondary dentin, dentinal bridges, and pulpal obliteration. Pulp stones radiographically appear as round or oval opacities within the pulp. Little or no significance is attached to such stones unless they create a problem in endodontic therapy. Typical pulp stones are shown in Fig. 15-39.

Secondary dentin reduces the size of the pulp chamber. It appears to be a normal aging phenomenon as well as a defense mechanism. Calcification within the primary dentin is often incorrectly called secondary dentin. Both mechanisms are apparently a response to pathologic change. Secondary dentin appears radiographically as complete or partial obliteration of the pulp chamber or pulp canal.

Dentinal bridges occasionally develop between normal pulp tissue and a large carious lesion. They are frequently associated with the successful use of calcium hydroxide; the latter is used as either a pulp-capping material or as a subbase. A typical dentinal bridge is depicted in Fig. 15-40.

Pulpal obliteration is associated with aging and degenerative pulp changes. It is also a frequent sequela of a traumatic experience. Radiographically, the pulp may appear very small or may be completely obliterated. A completely obliter-

Text continued on p. 344.

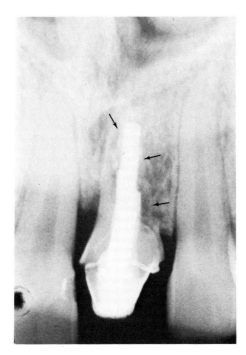

Fig. 15-37. Root resorption frequently occurs in teeth that are replanted. A rather typical type of resorption is shown.

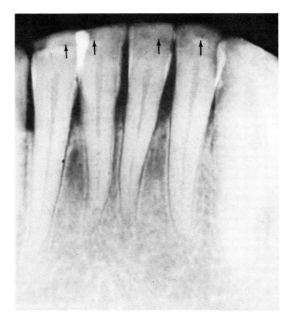

Fig. 15-38. Hypoplastic defects are apparently associated with acute infectious processes that occur during the time of enamel development. Defects running linearly across the upper portions of the crowns of the mandibular incisor teeth are shown. A similar defect was observed in Fig. 15-11.

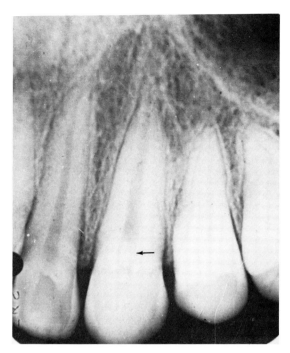

Fig. 15-39. Typical pulp stone can be observed in the coronal portion of the root canal in the maxillary cuspid tooth. Multiple pulp stones are also observable in the mandibular first molar in Fig. 15-20.

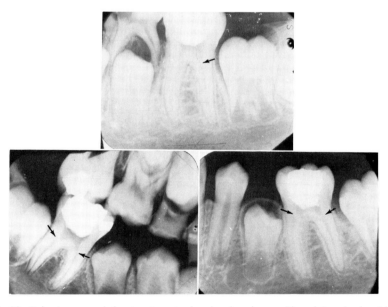

Fig. 15-40. Pulpotomy and the treatment of pulp chambers with calcium hydroxide result, when successful, in the creation of a dentinal bridge. Such bridges are difficult but possible to observe radiographically. The arrows point to a bridging of the canal with secondary dentin. (Courtesy Dr. S. B. Finn.)

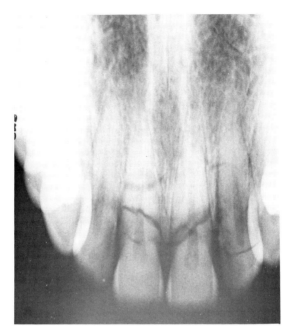

Fig. 15-41. Tooth fractures vary considerably in appearance. Care must be taken to be certain that the supposed fracture line is neither an artifact nor an anatomic entity in the bone such as a nutrient vessel that is superimposed on tooth structure. Typical multiple fractures are shown.

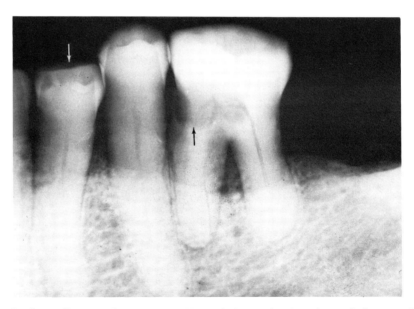

Fig. 15-42. Radiogram illustrating attrition of the occlusal surface of the mandibular first bicuspid because of function (white arrow). Note that the second bicuspid and the first molar have extruded because of the absence of opposing teeth. Buccal erosion can be observed on the first molar. This erosion was due to overvigorous use of a hard bristle toothbrush.

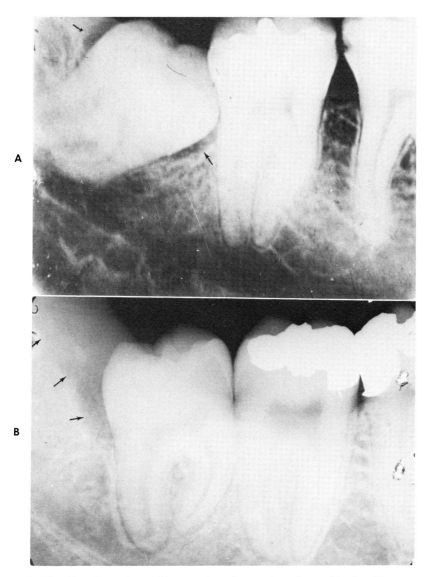

Fig. 15-43. Chronic pericoronitis can be observed radiographically. However, acute stages of pericoronitis that have not been preceded by a chronic destructive process are ordinarily not observable radiographically. **A,** Impacted third molar with a normal-appearing pericoronal space. The patient's symptoms were acute. **B,** Chronic lesion that has resulted in considerable destruction of bone distal to the mandibular molar.

ated canal is shown in Fig. 15-23, *A*. Such teeth are usually nonvital and asymptomatic. They create a difficult endodontic situation when such therapy becomes necessary.

Tooth fractures

Radiograms are useful in locating tooth fractures. More than one view of a suspected tooth should be obtained. A fracture line and discontinuity in the outline of the tooth are the most usually observed signs of fracture. It must be remembered that the radiogram can have an appearance that simulates a fracture, and fractured segments can be superimposed in a manner that hides the fracture. Multiple views of the questionable area ordinarily resolve such difficulties. A typical tooth fracture is shown in Fig. 15-41.

Erosion, abrasion, and attrition

Loss of tooth structure, whether physiologic or pathologic, can be observed radiographically. However, clinical observations of these conditions are more informative. Radiograms are useful in evaluating the size of the pulp and the thickness of tooth structure between the pulp and the tooth surface. Attrition and buccal erosion are illustrated in Fig. 15-42.

Pericoronitis

Primary acute pericoronal infections do not ordinarily demonstrate radiographic change. However, acute exacerbation of chronic pericoronal infections or quiescent asymptomatic chronic conditions do demonstrate radiographic alterations. The space that represents the normal enamel follicle around the crown of partially or completely unerupted teeth is enlarged as a result of pericoronal infection; its periphery is usually rough and irregular. The amount of bone loss is related to the duration and severity of the infectious process. The radiographic appearance of two stages of pericoronal infection is demonstrated in Fig. 15-43.

Dry sockets and pulpitis

The two conditions of dry socket and pulpitis are discussed together because neither demonstrates significant radiographic change. They are common conditions encountered in the dental office and are included for purposes of completeness.

CHAPTER 16

Diseases of radiographic importance

Many disease entities cause alterations in osseous tissue, and these changes may result in radiographic manifestations. The radiographic appearance of the pathologic condition will often vary, depending on the lesion's stage of development and on other factors peculiar to the pathologic process. The material to be covered in this chapter could readily be expanded into a full-size text. To expand would unnecessarily complicate a book written primarily for the dental student and the general practitioner. Since many of the included disease entities are rarities—particularly from the general practitioner's viewpoint—some consideration was given to omitting topics that would concern the average practitioner only minimally, but this idea was discarded. If no other purpose is accomplished, the listing of diseases that can produce changes in the mandible and maxilla gives the beginner an appreciation of radiology's role in diagnosis; similarly, it helps the more sophisticated diagnostician develop a differential interpretation of a questionable lesion. Thus a desire for completeness and a belief that even superficial coverage of rare disease manifestations is helpful resulted in the approach used in the following pages. As mentioned in the Preface, "To fully comprehend the subject of dental radiology, students will need to attend the lectures of their teachers and read the works of other authors, which will supplement most chapters by providing information on some aspects of the field not mentioned in this text."* The reader is cautioned that the illustrations tend to portray advanced radiographic manifestations; the practitioner must be watchful for less obvious signs of beginning osseous alterations.

A study of oral pathology shows that radiography does not play a part in the diagnosis of all disease processes affecting oral structures. Since oral radiology is the subject of this text, the content of this chapter is limited to those diseases wherein radiography is a valuable diagnostic tool. The discussion, in the main,

---

*The reader's attention is redirected to the statements above. The text has been criticized for brevity of coverage in this chapter. The reasons for brevity are given here and in the Preface.

345

is confined to radiographic findings. It is to be remembered that basically the oral diagnostic radiogram shows changes in the calcified tissues or, more specifically, the calcified portions of tissues. The radiogram also shows calcifications within soft tissues and changes that can be visualized through the use of contrast media. Note also that radiograms showing changes are not the only ones of importance; negative radiographic findings are equally significant in the evaluation of oral disease.

Oral disease can be classified in several different ways. The system used in this chapter is based on etiology; it is hoped that this method will permit easy reference with standard texts on oral pathology. The diseases, other than those discussed in Chapter 15, that are of radiographic significance are discussed in the following order: (1) developmental disturbances; (2) diseases caused by biologic agents; (3) pathologic change caused by physical agents; (4) cysts; (5) neoplasms; (6) hormonal, nutritional, and metabolic disorders; and (7) miscellaneous pathologic conditions.

DEVELOPMENTAL DISTURBANCES

Many developmental disturbances affect oral structures. Not all of these disturbances produce variations in teeth and/or bone. Developmental disturbances can be divided into local and generalized conditions. Local disturbances are those that affect oral and/or cranial structures. Generalized disturbances are those wherein the oral changes are related to disturbances in other parts of the body. Developmental disturbances of radiographic importance are listed as follows:

Local disturbances

Amelogenesis imperfecta
Dentinogenesis imperfecta
Dentinal dysplasia
Odontodysplasia
Dens in dente
Fusion, gemination, and concrescence
Taurodontism
Macrodontia and microdontia
Supernumerary teeth
Missing teeth
Malpositioned teeth
Palatal and mandibular clefts
Pierre Robin syndrome
Facial gigantism
Facial hemiatrophy

Cherubism
Agnathia
Microcephalus and hydrocephalus
Craniostosis
Craniofacial dysostosis

Generalized disturbances

Osteogenesis imperfecta
Ectodermal dysplasia
Cleidocranial dysostosis
Achondroplasia
Osteopetrosis
Sickle cell anemia
Thalassemia

Amelogenesis imperfecta

Basically, only two types of enamel hypoplasia present different radiographic appearances. In the hypoplastic type, the enamel fails to achieve its proper thickness. The radiogram shows the enamel to have a normal film density; the thickness of the enamel is reduced. The enamel may be smooth or may have pitted hypoplastic areas. In the hypocalcification type of amelogenesis imperfecta, the correct amount of enamel is formed but the enamel is not properly calcified. The radiogram shows an enamel layer of correct dimensions but with greater film density. The enamel density, in a classic case, is almost the same as the dentin, and the dentinoenamel junction is therefore undiscernible on the radiogram. Examples of amelogenesis imperfecta are shown in Fig. 16-1.

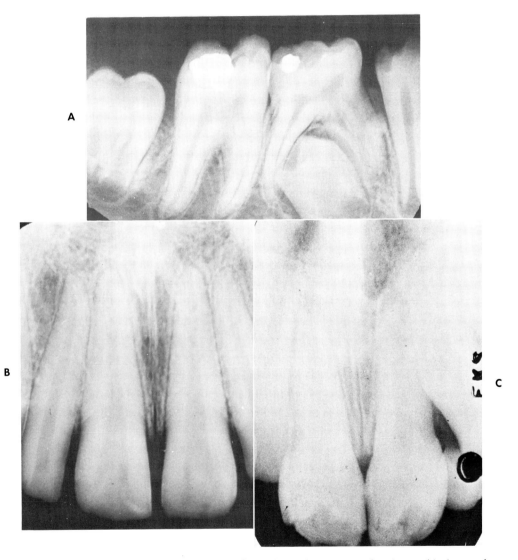

Fig. 16-1. A and **B,** Amelogenesis imperfecta, hypoplastic type, showing a thin layer of well-formed enamel covering the crowns of the teeth. **C,** Amelogenesis imperfecta, hypocalcification type, showing a more radiolucent enamel layer, an indistinct dentoenamel junction and early wear, and fracture of the incisal enamel.

Dentinogenesis imperfecta

Dentinogenesis imperfecta, or hereditary opalescent dentin, is a developmental disturbance in dentin formation. Radiographically, the teeth have thinner, shorter roots, and the necks of the teeth appear to be constricted. The pulp chambers are wide in the early stages, but are often soon calcified and obliterated. The dentin is more radiolucent, and its image shows greater film density. The observer notes a rather high film contrast between the crowns and the roots of the teeth. One or more teeth are sometimes missing, and the periodontal space is occasionally enlarged. Other findings that are more obvious clinically include chipped enamel and rapid wearing away of the tooth crowns. The radiographic appearance of dentinogenesis imperfecta is shown in Fig. 16-2.

Dentinal dysplasia

Dentinal dysplasia is a relatively rare but severe disturbance of dentin formation. The permanent teeth show very little root formation. The apices of multirooted posterior teeth are bunched together. The teeth show little or no pulp chambers. Clinically, the teeth usually appear normal. Early loss of some teeth is a frequent finding (Fig. 16-3).

Odontodysplasia

Odontodysplasia is a relatively rare developmental anomaly in tooth formation. Both dentin and enamel are affected. The condition tends to affect teeth in only one quadrant of the dentition and is sometimes referred to as localized, arrested tooth development. Odontodysplasia can occur in the deciduous or permanent dentition, and the affected teeth tend to be embedded in the bone. No etiology has been identified, and there is no evidence of any familial connection or of a relationship to sex or race. Radiographically, the affected teeth have a ghostlike appearance (Fig. 16-4).

Dens in dente

Dens in dente, sometimes described as a tooth within a tooth, is actually an invagination of the calcified layers of the tooth into the body of the tooth. In the crown the invagination often forms an enamel-lined cavity projecting into the pulp. The cavity is usually connected to the outside of the tooth, and defects in the wall of the cavity often associate this condition with pulpal and periapical infection. Two examples of dens in dente are shown in Fig. 16-5.

Fusion, gemination, and concrescence

Fusion (Fig. 16-6, A and B) is a condition in which two teeth are joined together early in their development to form a single, large tooth. Usually, a single large crown and two root canals are seen. Gemination (Fig. 16-6, C) is the condition in which a single tooth germ splits and usually results in a single root with two crowns. When the possibility of supernumerary tooth formation and subsequent fusion is considered, it is often difficult to distinguish between fusion

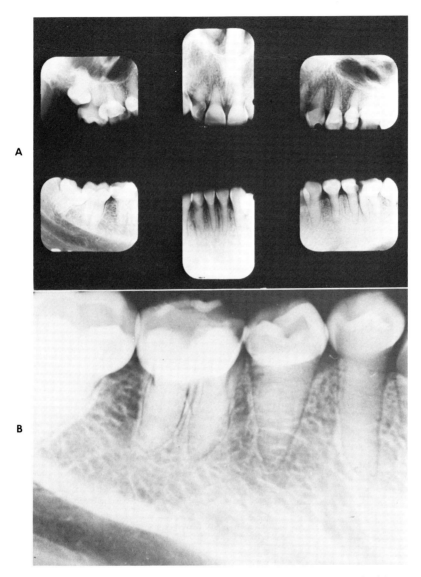

Fig. 16-2. Dentinogenesis imperfecta. The thinner, shorter roots and obliterated pulp chambers of the teeth are demonstrated. The dentin is relatively radiolucent, and the necks of the teeth appear constricted. (Courtesy Dr. S. B. Finn.)

and gemination. Concrescence is a condition in which two well-formed teeth are joined together by their cementum layers (Fig. 16-6, *D*).

Taurodontism

Taurodontism refers to teeth that have large bodies and pulp chambers with very little root formation. This condition is thought to be due to a retrograde evolutionary process. An example of this condition is shown in Fig. 16-7.

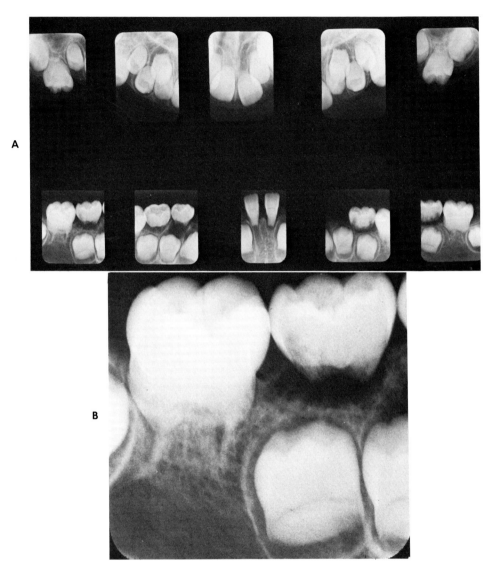

Fig. 16-3. Intraoral radiograms of dentinal dysplasia. The teeth show very little root formation and no pulp chambers. The shape of the crowns is within normal range. (Courtesy Dr. T. S. Grant.)

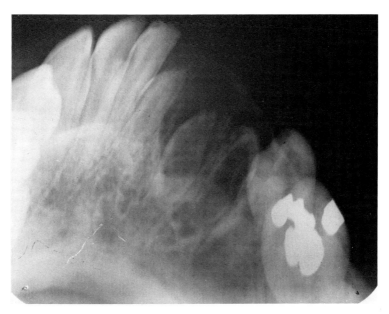

Fig. 16-4. Odontodysplasia. The affected teeth have a ghostlike appearance.

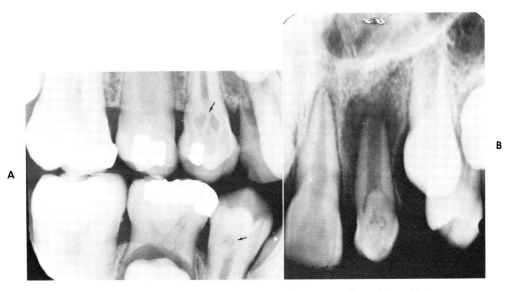

Fig. 16-5. A, Dens in dente of both first bicuspids. The maxillary bicuspid demonstrates two invaginations. The radiolucent invaginations are lined with a thin layer of radiopaque enamel. **B,** More bizarre form of dens in dente affecting an upper lateral incisor. Periapical disease and incomplete root formation are associated with the tooth malformation.

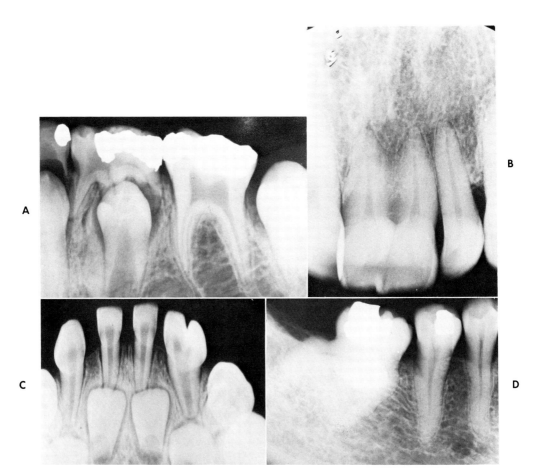

Fig. 16-6. A, Fusion of two deciduous molars. A single amalgam restoration is seen in the joined crowns. **B,** Another example of fusion. **C,** Gemination of lower deciduous incisors. **D,** Concrescence involving two teeth in the mandibular molar area. (**D,** Courtesy Dr. E. C. Stafne.)

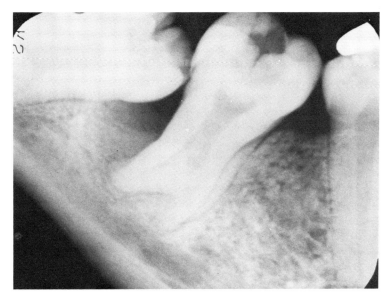

Fig. 16-7. Example of taurodontism. Note the large body and pulp chamber and relatively short roots.

Macrodontia and microdontia

Macrodontia refers to a large tooth and microdontia, to a small tooth. In microdontia of the entire dentition, the spaces between the teeth are usually greater than normal.

Supernumerary teeth

A supernumerary or extra tooth can be a well-formed or a malshaped tooth. Supernumerary teeth tend to be shaped like the teeth in the area where they occur. Supernumerary teeth occurring between the maxillary central incisors are called mesiodentes. Since many supernumerary teeth fail to erupt, routine radiographic surveys play an important part in discovering the number and position of these teeth. Radiograms also show if these teeth are being resorbed; if they are associated with dentigerous cysts, ameloblastomas, or other odontogenic neoplasms; if they are preventing the eruption of normal teeth; or if they are the cause of malocclusion. Examples of single and multiple supernumerary teeth are shown in Fig. 16-8.

Missing teeth

Missing teeth can be a local condition or part of a generalized condition. As an example of the latter, oligodontia (partial absence of teeth) is very often associated with ectodermal dysplasia. Missing teeth can range from a single missing tooth to anodontia (complete absence of teeth). Third molars are the most frequently missing teeth and are followed in order by mandibular second bicuspids, maxillary lateral incisors, and maxillary second bicuspids. When the permanent successor of a deciduous tooth is missing, the deciduous tooth may remain in the arch for many years. If such a deciduous tooth becomes ankylosed to the bone in childhood, the bone may continue to develop as the permanent teeth erupt. The deciduous tooth becomes located at a different level from the occlusal plane. Such a tooth is called a submerged tooth. Examples of missing and submerged teeth are shown in Fig. 16-9.

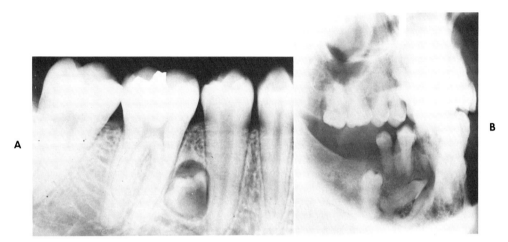

Fig. 16-8. A, Patient with a clinically good dentition showing a developing supernumerary lower bicuspid on radiographic examination. **B,** Radiogram of a patient with multiple supernumerary teeth.

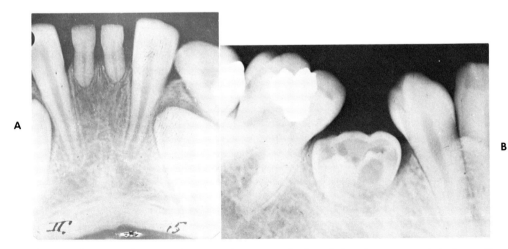

Fig. 16-9. A, Radiogram demonstrating congenitally missing lower central incisors. **B,** Submerged second deciduous molar, probably resulting from a missing second permanent bicuspid and ankylosis of the deciduous tooth.

Malpositioned teeth

A malpositioned tooth is one that does not achieve its normal position in the dental arch. This is usually due to a lack of space in the arch or to an obstruction in the eruptive pathway of the tooth. Obstructions include cysts, supernumerary teeth, odontomas, and tumors. In some instances, a tooth simply fails to erupt. Such a tooth is called an embedded tooth. Multiple embedded teeth are sometimes seen in association with some systemic conditions. Infection and other forms of trauma may cause ankylosis and the retention of teeth in an abnormal position. A tooth may develop with its crown pointed in the wrong direction. In some instances, two adjacent teeth may develop in each other's position in the arch; these are called transposed teeth. The radiogram plays a very important part in the diagnosis of malpositioned teeth and in establishing their position relative to other anatomic structures. Some examples of this condition are shown in Fig. 16-10.

Palatal and mandibular clefts

Clefts of the palate can involve the soft palate, the hard palate, or both. The cleft in the upper anterior region can be unilateral or bilateral in the canine–lateral incisor region. A median cleft can occur between the central incisors;

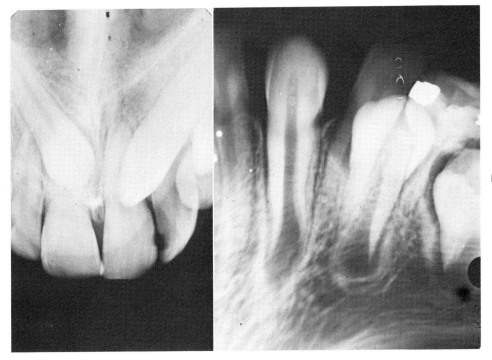

Fig. 16-10. A, Radiogram demonstrating bilaterally impacted maxillary canines. **B,** Transposed lower cuspid and lateral incisor teeth.

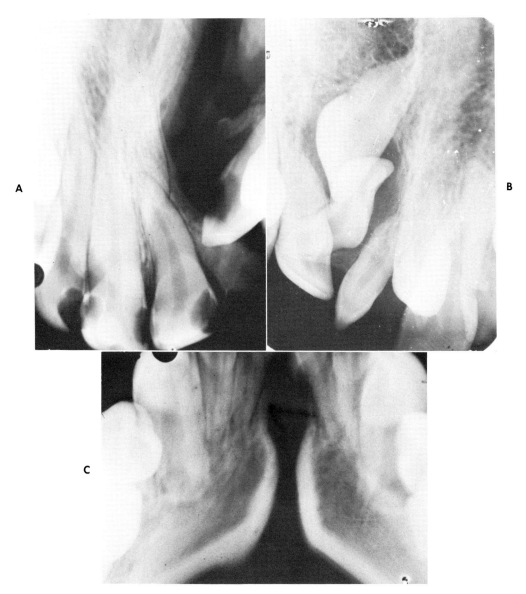

Fig. 16-11. **A** and **B**, Examples of cleft palates showing the bone defect and malposed and supernumerary teeth. **C**, Radiogram of cleft mandible showing complete lack of bone union in the midline. (Courtesy Dr. C. E. Crandell.)

this condition is rare. Clefts of the palate often disturb the dental lamina in the area, and it is not uncommon to find supernumerary, missing, or malpositioned teeth associated with such clefts. Radiograms are very helpful in determining the position of such teeth and the amount of bone present in the area. Examples of cleft palates are given in Fig. 16-11, *A* and *B*.

Clefts can occur in the midline of the mandible; however, these are very rare (Fig. 16-11, *C*).

Pierre Robin syndrome

Pierre Robin syndrome associates a cleft palate, micrognathia, and ptosis of the floor of the mouth.

Facial gigantism

Enlargement of the facial tissue can be unilateral or bilateral. Facial gigantism can be of developmental or pathologic origin.

Facial hemiatrophy

Atrophy of one side of the face may be congenital or acquired.

Cherubism

Cherubism, or familial intraosseous swelling of the jaws, occurs in childhood. The condition is bilateral, and the site is usually the area of the angle of the mandible. The lesion may appear radiographically as bilateral polycystic or multilocular cystlike areas, or they may resemble the ground-glass appearance of fibrous dysplasia. Cherubism may also produce tooth resorption and tooth migration (Fig. 16-12).

Agnathia

Failure of jaw development can be visualized radiographically.

Microcephalus and hydrocephalus

The skull is at times underdeveloped or pathologically enlarged. Radiograms are useful in showing the relative size of the face and cranium and the severity of these conditions. The degree of severity varies widely.

Craniostosis

Radiograms show the closure of the various sutures of the skull and the changes in the shape of the skull caused by early synostosis of the sutures.

Craniofacial dysostosis

Craniofacial dysostosis, or Crouzon's disease, shows the same radiographic findings as cleidocranial dysostosis, with the exception of the defects in the clavicle. The skull findings include delayed closure of the fontanelles and cranial

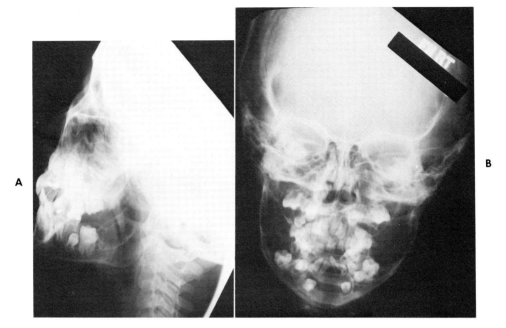

Fig. 16-12. A, Lateral jaw radiogram of cherubism showing the lesion distal to the molar teeth. The lesion appears cystlike and shows expansion of the bone in the retromolar and ramus areas. **B,** Posteroanterior radiogram showing bilateral expansion of the mandible. The lesions are situated at the angles of the mandible and extend into the ramus and body on both sides. (Courtesy Dr. K. W. Bruce.)

sutures, an increased number of wormian bones, a relatively small upper face, delayed eruption of teeth, and the presence of supernumerary teeth. Skull changes are shown in Fig. 16-15.

Osteogenesis imperfecta

Osteogenesis imperfecta, fragilitas ossium or Lobstein's disease, is a developmental disturbance of mesenchymal tissues. Patients tend to have blue sclerae, osteoporosis, and loose ligaments; osteosclerosis is sometimes seen. Development of bone and dentin is poor. The oral radiographic findings are essentially the same as those for dentinogenesis imperfecta with the addition of osteoporosis of the bones (Fig. 16-13).

Ectodermal dysplasia

Ectodermal dysplasia is a developmental disturbance of ectodermal tissues. There is lack or total absence of some structures of ectodermal origin. These structures include hair, fingernails, sweat glands, and teeth. The significant oral radiographic finding is partial dental aplasia (oligodontia) or anodontia. The dental radiogram of a patient with ectodermal dysplasia is shown in Fig. 16-14.

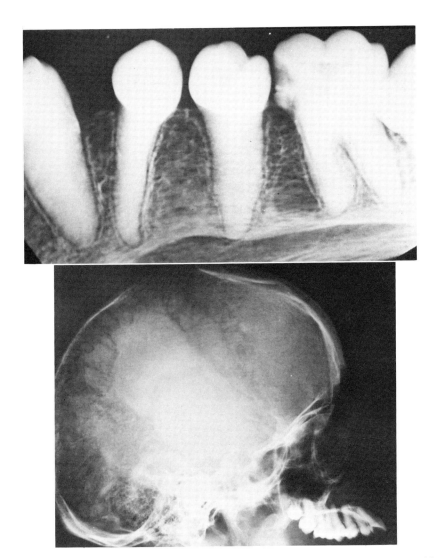

Fig. 16-13. Osteogenesis imperfecta. The teeth show narrow constricted roots with ob-literated root canals. The alevolar bone and skull demonstrate generalized osteoporosis. (Courtesy Dr. E. Cheraskin.)

Cleidocranial dysostosis

Cleidocranial dysostosis, or Sainton's disease, is a developmental disturbance affecting the skull and clavicles. One or both clavicles are partially or completely missing. The skull findings are the same as those seen in craniofacial dysostosis. An example of cleidocranial dysostosis is shown in Fig. 16-15.

Achondroplasia

Achondroplasia is a disturbance in cartilage development. The marked skeletal changes that may produce dwarfism are characteristic. The skull findings include a shortened cranial base, retarded or nonerupted teeth, a relatively enlarged calvarium, and a prognathic mandible and retruded maxilla that result in a saddle-nose profile.

Osteopetrosis

Osteopetrosis, or Albers-Schönberg disease, is a rare hereditary disease characterized by sclerosis of the skeleton (marble bones), fragility of bones, and secondary anemia. Bone formation is normal, but bone resorption is reduced. The individual bones may show patchy areas of sclerosis. There is a bilateral symmetrical sclerosis of all bones. Sclerotic areas in the bones of the hands may produce a "bone-in-bone" appearance. The end result is uniformly dense radiopaque bones. The teeth may be deformed and may show delayed eruption or failure of eruption. Impingement on nerves, glands, and so forth, can produce blindness, deafness, diabetes insipidus, facial palsy, and so forth. An example of osteopetrosis is shown in Fig. 16-16.

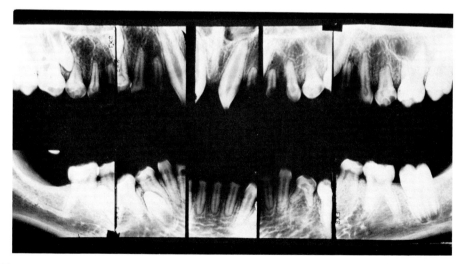

Fig. 16-14. Radiographic survey of a patient with ectodermal dysplasia. Note the failure of development of many permanent teeth.

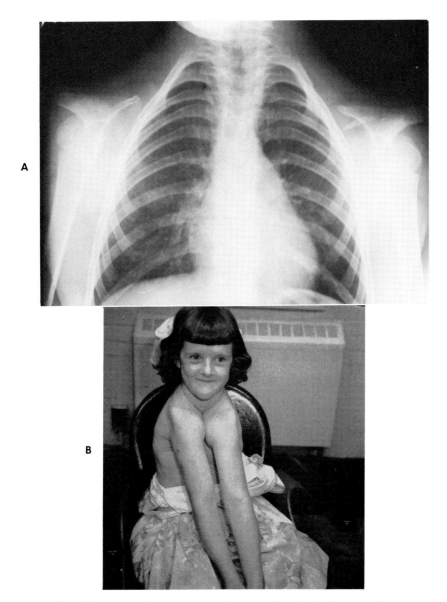

Fig. 16-15. Cleidocranial dysostosis in a 9-year-old girl. **A,** Chest radiogram shows the complete absence of both clavicles. **B,** Patient is able to bring the shoulders together.

Continued.

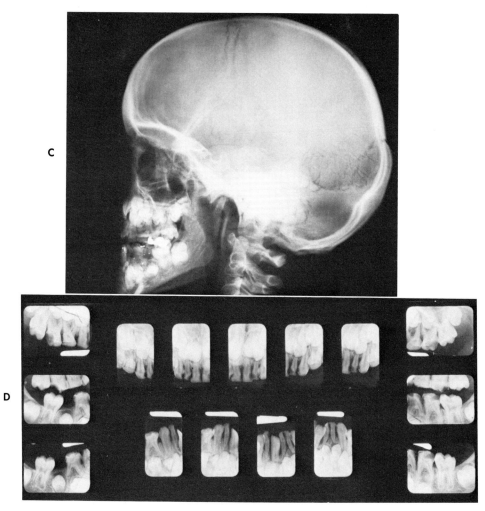

Fig. 16-15, cont'd. C, Skull radiogram demonstrates the small upper face, delayed closure of sutures, and many wormian bones. **D,** Dental survey shows many supernumerary teeth and failure of eruption of almost all the permanent teeth.

Sickle cell anemia

Sickle cell anemia is a hereditary, chronic, hemolytic anemia. This condition appears to be associated with blacks. Radiographic examination shows generalized osteoporosis. However, the lamina dura is not affected. The trabeculae in in the mandible may be coarse and have a "stepladder" appearance. The skull findings include, in addition to osteoporosis, generalized thickening of the bones and an indistinct outer table. There can also be a granular appearance of the cranium or alternate radiolucent and radiopaque lines radiating outward from the inner table. The last mentioned sign gives the radiographic image of the skull a hair-on-end appearance that, when seen in a black person, is highly indicative of sickle cell anemia. Skull and mandibular bone findings are shown in Fig. 16-17. The radiographic findings of this condition are not unlike those seen in thalassemia and some deficiency anemias.

Thalassemia

Thalassemia, also known as Cooley's or Mediterranean anemia, is a hereditary, chronic, progressive anemia. This condition is more prevalent among people living in or originating from the lands around the Mediterranean Sea. Radiographic examination shows generalized osteoporosis in the early stages and osteosclerosis in the late stages. The skull examination shows a wider diploe. The bone may have a granular appearance or may show radiolucent and radiopaque lines between the two tables of the cranium that give the calvarium a hair-on-end appearance. The radiographic signs are similar to those seen in sickle cell and some deficiency anemias.

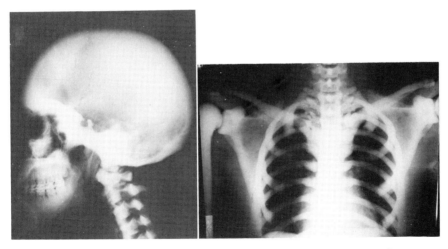

Fig. 16-16. Radiograms of a patient with a long history of osteopetrosis. The marrow of all the bones is almost completely replaced by calcified bone.

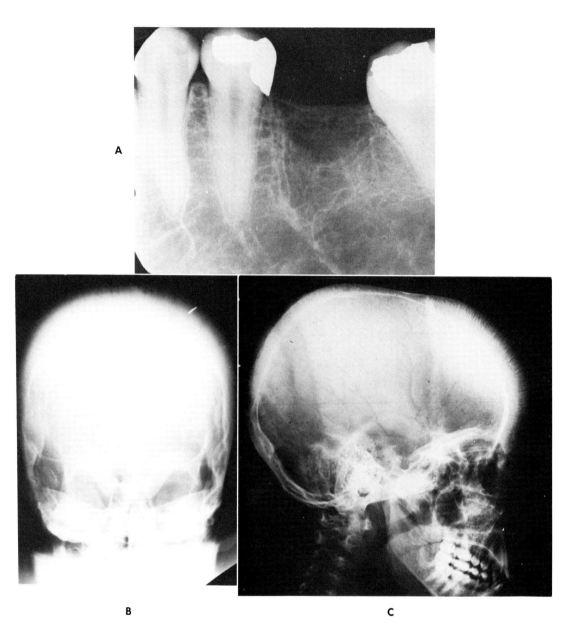

Fig. 16-17. A, Dental radiogram of a patient with sickle cell anemia. The bone is osteoporotic with fewer, coarser trabeculae. **B,** Skull radiograms of a patient with sickle cell anemia. The outer table is absent, and the diploe is markedly enlarged. The cranial vault is much thicker than normal and has a hair-on-end appearance. **C,** Skull radiogram of a patient with thalassemia. The changes are similar to those in **B.**

DISEASES CAUSED BY BIOLOGIC AGENTS

Many pathologic oral conditions are caused by the invasion of biologic agents. These agents may be bacteria, fungi, viruses, or parasites. Rarely does the radiogram play a part in the identification of the injurious agent. Note that other lesions, secondarily infected by biologic agents, will very often present the radiographic signs of infection. Since the radiogram shows mainly calcified tissues and these calcified tissues take relatively long periods of time to be deposited or resorbed, the time of onset of the condition must be considered in the radiographic diagnosis of infectious lesions. No radiographic signs are seen in the early stages of an infection, when pain, fever, and swelling may be most evident. When enough bone destruction occurs, a radiolucent lesion is seen. Overproduction of bone can also occur and can produce a radiopaque area (sclerosing osteitis); such is the case in infections of low virulence or at the borders of a long-standing abscess. In the main, chronic infections produce more radiographic signs than do acute infections.

Pulpal and periodontal infection

Pulpal and periodontal infections are discussed in Chapter 15.

Osteomyelitis

Osteomyelitis means inflammation of bone and marrow. However, the term is commonly used to indicate a progressive suppurative and/or sclerosing condition that can involve a complete bone. The early phase of osteomyelitis shows no radiographic sign. In 10 to 14 days enough bone resorption may take place to show irregular radiolucent areas within the bone. When the body defenses localize the condition, a border of condensing or sclerosing osteitis may wall off the area; this is called involucrum formation. If the affected area is great, a sizable piece of necrotic bone or sequestrum may be visible within the radiolucent area. The sequestration may be complete or incomplete and may absorb calcium salts from its surroundings, becoming rather dense; thus a radiopaque image that has less film density than the normal bone in the area may be produced. When the infection spreads unevenly and the necrotic bone assumes irregular shapes within a diffuse area of bone destruction, the radiographic image presents a worm-eaten appearance. The radiographic appearance of osteomyelitis varies with the virulency of the invading organism and with the defensive and reparative ability of the bone. Radiograms are also useful in locating the original site of the infection, such as an infected tooth, a fracture, or sinusitis. The use of antibiotics may abort the infectious process; consequently, the expected radiographic changes may not materialize. Classic examples of suppurative osteomyelitis and an example of sclerosing osteomyelitis are shown in Fig. 16-18.

In some instances, more often in children, the periosteum reacts to injury, infectious or otherwise, by producing bone. This condition is called periostitis

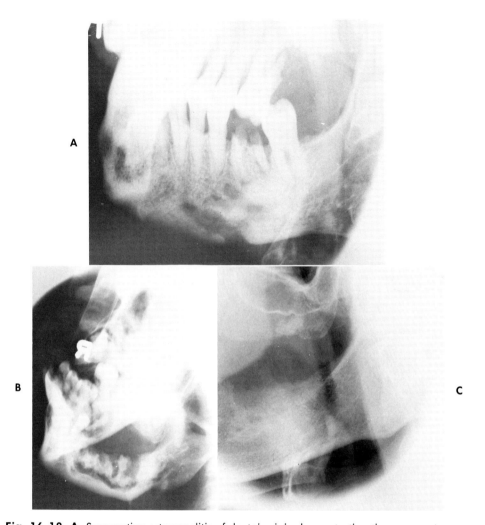

Fig. 16-18. A, Suppurative osteomyelitis of dental origin demonstrating the worm-eaten appearance of the bone, with perforation of the cortical plate at the lower border of the mandible. **B,** Suppurative osteomyelitis of the body of the mandible showing involucrum formation and a large sequestrum. **C,** Nonspecific infection producing chronic osteomyelitis of the body of the mandible. The patient complained of periodic suppurative discharges. The radiogram demonstrates mainly osteosclerosis with many fine trabeculae. Two small radiolucent areas can be seen in the bicuspid region.

ossificans and is seen more often in the mandible than in the maxilla. A common etiologic factor is the chronic periapical abscess that penetrates the cortical plate of the mandible and affects the periosteum. An example of periostitis ossificans is shown in Fig. 16-19. A similar increase in bone dimension can result from trauma. Periostitis ossificans associated with a sclerosing osteomyelitis is called Garré's osteomyelitis.

Temporomandibular joint infections

Infections involving the temporomandibular joint may cause ankylosis of the joint. Ankylosis can also result from inflammatory conditions caused by other etiologic agents, for example, trauma. In children, joint ankylosis results in underdevelopment of the jaw. Unilateral joint involvement produces facial asymmetry. Radiograms are useful in evaluation of these conditions. Facial asymmetry is illustrated in Fig. 16-28.

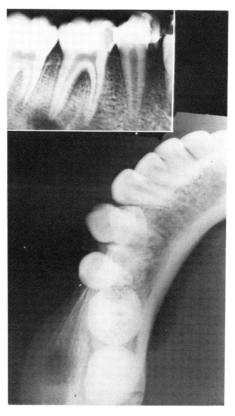

Fig. 16-19. Periostitis ossificans of the buccal surface of the mandible caused by periapical infection of the first molar. The occlusal cross-sectional view demonstrates the buildup of bone that changes the contour of the outer surface of the mandible.

Ludwig's angina

Ludwig's angina is cellulitis of the floor of the oral cavity. The infection causing this condition often originates from the lower molar area. Radiograms are useful in the diagnosis of absence or presence of abscessed teeth and perforations of the cortical plate of the mandible.

Sinusitis

Maxillary sinusitis can result from the extension of infections, especially those located in and around the maxillary teeth. The sinuses can also be directly infected via the nasal passages. Sinusitis can also result from trauma and is associated with some allergic states. Radiograms are helpful in determining the possible source of sinusitis, such as a periapical abscess or a root tip or foreign body in the sinus. Connections between the oral cavity and the maxillary sinus can be traced radiographically with radiopaque probes. Sinus radiograms may show a cloudy, slightly radiopaque sinus that can be caused by the presence of thickened sinus mucosa, granulomatous tissue, and fluid secretions or pus within the sinus. Generally speaking, the orbits and maxillary sinuses normally show the same density in a sinus radiogram. A comparison of the density of the right and left maxillary sinuses, and subsequently a comparison of the two sinuses with the orbits, usually shows whether one or both sinuses are affected. Intraoral radiograms that compare the right and left maxillary sinuses may show an appreciable difference in density, which indicates the possible presence of sinusitis in one of the sinuses. Sinusitis involving one antrum is shown in Fig. 16-20.

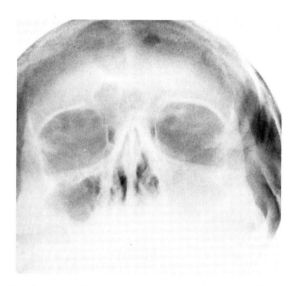

Fig. 16-20. Sinusitis of one maxillary sinus seen on a posteroanterior sinus radiogram. The affected sinus shows appreciably greater radiopacity, whereas the unaffected sinus has approximately the same film density as the orbits.

Infective granulomatous diseases

Chronic granulomatous conditions that affect bone include tuberculosis, syphilis, yaws, bejel, actinomycosis, and blastomycosis. Invasion of the bones of the jaws by organisms that produce chronic granulomatous conditions results in irregular osteolytic radiolucent areas or sclerosed radiopaque areas. Periostitis ossificans can also occur and change the contour of the bone. In tuberculosis, the lymph nodes may become calcified, and radiograms may depict such calcifications. Involvement of bone in tuberculosis and actinomycosis is shown in Fig. 16-21.

Congenital syphilis often produces central and lateral incisors that have screwdriver-shaped crowns and a notch in the incisal edge. These teeth are called Hutchinson's incisors; the tooth most often affected is the maxillary central incisor. Examples of Hutchinson's teeth are shown in Fig. 16-22. The first permanent molars may show constricted crowns and cusps and relatively short roots; these molars are called mulberry molars. In the late stages, syphilitic gummas

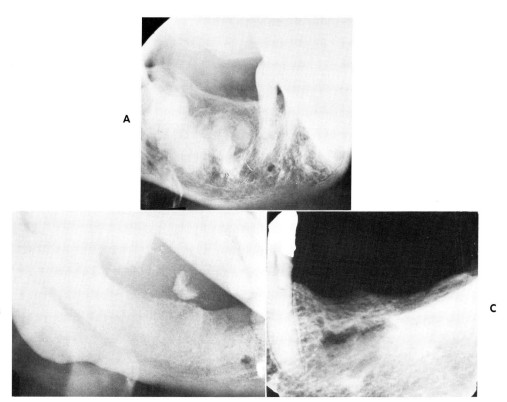

Fig. 16-21. A, Lateral jaw radiogram showing osteosclerotic areas within the body of the mandible of a patient with long-standing tuberculosis. **B,** Lateral jaw radiogram showing the osteosclerosis produced in actinomycosis. **C,** Intraoral film showing an osteolytic radiolucent area in actinomycosis. (**C,** Courtesy Dr. D. T. Waggener.)

can destroy bone and produce localized osteitis or widespread osteomyelitis. The hard palate is frequently involved and can be perforated by syphilitic gummas.

Lymphadenitis

Some infections of lymph nodes can result in calcification of the affected nodes. Calcified nodes in the submaxillary area are shown in Fig. 16-23. Such

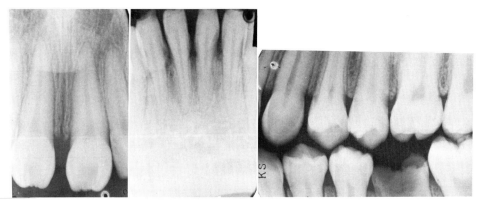

Fig. 16-22. Congenital syphilis with Hutchinson's teeth. The incisors show the typical screw-driver shape and notched incisal edges. The upper first molar demonstrates a mulberry-shaped crown.

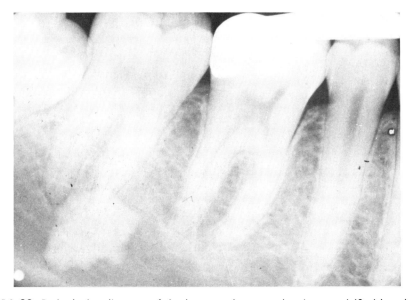

Fig. 16-23. Periapical radiogram of the lower molar area showing a calcified lymph node situated in the buccal soft tissue, superimposed on the apex of the second molar (see also Fig. 10-5).

calcifications seen on periapical radiograms can be mistaken for changes within the mandible if they are not properly localized. (See also Fig. 10-5.)

Sialadenitis

Infections of the major salivary glands can produce destruction of areas within the gland. Sialograms made after a radiopaque material is injected into the ductal system of the gland will depict the cavities within the gland. When mumps is the cause of sialadenitis, negative findings on regular diagnostic radiograms of the salivary glands are of importance.

Exanthematous fevers

Infectious diseases that produce prolonged fevers can also produce hypoplastic defects in the teeth. Radiograms are useful in showing these defects in unerupted teeth. (See discussion of hypoplastic teeth, Chapter 15.)

Cysticercosis and trichinosis

In cysticercosis, the calcified encysted larvae in the muscles are sometimes visualized in radiograms. These appear as multiple ovoid radiopaque masses within the soft tissues (Fig. 16-24). The masses vary in size; they may be irregularly calcified and may show a more radiolucent center when viewed longitudinally. The oval masses within muscles tend to have their long axes parallel with the muscle fibers. The radiographic appearance of trichinosis is similar to cysticercosis except that the larvae are smaller.

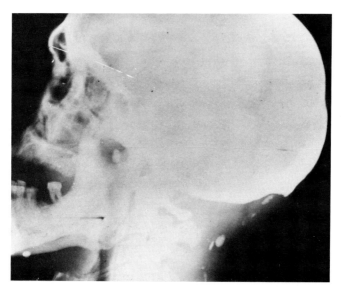

Fig. 16-24. Radiogram of a patient with cysticercosis. The calcified encysted larvae are clearly seen in the soft tissues. Note the single calcification in the area of Wharton's duct that can be easily mistaken for a sialolith on intraoral films. (Courtesy Dr. E. Cheraskin.)

PATHOLOGIC CHANGE CAUSED BY PHYSICAL AGENTS

Trauma denotes injury arising from all causes. Injury to oral structures because of agents that enter the body can be divided into those caused by biologic agents and those caused by physical agents. This discussion is devoted to conditions that arise from trauma from physical agents. Physical agents may produce injury by the application of thermal, electrical, radiant, chemical, and mechanical energy. Some conditions caused by physical agents are of radiographic importance; these mainly pertain to injury caused by radiation, chemicals, and force.

Radiation injury

The biologic effects, hazards, clinical signs and symptoms, and significance of exposure to ionizing radiation are discussed in Chapter 4. Radiographic findings are useful in the diagnosis of radiation injury. The patient's history usually provides an estimate of the patient's age at the time of exposure to ionizing radiation. Exposed teeth that were developing at the time of exposure may show

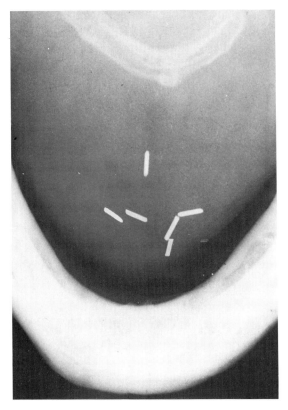

Fig. 16-25. Radon seeds implanted in the floor of the mouth for radiation treatment of a malignancy. The damage to the bone (osteoradionecrosis) is not seen radiographically until trauma or infection is superimposed on this condition and causes breakdown of the calcified elements of the bone.

defects ranging from imperceptible hypoplasia to failure of tooth development. Radiograms show very little bone change unless the radiation dose was so great that the exposed tissues could not maintain their integrity; in this instance, the patient is usually still under the care of a radiotherapist or physician. The condition most likely to be seen in the dental office is that of a patient who has had radiation therapy some time in the past. Depending on the dose of radiation absorbed, the irradiated tissues have reduced ability to repair themselves, and radiograms may show some areas of slight osteoporosis. Because of their impaired vitality, the irradiated tissues are very susceptible to infections, and fulminating osteomyelitis is often the result when irradiated bone is subsequently damaged. When osteoradionecrosis (noninfected necrotic bone) or osteomyelitis occurs, the sequestrum of bone may assume the shape of the beam of radiation used during radiotherapy. Sclerosing osteitis, if present, is seen in the radiogram at the borders of the irradiated area. If radon seeds, needles, or other radiation-applying devices are left within the soft tissues after therapy, they may be identified as foreign bodies in the diagnostic radiograms. Osteoradionecrosis is shown in Fig. 16-25.

Attrition, abrasion, erosion, hypercementosis, and root resorption

These conditions are discussed in Chapter 15.

Dilaceration

A deformed tooth caused by injury during development is called a dilacerated tooth. Dilaceration is most often due to mechanical trauma. The deformity may affect the crown or root of the tooth, or both. The pulp chamber assumes the shape of the tooth. Observation of the pulp shape on the radiogram is important in some instances in differentiating the dilacerated root from a normally shaped root that is undergoing root resorption. Examples of dilacerated teeth are shown in Fig. 16-26.

Dislocation

Dislocation, or luxation, occurs in the temporomandibular joint and between the teeth and their supporting structures. Radiograms are valuable in differentiating fractures from dislocations. In dislocations of the temporomandibular joint, radiograms show the position of the condylar head to be anterior to the articular eminence in some cases and positioned overly superior and posterior in the glenoid fossa in other instances. Dislocation of teeth is clearly seen radiographically by observing the width of the periodontal space around the roots of the affected teeth. Gross dislocations affecting teeth or temporomandibular joints are easily identified radiographically. It is important that radiograms be made when a child with a missing tooth complains that the tooth came out from a blow and that the tooth could not be found. Radiograms often show the missing tooth pushed into the jaws, out of sight clinically, and located under a blood clot. An example of a tooth dislocation is shown in Fig. 16-27.

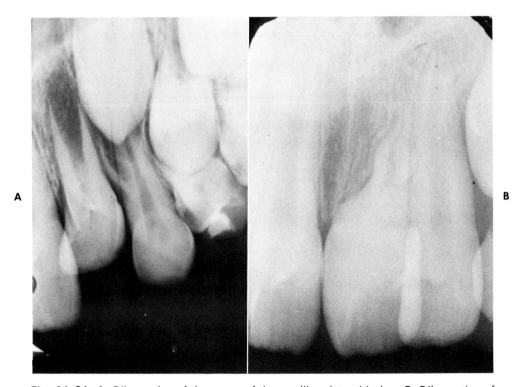

A

B

Fig. 16-26. A, Dilaceration of the crown of the maxillary lateral incisor. **B,** Dilaceration of the root of a maxillary central incisor. Note that the pulp chamber conforms to the shape of the root; this is important in differentiating dilaceration from root resorption. (**A,** Courtesy Dr. S. B. Finn.)

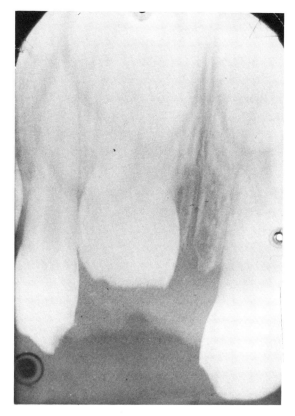

Fig. 16-27. Radiogram of a child who received a blow to the face and appeared with a clinically missing deciduous central incisor. This radiogram shows that the tooth was completely pushed up into the maxilla. (Courtesy Dr. S. B. Finn.)

Costen's syndrome

Signs and symptoms affecting the temporomandibular joint are associated with Costen's syndrome; unbalance in mechanical forces is often mentioned as an etiologic factor. Serial radiograms of both temporomandibular joints are often made to show the relationship of the head of the mandibular condyle to the glenoid fossa when the mandible is in the occlusal, rest, and open positions. Radiograms play an important role in the observation of discrepancies in the position of the mandibular condyle. However, serial temporomandibular joint radiograms do not have sufficient diagnostic sensitivity to show slight malpositioning in the fossa-head relationship.

Teeth and joint ankylosis

Trauma can produce pericementitis in teeth and osteoarthritis in the temporomandibular joint. Ankylosis of teeth or joints can result from these conditions. The radiogram shows the extent of the affected area and the amount of bone production, especially in temporomandibular joint ankylosis. Radiograms do not usually show whether there is fibrous or a true bone union between the tooth

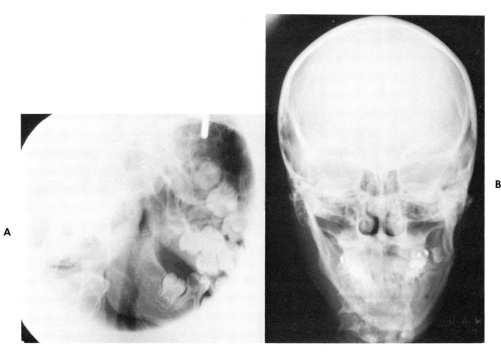

Fig. 16-28. Radiograms of a patient with long-standing ankylosis of one temporomandibular joint. **A,** Lateral jaw film shows the affected side. The fused area is seen plus a well-formed coronoid process and distorted sigmoid notch. **B,** Posteroanterior skull view shows the deviation of the mandibular midline toward the affected side caused by normal development of one side of the mandible and underdevelopment of the affected side. (Courtesy Dr. C. A. McCallum, Jr.)

and alveolar bone or between the condyle and the temporal bone. When tempo-romandibular joint ankylosis occurs in a child, skull radiograms (especially the posteroanterior skull projection) are valuable in showing the subsequent under-development of the mandible on the affected side (Fig. 16-28). Tooth ankylosis is shown in Fig. 15-25. Temporomandibular radiographic technics are discussed in Chapter 7.

Fractures

Fractures of teeth and jaws occur. Fractures usually result from excessive mechanical force; however, normal forces applied to weakened teeth and bone also produce fractures. Radiograms are valuable in the evaluation of fractures. Radiograms show whether the patient has a single fracture, mutiple fractures, a comminuted fracture, or a complicated fracture. Radiograms show the loca-tion of the fracture, the amount of separation between parts of the involved structure, and the size of the fragments in a comminuted fracture. Examples of fractures are shown in Fig. 16-29.

To properly survey a fracture patient radiographically, one must know the patient's history and the findings of the clinical examination. One must also be aware of the association of certain types of fractures with others, of the effect of muscles pulling on the various parts of affected bones, and of the effect of ligaments and fascia on the position of bone fragments. It is important to remember that, when the x-ray beam is directed more or less at right angles to the plane of the fracture, the fracture is sometimes not seen in the radiogram. The amount of separation shown in the radiogram between the parts of the involved structure is minimal, not maximal. An awareness of possible optical illusions and a knowledge of the skull sutures are also of importance; the viewer may misinterpret these usual images as fractures.

Radiograms are not only valuable in the diagnosis of fractures but are also needed to show the reduction of fractures during treatment and the production of new bone during the healing process.

Traumatic cyst

The traumatic cyst, or intraosseous hematoma, is not an epithelium-lined sac but a pseudocyst. Radiographically, it often resembles a cyst. Like cysts, this condition is usually asymptomatic and is often discovered through routine x-ray examination. The lesion is radiolucent and tends to assume the shape determined by the cortical plates of bone and the roots of teeth in the area. Its borders are irregular or notched and tend to be less well defined than the borders of a true cyst. Traumatic cysts are seen most frequently in younger persons and are most often situated in the body of the mandible. Traumatic cysts are usually solitary lesions; however, those shown in Fig. 16-30, *A,* are multiple. Traumatic cysts result from the extravasation of blood into bone. Radiograms are also use-ful in the diagnosis of cases in which blood fills body cavities such as the sinuses.

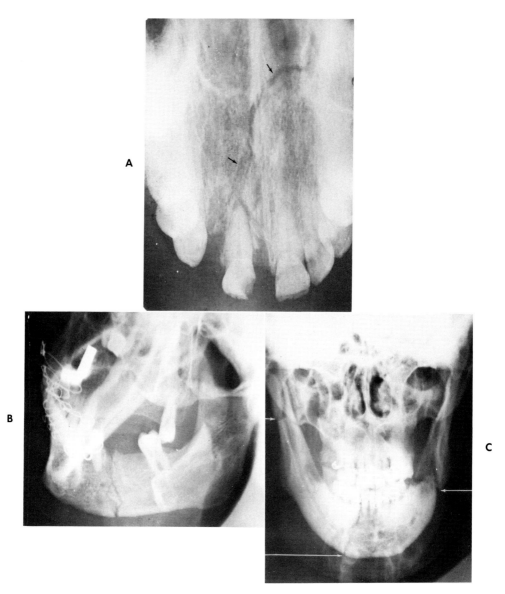

Fig. 16-29. A, Occlusal radiogram showing a fracture of the maxilla that crosses the midline. Bone fragments, one containing a central incisor, are clearly seen in this projection. **B,** Lateral jaw radiogram showing a fracture through the body of the mandible. Separation of the two segments has been reduced by intermaxillary wires. **C,** Posteroanterior mandibular view demonstrating fractures of the mandible at the angle, near the symphysis, and in the condylar neck.

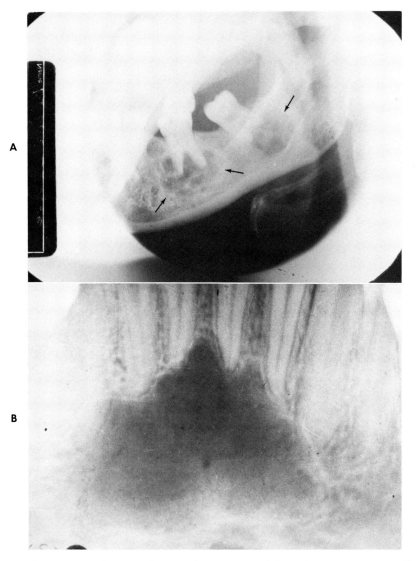

Fig. 16-30. A, Lateral jaw radiogram showing two of three lesions in an unusual case of multiple traumatic cysts. **B,** More conventional type of intraosseous hematoma showing the cystlike appearance that gives rise to the name "traumatic cyst." The lesion is located at the apices of the mandibular anterior teeth.

Sialolithiasis

Radiograms are useful in detecting and localizing salivary stones in the major salivary glands and their ducts. The radiograms are made with less exposure time than would be used for examination of the jaw bones. Sialoliths within the glands tend to have a spherical shape with irregular borders, whereas those within the ducts tend to be oval. Sialoliths are shown in Fig. 16-31.

Phleboliths

Calcified masses in blood vessels are sometimes seen in dental radiograms. They are most commonly found in the cheek and are often associated with hemangiomas. They tend to have ovoid shapes, may be unevenly calcified, and have a laminated appearance. Phleboliths are shown in Fig. 16-32.

Chemical pericementitis

Arsenical compounds, if used in endodontic therapy, may reach the periodontal tissues. Silicate restorations placed in deep cavities without protective bases can also indirectly injure the periapical tissues. In both instances, pericementitis and a radiolucent periapical area result. Chemical pericementitis can also be caused by pulp necrosis resulting from phenol, eugenol, and other chemical agents used in dental therapy.

Phosphorus and mercury intoxication

Phosphorus- and mercury-containing compounds can produce poisoning if ingested in excessive amounts. Radiograms may show the chronic progressive osteitis, periostitis, or osteomyelitis that accompanies such cases.

Foreign bodies

Radiograms are very helpful in identifying and locating foreign bodies. However, radiolucent objects, such as wood splinters and silk sutures, cannot be visualized radiographically. It should be remembered that translucent objects, such as glass, are not necessarily radiolucent. An example is leaded glass. Radiopaque objects entering the oropharynx can be traced with radiograms to determine if they were swallowed or aspirated. Examples of foreign bodies are shown in Fig. 16-33.

Postsurgical defects

Surgical intervention of oral pathologic processes often produce unusual radiographic findings. Examples of postsurgical defects are shown in Fig. 16-34.

CYSTS

Cysts are epithelium-lined sacs that are often filled with fluid. Equal pressure is exerted on the walls of the cyst from within; the cyst tends to be spherical except when unequal resistance to its growth is encountered. The cyst is thus

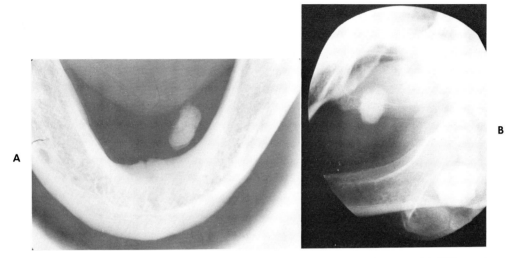

Fig. 16-31. A, Cross-sectional occlusal radiogram showing a sialolith situated in Wharton's duct. **B,** Lateral jaw radiogram of bilateral sialolithiasis of the submandibular glands. A single large sialolith can be seen in each gland.

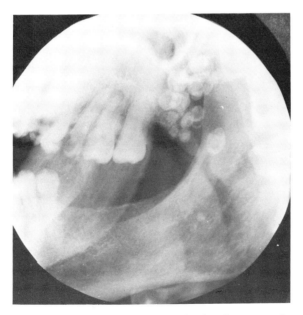

Fig. 16-32. Phleboliths in a hemangioma of the cheek adjacent to the coronoid process. The outine of the hemangioma cannot be seen.

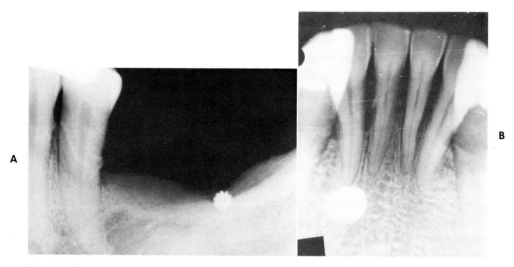

Fig. 16-33. A, Radiogram demonstrating a dental bur head within the body of the mandible. **B,** Radiogram of a spherical lead pellet situated in the anterior mandibular region.

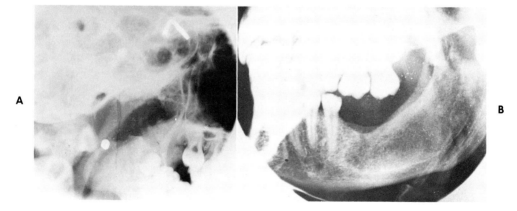

Fig. 16-34. A, Postoperative radiogram of a partially resected mandibular ramus. The opaque objects are temporary localization markers. The anatomic structures of the mandible in this area are now permanently missing. **B,** Postoperative radiogram of a healed cyst. The original outline of the cyst involving the body and ramus of the mandible is still observable. The new bone has a finer trabecular pattern. Note the displacement of the mandibular canal and unclear posterior border of the coronoid process caused by the original displacement and distortion produced by the cyst.

shaped by the obstructions it encounters in growing. Cysts are relatively slow growing lesions and tend to push aside structures such as teeth; teeth are sometimes resorbed. Cysts also tend to expand instead of perforating the cortical plates of bones; in this manner, they produce bone enlargement.

Cysts, being soft tissue sacs filled with fluid, cast radiolucent images of homogeneous density on the radiogram. Cysts within soft tissues do not produce definite radiographic shadows; such cysts are made radiographically visible through the use of contrast media. A cyst within bone has a well-defined border of bone whose appearance on the radiogram often resembles the lamina dura around the root of a tooth. The bone outside the border of the cyst radiographically appears quite normal.

Cysts can be unilocular or multilocular. The multilocular appearance of a cyst in a radiogram can be due to two or more separate cysts encroaching on each other or to a single cavity with invaginations. Multilocular cysts often show thin bony septa separating the multiple cystic areas.

Cysts are of epithelial origin and arise whenever epithelium or the remnants of epithelium are likely to be found. A knowledge of the sites of origin of cysts in and around the jaws is important from a diagnostic standpoint. Also, therapy may vary for the different types of cysts. The association of cysts with other structures must be noted on the radiogram. Cysts will be listed as being of odontogenic origin, nonodontogenic origin, or unknown origin.

Odontogenic cysts

Odontogenic cysts arise from epithelial cells associated with the development of a tooth. The enamel organ is of epithelial origin, and odontogenic cysts arise from this organ or its remnants. A source of epithelium of odontogenic origin is the epithelial remnants (the rests of Malassez) found in the periodontal membrane.

Periodontal cyst (radicular). The radicular cyst is a periodontal cyst arising in the periodontal membrane. It is usually of inflammatory origin and is often associated with a periapical abscess or granuloma. The radiographic characteristics of this cyst are discussed in Chapter 15. Radicular cysts occur most commonly at the apices of teeth; when situated there, they are called apical radicular cysts. When located at the side of the root, they are called lateral radicular cysts. Like the apical radicular cyst, the lateral radicular cyst is usually of inflammatory origin. The radiographic characteristics of radicular cysts vary widely.

Follicular cyst. Cysts arising from the dental lamina or enamel organ are called follicular cysts. These cysts are of developmental origin and are sometimes further classified into primordial cysts and dentigerous cysts.

Primordial cyst. The primordial cyst arises from the tooth follicle and is often called a simple follicular cyst. The cyst arises before the odontogenic epithelium has differentiated. If the cyst develops from a normal enamel organ, it will be seen in an area where a tooth did not develop (Fig. 16-35). The cyst can also be found in an area where no tooth is missing if it arises from a supernumerary tooth bud.

Dentigerous cyst. A dentigerous cyst is one that develops from the enamel organ and is associated with the crown of a tooth. The teeth most often involved are third molars, canines, and embedded teeth. The crowns of the tooth can project into the cyst cavity, or the cyst can be attached to the side of the enamel organ. These cysts tend to develop in the early decades of life and often achieve great size. The associated tooth is sometimes significantly displaced, and the cortical plates of the bones of the jaw may be expanded. Examples of dentigerous cysts are shown in Fig. 16-36. Dentigerous cysts should be examined very carefully because these cysts sometimes give rise to ameloblastomas.

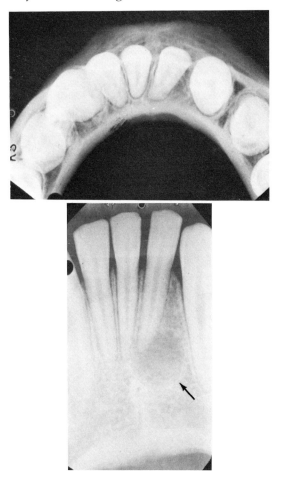

Fig. 16-35. Primordial cyst that has developed between the mandibular cuspid and central teeth. The lateral incisor had failed to develop. All teeth were vital. (Courtesy Dr. D. T. Waggener.)

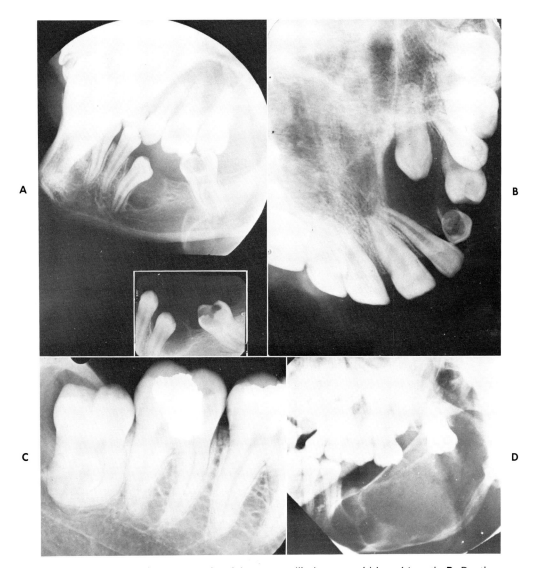

Fig. 16-36. A, Dentigerous cyst involving a mandibular second bicuspid tooth. **B,** Dentigerous cyst involving a maxillary cuspid tooth. The deciduous cuspid is still present. **C,** Dentigerous cyst (lateral type) involving a mandibular third molar. **D,** Extremely large dentigerous cyst involving the entire ramus. (**C,** Courtesy Dr. E. C. Stafne.)

Nonodontogenic cysts

Nonodontogenic cysts arise from epithelium other than that associated with tooth formation. In the development of the human embryo, the jaws are formed by various embryonic arches. Embryonic arches and processes join at various fissures; cysts may arise at these junctions. Such cysts are sometimes collectively called fissural or cleft cysts. Since the embryonic arches form definite parts of the face, the fissural cysts occur at specific locations in the adult human being (Fig. 14-1). A knowledge of these locations is beneficial in the diagnosis of nonodontogenic cysts. A few nonodontogenic cysts, not of fissural origin, are also of interest to the oral diagnostician. A significant radiographic finding is that nonodontogenic cysts are not connected to teeth.

Median cyst. Median cysts are fissural cysts that occur in the midline of the mandible (median mandibular cysts) or maxilla (median maxillary cyst). The maxillary cyst is sometimes further categorized into median alveolar and median palatine cysts. A median mandibular cyst and a median palatine cyst are shown in Fig. 16-37; the latter occurs with considerably greater frequency than either the median mandibular cyst or the median alveolar cyst.

Globulomaxillary cyst. The globulomaxillary cyst is a fissural cyst. It is seen between the maxillary cuspid and lateral incisor teeth. The cyst often pushes apart the apices of the cuspid and lateral teeth and assumes the shape of a pear with the bulbous portion situated superiorly. A globulomaxillary cyst is shown in Fig. 16-38.

Nasoalveolar cyst. The nasoalveolar cyst is a fissural cyst that occurs at the base of the nose where the wing of the nose, the cheek, and the upper lip meet. This cyst usually occurs in the soft tissue. However, it can create a depression in the buccal surface of the maxilla that is often visible in the intraoral radiographic survey. A lateral or tangential view of the area will also show this depression. The withdrawal of some of the cyst fluid and the injection of contrast medium are very helpful in radiographically localizing the boundaries of this cyst. An example of the nasoaveolar cyst is shown in Fig. 16-39.

Nasopalatine cyst. The nasopalatine cyst is a cyst that occurs in the incisive canal or in the incisive papilla. These cysts are sometimes subdivided into incisive canal cysts and cysts of the incisive papilla. The cyst of the incisive papilla occurs in soft tissue, and radiography is of little value in its diagnosis. However, incisive canal cysts are of radiographic importance. When the cyst occurs high up in the canal or in an edentulous jaw, it tends to assume a spherical or ovoid shape. When the cyst occurs low in the canal and the upper central incisors are present, it is shaped by the roots of the incisor teeth and by the nasal septum. In this latter case, the cyst may assume the shape of a heart. A cyst of the incisive canal is shown in Fig. 16-40.

Thyroglossal cyst. The thyroid gland develops from the same epithelium that goes into the formation of the oral cavity. The path of development of the gland lies in the midline of the neck from the foramen cecum of the tongue to the

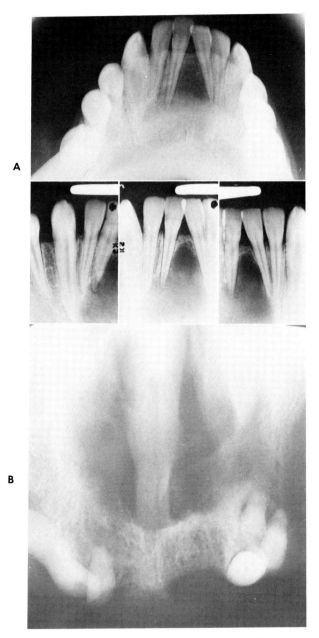

Fig. 16-37. A, Median mandibular cyst separating the mandibular central incisors as seen on periapical and occlusal radiograms. **B,** Large median maxillary cyst involving the palate as seen on a topographic occlusal radiogram.

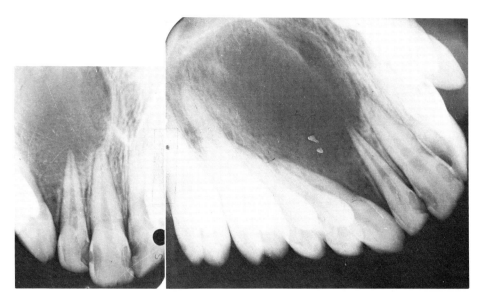

Fig. 16-38. Radiograms of a globulomaxillary cyst. The separation of the lateral incisor and cuspid teeth by the radiolucent lesion is depicted in these projections.

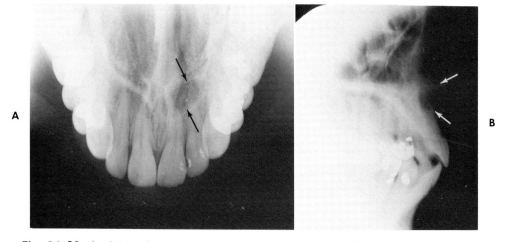

Fig. 16-39. A, Occlusal radiogram of a nasoalveolar cyst showing the radiolucency produced by a depression in the outer surface of the maxilla caused by the cyst. **B,** Tangential projection of the maxilla in the lateral incisor area of the affected side, showing the depression in the surface of the maxilla and elevation of the anterior nasal spine.

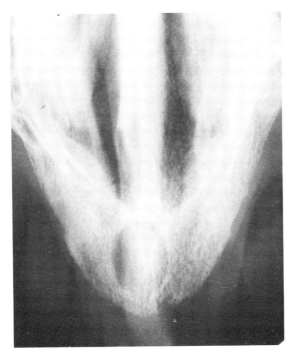

Fig. 16-40. Nasopalatine cyst occurring in the incisive canal. With no great obstruction in its path of growth, this particular cyst has assumed a spherical shape.

gland. The thyroglossal cyst lies within soft tissue. Radiography is helpful if done for the soft tissues. The displacement of the hyoid bone is sometimes shown on lateral projections of the neck, and displacement of the larynx can be visualized when contrast medium is used.

Branchial cyst. The branchial cyst occurs at the side of the neck along a vertical line just posterior to the posterior border of the ramus of the mandible. Radiopaque media trace the borders and/or fistulas of this cyst.

Mucous cyst. The mucous cyst, or mucocele, is a retention cyst that can occur wherever there is mucous membrane. These cysts are not usually seen on radiograms. However, when they occur in the mucous membrane of the maxillary sinus, the cyst may cast a faint dome-shaped shadow into the radiolucent image of the maxillary sinus. A mucous cyst as it appears on an intraoral radiogram is shown in Fig. 16-41.

Cysts of unknown origin

Residual or retained cyst. A residual cyst is the name given to any cyst in the jaws that is not associated with a tooth and is not situated at the site of any fissural cyst. It should be noted that, if the cyst is the result of an odontogenic cyst's being left in the jaw after the extraction of a tooth, it may be secondarily infected. Sclerosing osteitis often occurs at the periphery of an infected cyst; this type of osteitis is seen radiographically. Examples of residual cysts are shown in Fig. 16-42.

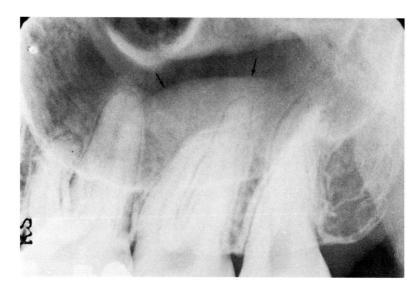

Fig. 16-41. Mucous cyst located in the floor of the maxillary sinus and seen in a periapical radiogram.

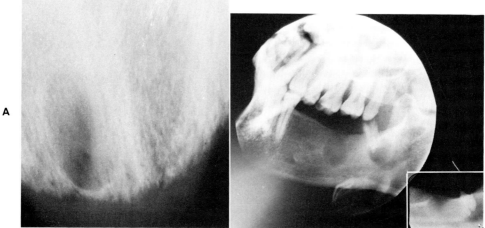

Fig. 16-42. A, Periapical radiogram of a residual cyst in the alveolar process of an edentulous patient. The cyst is situated in the maxillary central area. **B,** Lateral jaw and periapical radiograms showing a residual cyst in the mandibular first molar area and a radicular cyst of the mandibular third molar.

NEOPLASMS

Radiography is very helpful in the diagnosis of neoplasms that affect bone and teeth. Radiograms show the area involved and its position, whether the patient has single or multiple lesions, whether the neoplasm forms calcified material, and whether this calcified material is well organized, for example, in the form of small teeth. Radiograms do not show signs characteristic of *specific* neoplasms; however, some broad inferences can be made about neoplasms in general from radiographic data. It must also be realized that nonneoplastic lesions can produce radiographic signs similar to those of neoplasms.

Expansive tumors tend to form smooth borders, whereas invasive tumors tend to form jagged borders. Slowly growing tumors tend to push teeth and cortical bone plates out of their way and tend to show a thin layer of cortical bone or bone sclerosis at their borders. Rapidly growing neoplasms show mainly bone destruction; the lesions surround the roots of teeth. Tumors that are aggressive but not growing extremely rapidly tend to produce root resorption when teeth obstruct their path of growth. The radiogram is extremely useful in detecting the number of lesions present and in depicting the amount of bone involvement. This information is valuable since a neoplasm may appear as a small lesion clinically and yet show massive involvement of the underlying bone radiographically. Radiography is also useful in showing the course of treatment and postoperative healing.

Radiograms do not show whether a tumor is benign or malignant. Radiograms also generally do not show the type of tissue involved, for example, epithelial or mesenchymal tissue. Radiograms show only changes in calcified tissues; they cannot show the borders of a rapidly invading neoplasm, because these changes in the calcified tissues take time to appear on radiograms. Clinical, radiographic, microscopic, and sometimes biochemical findings are all necessary in the diagnosis of neoplasms.

Neoplasms of dental importance are generally classified into odontogenic and nonodontogenic tumors. Regardless of origin, tumors present similar radiographic findings and are therefore discussed collectively. Only neoplasms of oral radiographic importance are discussed; consideration of hyperplasias and hamartomas is included in the general discussion of neoplasms.

It is recommended that radiographic examination of the chest and spine be requested when oral malignancies are discovered. The reason is that a metastatic rate as high as 20% has been reported for malignancies arising in the head and neck.

Ameloblastoma

The ameloblastoma, or adamantinoma, presents various microscopic appearances; for example, there are solid and cystic types. The radiographic appearance of this neoplasm also varies greatly. It may resemble a single small or large cyst. It may resemble a multilocular cyst or many small cysts, with a soap bubble or honeycomb appearance. The ameloblastoma is more a benign than a malignant lesion; however, it has no capsule and can cause great bone destruction. These characteristics tend to produce a lesion that radiographically shows a single area whose overall shape is like a cyst or an expansive lesion. Close examination shows the border of the lesion to be indistinct and sometimes notched. The lesion tends to surround the roots of teeth or to produce tooth resorption. An ameloblastoma may present one or more of these radiographic findings at the same time in different areas of the neoplasm. Examples of ameloblastomas are shown in Fig. 16-43. Ameloblastic cells are sometimes seen in other odontogenic tumors such as fibromas, sarcomas, odontomas, and dentigerous cysts. Proliferation of the ameloblastic component may change the radiographic characteristics of the original tumor.

Enameloma

Most enamelomas, or enamel pearls, are asymptomatic and are usually discovered on routine x-ray examination of the dentition. They are usually small and are often attached to the roots of teeth near the cementoenamel junction. Because of its high degree of calcification, an enameloma appears as a distinct radiopaque mass (Fig. 16-44).

Dentinoma

The dentinoma is a rare tumor situated in the alveolar bone and is composed entirely of dentin. Radiographically, the dentinoma may be seen as a radiopaque mass surrounded by a radiolucent line and possibly by an outer radiopaque lamina or border of bone (Fig. 16-45). However, the dentinoma may blend into the surrounding bone without any interposed line or border.

Cementoma

Cementomas occur most often at the apices of teeth; they are frequently observed in the mandibular anterior region and most often in women. In the proliferative phase of the cementoma (cementoblastoma), the periapical bone is resorbed, and the lesion appears as a radiolucent area similar to a periapical abscess or granuloma. In the calcification stage, an unevenly calcified radiopaque mass appears within the radiolucency. The mature cementoma appears radiographically as a fairly uniform radiopaque mass, surrounded by a radiolucent line suggestive of a capsule. It is sometimes bordered by a radiopaque line indicative of a bone wall. The various stages of cementoma formation are shown in Fig. 16-46.

Odontoma

Odontomas can appear as either radiopaque or radiolucent masses. They are usually seen as well-defined radiolucent areas within bone that contain varying amounts of calcified material. They may or may not be associated with a cyst

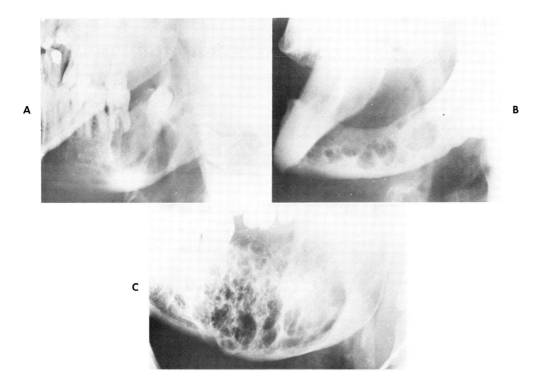

A

B

C

Fig. 16-43. A, Ameloblastoma presenting a radiographic picture very similar to a cyst. **B,** Ameloblastoma presenting a polycystic appearance. **C,** Ameloblastoma showing a honey-comb or soap-bubble appearance. (**A,** Courtesy Dr. E. Cheraskin; **B,** courtesy Dr. M. H. Jacobs.)

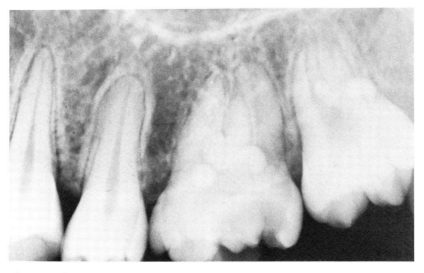

Fig. 16-44. Radiogram of the maxillary molar area showing radiopaque spherical enamel pearls attached to the roots of the molar teeth.

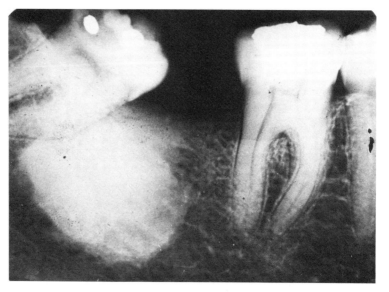

Fig. 16-45. Opaque mass anterior to the mandibular third molar was reported histologically to be a dentinoma. Massess of this type are more often sclerotic bone.

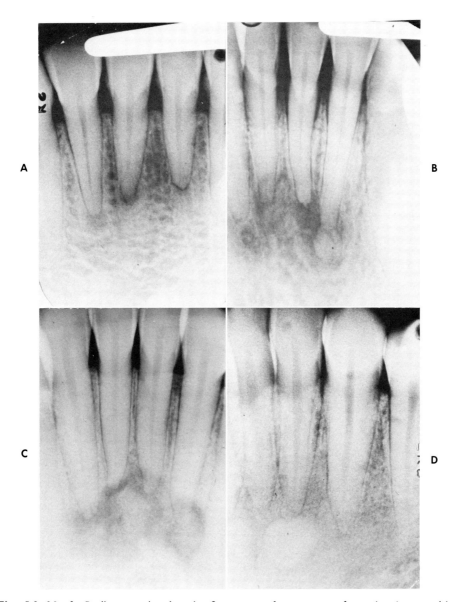

Fig. 16-46. A, Radiogram showing the first stage of cementoma formation (cementoblastoma). The lesion appears as a small radiolucency at the apex of the tooth. This radiogram shows the condition affecting lower incisor teeth. **B,** Radiogram of lower anterior teeth showing a cementoma in the matrix and early calcification stage. The border of the radiolucency is ill defined. Nonhomogeneous, ill-defined calcifications can be seen within the radiolucency. **C,** Cementoma showing a great deal of calcified material within the lesion. The radiolucency is fairly well defined. **D,** Final stage of cementoma.

(cystic odontoma). Odontomas are slow-growing lesions that are usually encapsulated. Two odontomas of importance are the complex composite and compound composite odontomas.

The complex composite odontoma shows varying amounts of nondescript calcified masses within the tumor. The compound composite odontoma shows many denticles or small teeth in various stages of formation. Composite odontomas mature to show densely calcified masses surrounded by a radiolucent line and bounded by a radiopaque border suggestive of a defensive bone wall. Radiograms of composite odontomas are shown in Fig. 16-47.

Enostosis, exostosis, and torus

Localized overgrowths of bone occur on the inner or outer surfaces of the bone plates of the jaws. Periapical radiograms show diffuse radiopaque shadows within the jawbones; the radiopacity depends on the size and degree of calcification of the growth. Exostoses and tori are easily identified when both radiographic and clinical findings are considered. On the other hand, enostoses are difficult to identify because they present no clinical findings. Enostoses produce irregular radiopaque shadows without radiolucent lines around them; they resemble areas of osteosclerosis within the jaws. Examples of enostoses and exostoses are shown in Fig. 16-48.

Osteoma

Osteomas may produce radiolucent or radiopaque tumors. The relatively rare radiolucent type (osteoid osteoma) appears as an irregular radiolucent area in the bone surrounded by bone lamina of increased radiopacity. The more common radiopaque type shows various degrees of radiopacity, depending on the type of bone being formed and the degree of calcification. The well-calcified osteoma appears as a very radiopaque mass surrounded by a radiolucent border and bounded by a radiopaque line. Osteomas projecting from the surface of a bone resemble tori and are clearly visualized in radiograms made with the x-ray beam directed parallel with the plane of the bone surface. Radiograms are useful in locating the site of attachment of the tumor to bone. Osteomas may be single or multiple. The well-formed bone spicules and basically normal architecture of the bone seen in an osteoma are indicative of a benign lesion. Radiograms of osteomas are shown in Fig. 16-49.

Fibroma

Fibromas can be of odontogenic or nonodontogenic origin. They can be located centrally (within bone) or peripherally. Fibromas may produce calcified material or bone (ossifying or osteofibroma). Radiographically, the centrally located fibroma in the initial phase appears as a radiolucent area surrounded by a white line, that is, very much like a cyst. When the lesion forms calcified spicules of bone, small bits or foci of radiopaque material appear within the

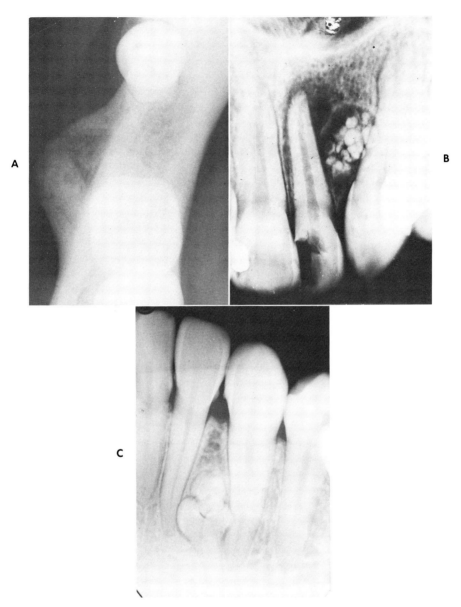

Fig. 16-47. A, Complex composite odontoma in the body of the mandible. The lesion shown here in a cross-sectional projection is expanding the buccal plate of the mandible. The opacity of the lesion is caused by the presence of a mixture of poorly calcified dental tissues within the lesion. **B** and **C,** Examples of compound composite odontomas seen radiographically as small, malformed teeth within a radiolucent area. In the maxillary odontoma, the outline of the lesion is still visible in spite of the infection around the apex of the lateral incisor.

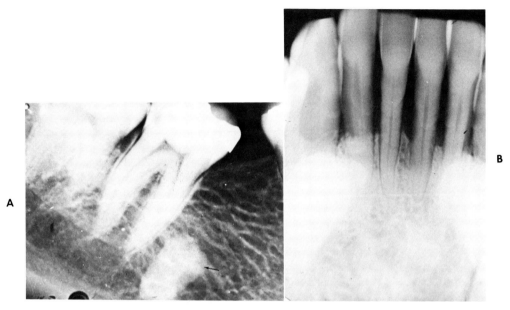

Fig. 16-48. A, Enostosis in the mandibular first molar area. **B,** Bilateral mandibular tori or exostoses on the lingual surface of the mandible in the bicuspid area, seen in a mandibular incisor periapical radiogram.

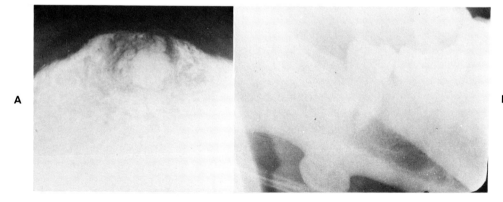

Fig. 16-49. Radiograms showing osteomas. **A,** Osteoma within bone surrounded by tissue having a radiolucent appearance. **B,** Osteoma projecting from the surface of the lower border of the ramus. (Courtesy Dr. E. Cheraskin.)

radiolucent area. The peripherally located fibroma shows essentially negative radiographic findings; however, if calcified, the calcification will be seen in the soft tissue areas of the diagnostic radiogram. Examples of fibromas are shown in Fig. 16-50.

Neuroma and neurofibroma

Neuromas and neurofibromas occurring within the jaws appear in radiograms as fairly well defined radiolucencies. An intimate relationship with the mandibular canal can usually be established by radiography. When these tumors arise within the mandibular canal, they tend to assume a bulbous or ovoid shape.

Hemangioma

Hemangiomas occurring within bone appear as cystlike areas of radiolucency within which may be seen radiopaque structures resembling large-course trabeculae. This pattern of the material within the radiolucency produces an image that has a somewhat honeycomb design.

Hemangiomas occurring in soft tissues essentially present no significant radiographic findings. However, these tumors often have phleboliths forming within them. Phleboliths appear as more or less spherical calcified masses of various small sizes. A radiogram of a hemangioma in the cheek is shown in Fig. 16-32.

Teratoma

Radiography is useful in the diagnosis of a teratoma, a dermoid cyst, and a tumor forming calcified structures. Radiograms may show well-formed teeth and bone within the soft tissue mass (Fig. 16-51).

Giant cell tumor

Giant cell tumors, giant cell reparative granulomas, and tumors containing a large number of giant cells present varied radiographic images. The tumor, when located within bone, may appear as a single radiolucent area or as a multilocular area and may even show polycystic radiolucencies. It may produce thin cortical plates and deform the shape of the involved bone. It may push teeth apart or resorb their roots. The varied radiographic appearance of the giant cell tumor makes it difficult to separate this lesion from many other lesions when a tentative clinical diagnosis is needed. An example of a giant cell tumor is shown in Fig. 16-52.

Myxoma

Myxoma of the jaws may be odontogenic or nonodontogenic in origin. The tumor appears on radiographic examination as a single area of radiolucency. A varying number of bony septa may appear within the tumor; a honeycomb appearance is sometimes seen. Expansion of the cortical plates and displacement of teeth may also be observed. The tumor may or may not be associated with an unerupted tooth (Fig. 16-53).

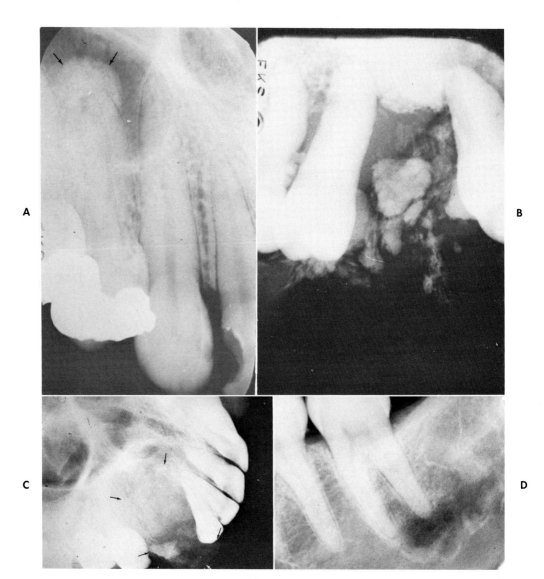

Fig. 16-50. Fibromas. **A,** Periodontal fibroma at the apex of a maxillary first bicuspid. The lesion is forming bone and projects into the maxillary sinus. **B,** Fibroma seen clinically as a soft tissue mass projecting into the vestibule. The radiogram shows the calcifications within the tumor. **C,** Fibroma demonstrating a ground-glass trabecular pattern that is clinically expanding the maxillary bone. **D,** Fibroma at the apex of a mandibular molar. The lesion is radiolucent and fairly well outlined by an uneven line of bone sclerosis. (**B,** Courtesy Dr. E. Cheraskin.)

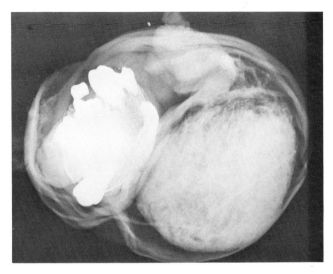

Fig. 16-51. Radiogram of a teratoma showing teeth and bone within the lesion. (Courtesy Dr. E. Cheraskin.)

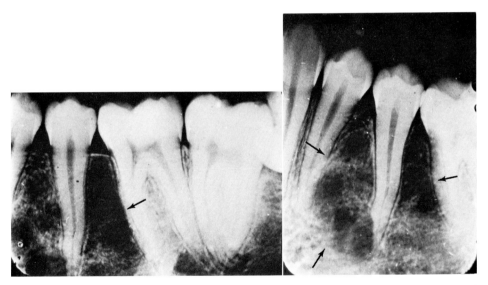

Fig. 16-52. Giant cell tumor radiographically seen as an ill-defined radiolucency around the mandibular second bicuspid. The tumor appears to be pushing the bicuspid teeth apart. (Courtesy Dr. D. T. Waggener.)

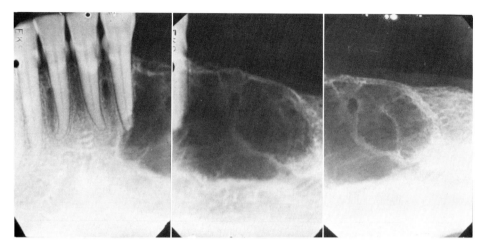

Fig. 16-53. Microscopic view of myxoma of the mandible containing a large fibrous component. (Courtesy Dr. D. T. Waggener.)

Carcinoma

The radiographic picture of a carcinoma invading bone is essentially one of bone destruction whether the tumor is squamous cell, basal cell, adenocarcinoma, or some other type. The radiolucent shadow of the tumor is pleomorphic, and the borders are very poorly defined. The cortical plates of bone, when involved, are resorbed and usually show erosion and penetration with little expansion of change in shape. Osteosclerosis around the lesion is not a common finding because of the relatively rapid growth of the tumor. Teeth in the area tend to be surrounded instead of being resorbed. Radiograms of carcinomas are shown in Fig. 16-54.

Sarcoma

Radiographically, sarcomas are of two basic types—those that consist only of soft tissue and those that produce calcified material. Sarcomas are malignant tumors and show radiographic images that depict bone destruction. Soft tissue sarcomas, for example, the fibrosarcoma, produce radiographic findings similar to those described for carcinomas. The osteogenic sarcoma and quite often the chondosarcoma produce calcified material that shows in the radiolucent image of the lesion as poorly defined patches of radiopacity. These two tumors may also produce thin projections of calcified material that radiate away from the cortex of the bone. This produces an x-ray image that is spoken of as having a sunray, sunburst, or fan-shaped appearance. Examples of sarcomas are shown in Fig. 16-55.

Ewing's tumor

The radiographic appearance of this tumor can be the same as that of the osteogenic sarcoma or chondrosarcoma. However, the cortex of the

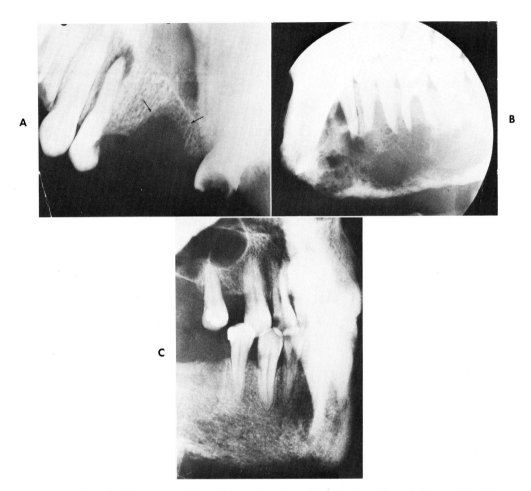

Fig. 16-54. A, Squamous cell carcinoma invading the alveolar ridge of the maxilla. The lesion destroys the bone as it progresses. **B,** Example of an aggressively invading squamous cell carcinoma of the mandible. The radiogram shows mainly bone destruction without signs of bone repair. The borders of the lesion are ill defined and ragged in general outline. **C,** Very aggressive squamous cell carcinoma of the mandible invading the bone so rapidly that the trabecular pattern and general outline of the bone are still identifiable.

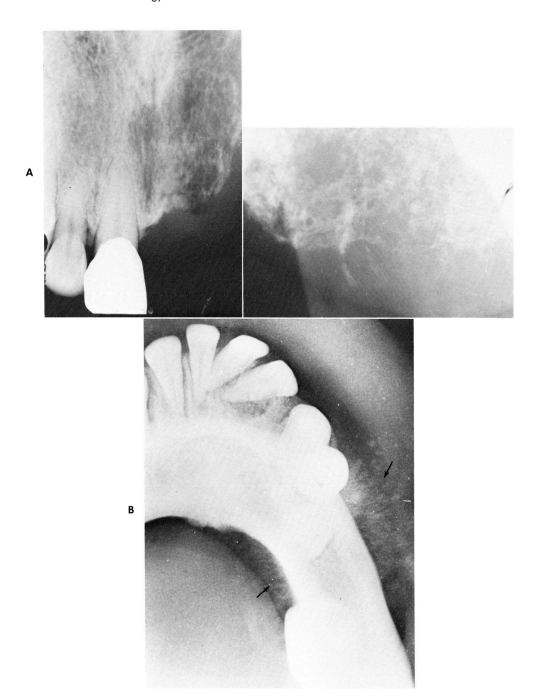

Fig. 16-55. A, Fibrosarcoma of the maxilla. There is no demarcation between the radiolucent lesion and the unaffected bone. All the teeth on the affected side have been lost. The calcified elements of the invaded area have not yet been completely resorbed and can still be observed radiographically. **B,** Osteogenic sarcoma of the mandible seen in a cross-sectional projection. The sun ray appearance is typical.

involved bone may be expanded and split; thus it will have an onionskin instead of the sunburst appearance. The displacement of the cortex is a significant finding.

Multiple myeloma

Multiple myeloma is a rapidly progressive disease and consists of many osteolytic lesions. The radiographic picture is one of many punched-out areas of bone. The radiolucent areas tend to be round in shape. There is no evidence of expansion and/or thinning of the cortical plates. The individual radiolucent lesion, though showing no definite border, is fairly well defined. Lesions in the cranium present more clear-cut radiographic characteristics than do those in the jaws. The solitary plasma cell myeloma appears radiographically like a single lesion of multiple myeloma. A case of multiple myeloma is shown in Fig. 16-56.

Metastatic tumors

The metastatic lesions of malignant tumors in oral structures may produce single or multiple lesions resembling the primary tumor. The primary sites of tumors that metastasize to the jaws are most often located in the kidney, lung, prostate, breast, thyroid, ovaries, and testes. The usual picture is one of multiple pleomorphic radiolucent areas within bone. Metastatic lesions of prostate or breast tumors may show calcifications resulting in multiple, diffuse radiopaque areas.

Peripheral tumors

A tumor may occur centrally (within bone) or peripherally (outside bone). Peripheral tumors may be primary or metastatic lesions; they may be lesions of tumors already discussed or of others that tend to form in the soft tissues. The radiographic picture of a peripheral tumor depends on whether the lesion is invasive or expansive. Invasive lesions cause irregular, ill-defined radiolucent shadows that are wider at the surface of the bone. Expansive lesions cause depressions in the surfaces of bones. Long-standing multiple expansive lesions can cause marked bone deformation. Radiograms are also useful in showing whether peripheral tumors form calcified structures. An example of peripherally located tumors is shown in Fig. 16-57.

Salivary gland tumors

Sialography is useful in the diagnosis of tumors of the major salivary glands. Sialograms show the ductal system of the gland. Deviation, distortion, compression, and destruction of the ducts can be visualized. Information can be gained indicating whether the tumor mass is within the gland or toward the side of the gland and/or whether the tumor mass destroys the ducts in its path, thereby creating cavities within the gland (Fig. 16-58).

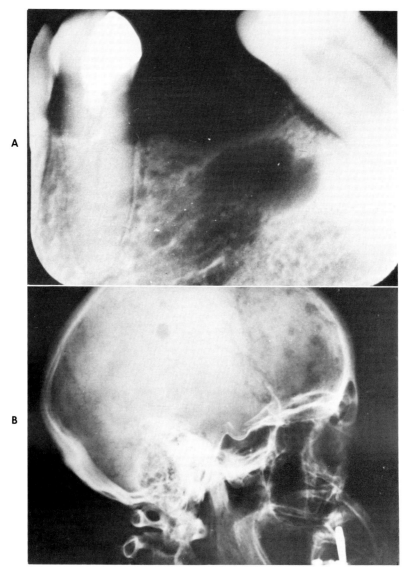

Fig. 16-56. A, Single lesion of multiple myeloma affecting alveolar bone. The finding is mainly one of bone destruction with the border of the lesion being ill defined. **B,** Skull radiogram of a patient with multiple myeloma showing fairly well demarcated, mainly spherical, radiolucent lesions in the cranial vault.

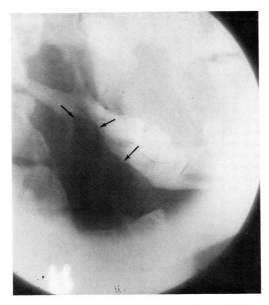

Fig. 16-57. Neurofibromatosis of very long duration. The multiple, expansive peripheral lesions have produced marked bone deformation as seen in this lateral jaw projection. The lesions cannot be seen.

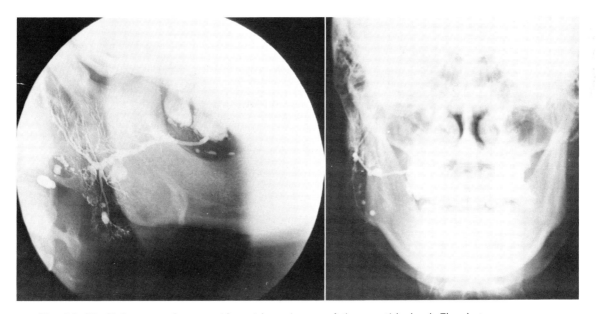

Fig. 16-58. Sialograms of mucoepidermoid carcinoma of the parotid gland. The destruction of the gland and the formation of cavity defects are seen in the lower part of the gland. (Courtesy Dr. H. D. Hall.)

HORMONAL, NUTRITIONAL, AND METABOLIC DISORDERS

Many hormonal, nutritional, and metabolic disorders affect bone and teeth; these diseases may show radiographic findings. The radiographic changes pertain mostly to bone density. Other significant findings include the presence of individual osteolytic lesions, changes in the shape of bones, and differences between the chronologic age and bone age of the patient. Radiographic findings may vary with the time of onset of the particular disorder.

Hyperpituitarism

Dental radiographic findings of hyperpituitarism are best seen on the lateral skull radiogram. In *hypophyseal gigantism*, the calvarium is thicker, the hypophyseal fossa (sella turcica) is enlarged, and the sinuses may appear unusually large. Dental findings include macrodontia and hypercementosis. The anterior teeth may show spaces between them.

In *acromegaly*, the skull is enlarged and possibly deformed, the hypophyseal fossa may be enlarged and changed in shape, and destruction of the clinoid processes may be visualized. The cranial vault is thick, and the sinuses are enlarged, as are the hands and feet. The mandible is larger, thicker, prognathic, and possibly osteoporotic. The antegonial notch may be absent. The mandibular teeth show widened interproximal spaces and possibly hypercementosis. Acromegaly is illustrated in Fig. 16-59.

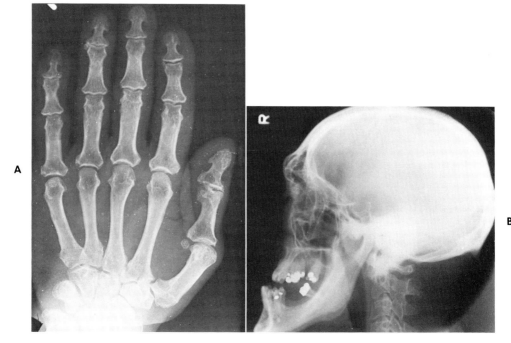

Fig. 16-59. Radiograms of acromegaly. **A,** Hand radiogram demonstrates the enlargement of the bones. **B,** Lateral skull view shows the patient to have a thicker cranical vault, a relatively large sella turcica, large sinuses, and an enlarged prognathic mandible.

Hypopituitarism

In hypophyseal dwarfism, the hypophyseal fossa is small. Usually, the relative proportions of bones are normal, but absolute sizes are small. Tooth size is not affected, and malocclusion is common. The sinuses are small and incompletely pneumatized. A carpal index shows the bone age to be less than the chronologic age of the patient. The teeth findings include retention of deciduous teeth, delayed eruption of permanent teeth, and crowding of the dentition.

Hyperthyroidism

Radiographic findings are not clear-cut; they include early eruption of permanent teeth, early loss of deciduous teeth, osteoporosis, and hypercementosis.

Hypothyroidism

In *cretinism,* the sinuses may be underdeveloped. Eruption of permanent teeth and exfoliation of deciduous teeth are delayed. The carpal index shows retarded osseous development. In *myxedema,* the x-ray findings are usually negative. However, osteoporosis or alveolar bone loss may be seen.

Hyperparathyroidism

Hyperparathyroidism, or osteitis fibrosa cystica generalisata, is characterized by defective bone formation. The condition may be secondary to kidney disease, that is, renal hyperparathyroidism or renal rickets. The radiogram shows osteoporosis and in some cases loss of the lamina dura. The teeth are not affected and stand out in contrast to the bone. In the later stages the bone trabeculae are replaced by fine, poorly calcified trabeculae that give the bone a mottled, granular, or ground-glass radiographic appearance. When the giant cell tumors of hyperparathyroidism occur, they produce poorly defined, cystlike radiolucent areas within the bone. Radiograms made of the skull and hand show the generalized nature of the condition. Radiograms are also useful in showing the return to normal density of the bone trabeculae and lamina dura and the apparent sclerosis of the finely trabeculated areas when treatment has been successful. Hyperparathyroidism is shown in Figs. 16-60 and 16-61.

Hypoparathyroidism

Hypoparathyroidism in early childhood can cause hypoplasia of the developing enamel and dentin and underdevelopment of the roots of forming teeth. There may be a generalized osteosclerosis.

Hypoinsulinism

Hypoinsulinism, or *diabetes mellitus,* is often associated with periodontal disease and alveolar bone loss. The finding of considerable alveolar bone loss and possibly osteoporosis in dental radiograms in the absence of a local causative factor is significant. Juvenile diabetes is shown in Fig. 16-62.

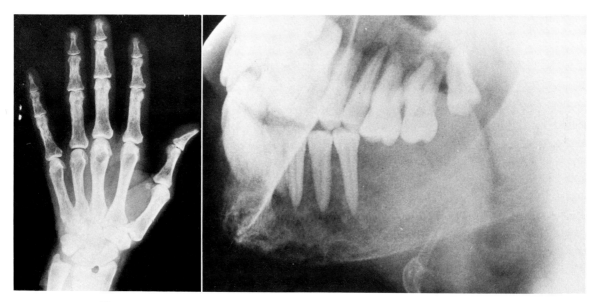

Fig. 16-60. Radiograms of hyperparathyroidism demonstrating the generalized osteoporosis. The mandible has a ground-glass appearance, and the lamina dura is absent. All cortical plates are thinned and show reduced bone opacity. (Courtesy Dr. C. A. McCallum, Jr.)

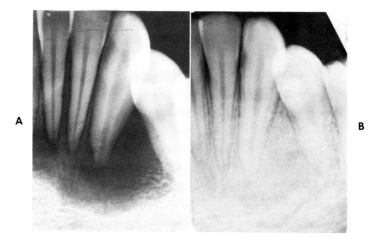

Fig. 16-61. Intraoral radiograms of a case of hyperparathyroidism. **A,** Radiolucent osteolytic appearance of a giant cell lesion. **B,** Repair of the area after treatment for the condition with reappearance of the lamina dura. (From Silverman, S., Jr.: Oral Surg. **26:**184, 1968.)

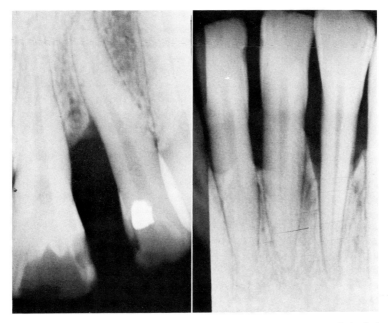

Fig. 16-62. Periapical radiograms of a 15-year-old girl with uncontrolled diabetes. The loss of alveolar bone is shown in these radiograms. Clinical examination and patient history indicate no abnormal local traumatic etiologic factors.

Hypergonadism and hypogonadism

There is usually a discrepancy in the relation of chronologic age to bone age or tooth eruption dates in patients who have either hypergonadism or hypogonadism. Dental radiograms are useful in showing the early or late eruption of teeth. Carpal index radiograms are useful in determining the bone age of the patient.

Avitaminosis D

The radiographic findings in *rickets* include delayed eruption of teeth and poorly calcified bones. Teeth may show rather large pulp chambers, open apical foramina, and enamel and dentin hypoplasia. The bones show osteoporosis and fewer trabeculae. The lamina dura may be indistinct or absent radiographically. Bone changes are seen more clearly in the rapidly growing bones. The hand and wrist radiogram shows indistinct outlines of the metaphyses and epiphyses of the radius and ulna. The ends of growing bones show cupping and spurring. Rickets is illustrated in Fig. 16-63.

Osteomalacia

Osteomalacia is a disease of adults. It can be caused by avitaminosis D, sprue, and other gastrointestinal disorders and by conditions causing excessive calciuria. Radiograms show osteoporosis with bones having thin cortical plates and fewer

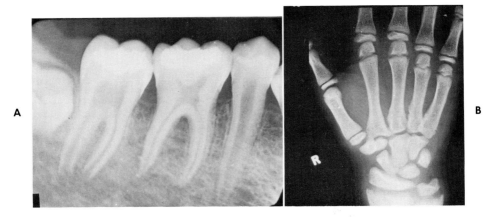

Fig. 16-63. Rickets. **A,** Intraoral radiogram shows osteoporosis and loss of the lamina dura. **B,** Carpal index shows the indistinct borders of the epiphyses of the long bones. (Courtesy Dr. E. Cheraskin.)

trabeculae. The lamina dura may be indistinct or missing. Remarkable rarefaction can occur in extreme conditions.

Emaciation and senility

Osteoporosis is a common finding in emaciated or aged people. Considerable resorption of the alveolar bone can occur.

Gaucher's disease

In Gaucher's disease, the radiologic findings are varied. Basically, generalized osteoporosis of the bones caused by the replacement of the marrow with Gaucher's cells is present. The bones may or may not show pseudocystic areas on the radiograms. Radiographic manifestations in Gaucher's disease are shown in Fig. 16-64.

Eosinophilic granuloma

Eosinophilic granuloma is seen mostly in children and may show single or multiple radiolucent lesions. The lesions tend to be round in shape with irregular margins. Although not sharply defined, they are clearly outlined. Lesions in the calvarium tend to have a punched-out appearance. Lesions in the jaws may resemble areas of infection, cysts, or metastatic tumors. Lesions in the alveolar bone tend to surround the roots of teeth and give the impression of floating teeth on the radiogram. Radiograms are useful in searching for lesions in other bones of the skeleton. Radiograms of eosinophilic granulomas are shown in Fig. 16-65.

Hand-Schüller-Christian disease

Eosinophilic granuloma and Hand-Schüller-Christian disease are thought to be variants of the same disease. The radiographic findings are similar in the two conditions. Extensive involvement of the calvarium produces a radiographic

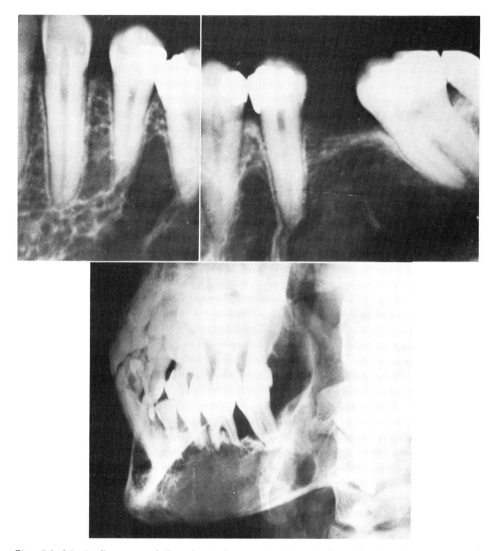

Fig. 16-64. Radiograms of Gaucher's disease showing the loss of trabecular structure of the jaws. The radiolucent areas present a pleomorphic, pseudocystic appearance. (Courtesy Dr. I. B. Bender.)

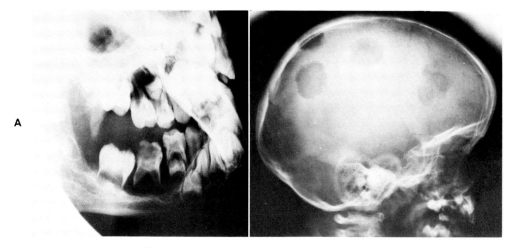

Fig. 16-65. Eosinophilic granuloma. **A,** Lateral jaw projection shows a lesion affecting the deciduous mandibular molar teeth. The bone loss around these teeth produced by the lesion gives the impression of floating teeth. **B,** Skull view shows more or less spherical radiolucent lesions in the cranial vault. The borders of the cranial lesions are rather sharp and present a punched-out appearance.

image similar to the land and sea areas seen on a map; this radiographic design is referred to as a *geographic skull.*

Letterer-Siwe disease

Letterer-Siwe disease, along with eosinophilic granuloma and Hand-Schüller-Christian disease, belongs to the group of diseases called histiocytosis X. Letterer-Siwe disease occurs in patients less than 2 years of age. The radiographic findings are the same as those in eosinophilic granuloma and Hand-Schüller-Christian disease; however, many more lesions are present.

MISCELLANEOUS PATHOLOGIC CONDITIONS

Many diseases or conditions of unknown cause may have radiographic signs but cannot be classified in any of the groups of diseases mentioned previously in this chapter. They are considered in the general discussion of miscellaneous pathologic conditions that follows.

Paget's disease

Paget's disease, or *osteitis deformans,* is characterized by destruction of bone and its replacement with finely trabeculated, poorly formed bone that may produce a ground-glass effect on radiograms. The new bone tissue may, in turn, be remodeled, and as a result the affected bones may be changed in size and shape. The overall radiographic picture is of diffuse areas of osteoporosis and osteosclerosis that give the affected area a cotton wool appearance. The disease may be either monostotic or polyostotic. The cortices of bone may be thickened, and when affected, the calvarium appears thicker; the jaws become enlarged, and the sinuses are encroached upon. Teeth may show root resorption or hypercementosis and may migrate to produce malocclusion. The lamina dura around tooth roots is destroyed in involved areas and does not reappear when the area recalcifies. The disease usually occurs in patients over 40 years of age; the long bones may show pathologic fractures. Radiograms show bone changes before deformation occurs. Paget's disease is shown in Fig. 16-66.

Fibrous dysplasia

Microscopically, fibrous dysplasia resembles ossifying fibroma or fibro-osteoma, cherubism, cementoma, reparative granuloma, and leontiasis ossea. Fibrous dysplasia presents three clinical forms: monostotic fibrous dysplasia, polyostotic fibrous dysplasia, and Albright's syndrome. The last form associates this condition with precocious sexual development in girls and with skin pigmentation. The polyostotic form is often associated with endocrine dysfunction.

The radiogram shows single or multiple lesions. The cortex of the affected bone is thin and possibly expanded. The architecture of the bone is changed. The lesion may present a radiolucent cystlike appearance with a definite or indefinite border. When calcifications occur within the lesion, they appear as mottled radiopaque areas. Fibrous dysplasia usually presents a mottled, ground-glass appearance that is more radiolucent than the surrounding bone. The lesion may show the same or greater density than the adjacent normal bone if it has expanded the bone in the affected area. There is no definite margin to the lesion; the affected area of fine spicules blends into the normal bone having larger trabeculae (Fig. 16-67). The lesion may cause root resorption and displacement of teeth. The lamina dura of teeth in the affected area may be absent. Involvement in the maxilla may result in obliteration of the sinuses. Skeletal involvement is often unilateral.

Leontiasis ossea

In leontiasis ossea, the affected bones become enlarged and dense. The absence of radiolucent areas in the affected bone is significant. Because of the increase in bone density, it is sometimes difficult to visualize the roots of teeth in the radiogram. The shape of the jaws, the temporomandibular joint, and the paranasal sinuses may be changed. The calvarium may be thickened, and megalocephalus is a possible finding.

Infantile cortical hyperostosis

Infantile cortical hyperostosis, or Caffey's disease, is a condition that occurs soon after birth and is characterized by thickening of the cortical plates and enlargement of the flat bones. The mandible is often involved. The affected bone increases in dimensions, and new bone tissue on the outer surface of the bone may be deposited in layers; the radiogram may show the bone to have a lami-

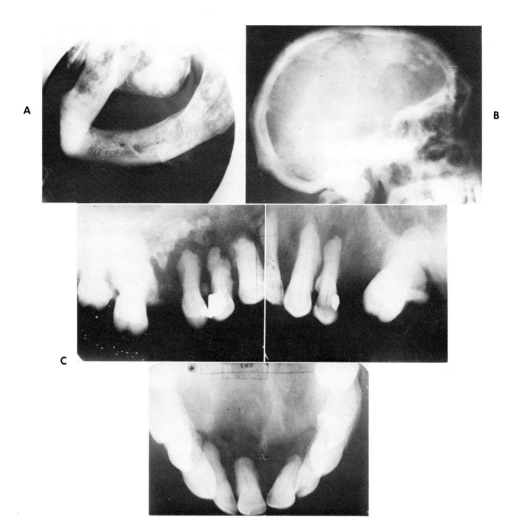

Fig. 16-66. A, Lateral jaw radiogram of Paget's disease showing osteosclerotic areas with a cotton wool appearance within the mandible and maxilla. Early deformation of the maxilla is evident. **B,** Skull view in Paget's disease showing areas of osteoporosis and osteosclerosis. The entire skull is affected, and the outlines of the bones are indistinct. **C,** Intraoral radiograms of Paget's disease. The normal trabeculae have been replaced by very fine trabeculae, giving the bone a ground-glass appearance. Hypercementosis of the teeth is seen in this case, which also demonstrates destruction of the lamina dura.

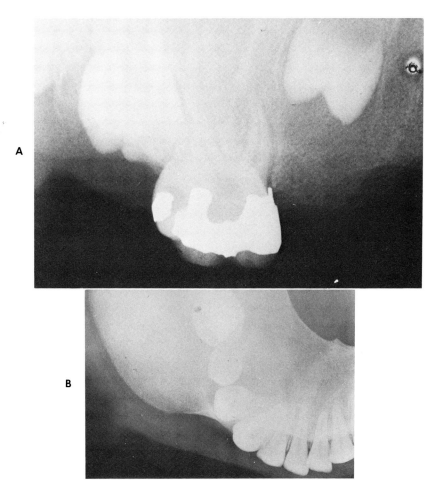

Fig. 16-67. A, Intraoral radiogram of fibrous dysplasia affecting the posterior maxilla of a 10-year-old girl. The bone is slightly enlarged and has a ground-glass appearance. The lamina dura around the first molar is faintly visible. The enamel organ of the second bicuspid is indistinct. **B,** Cross-sectional occlusal radiogram showing great enlargement of the body of the mandible in a case of fibrous dysplasia.

nated outer surface. Normal contour of the bone is restored during healing. Infantile cortical hyperostosis is illustrated in Fig. 16-68.

Myositis ossificans

The cause of calcification of muscles, ligaments, and tendons is unknown. There is often a history of trauma. Radiograms show diffuse radiopaque shadows within the affected soft tissues. Myositis ossificans in the face is shown in Fig. 16-69.

Calcification of arteries

The walls of arteries may be the site of calcium deposits in arterial disease and some other disorders. The radiogram of the facial area may show the artery as a wormlike, faintly radiopaque shadow bordered by two thin, parallel, slightly more radiopaque lines. Arterial calcification in the skull is shown in Fig. 16-70.

Rheumatoid arthritis

Rheumatoid arthritis causes joint changes that are visible in radiograms. The temporomandibular joint may show subluxation or reduction of the joint space; the condyle or fossa may show erosion of the articular surface, may be changed in shape, and may have osteolytic areas within the bone. Advanced conditions may show osteoporosis and considerable deformity of bone. A radiogram of the hand is very helpful in the diagnosis of rheumatoid arthritis. An example of rheumatoid arthiritis is shown in Fig. 16-71.

Scleroderma

Dental radiographic findings in scleroderma include a widened periodontal space and alveolar bone loss. Hand radiograms may show resorption of the distal phalanges (Fig. 16-72).

Sjögren's syndrome

Sjögren's syndrome is characterized by dryness of the eyes, mouth, and pharynx. The syndrome is more commonly seen in elderly women. Sialograms demonstrate the destruction of salivary acini (Fig. 16-73).

Mikulicz's disease and syndrome

Mikulicz's disease is a rare disorder involving the lacrimal, salivary, and sometimes oral mucous glands and lymph glands. Sialograms are useful in demonstrating the loss of acini and minor salivary ducts and the possible presence of filling defects.

Static bone cavity

A cavity within the mandible is sometimes seen in the area of the angle of the mandible (Fig. 16-74). Some of these cavities have been shown to open on

Text continued on p. 423.

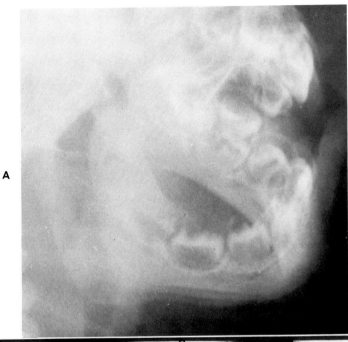

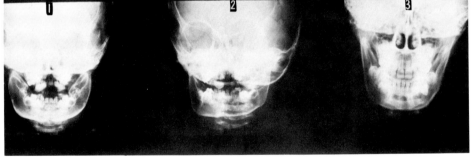

Fig. 16-68. A, Lateral jaw radiogram of infantile cortical hyperostosis showing the sub-periosteal proliferation of new bone. The lower border of the mandible is indistinct, and the laminations of new bone have an onionskin appearance. **B,** Radiograms demonstrating the residual mandibular asymmetry produced by infantile cortical hyperostosis. Patient is shown at (1) 8 months, (2) 16 months, and (3) 6 years, 11 months after the onset of the condition. (**A,** Courtesy Dr. H. Bethart; **B,** courtesy Dr. P. M. Burbank.)

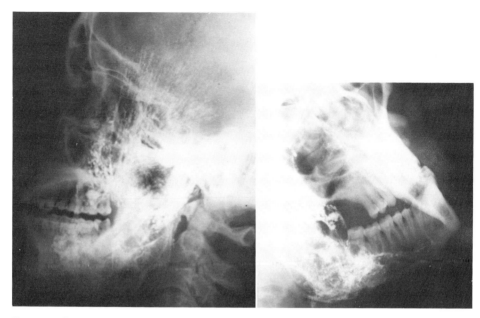

Fig. 16-69. Myositis ossificans in the masseter and temporalis. Note the fan-shaped calcifications in the temporalis seen in the lateral face radiogram. (Courtesy Dr. A. H. Shawkat; from Ennis, L. M., Berry, H. M., and Phillips, J. E.: Dental roentgenology, ed. 6, Philadelphia, 1967, Lea & Febiger.)

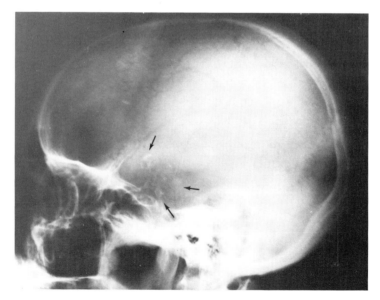

Fig. 16-70. Calcification of intracranial arteries. The involved arteries appear to be located in the midcranial fossa in the vicinity of the circle of Willis.

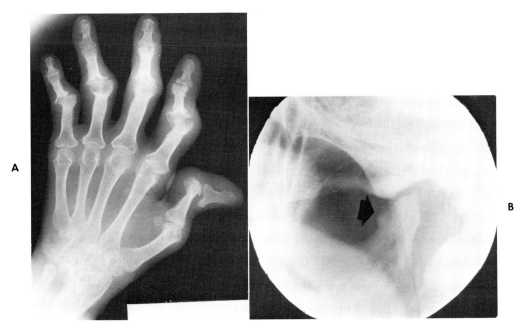

Fig. 16-71. Rheumatoid arthritis. **A,** Hand radiogram shows great destruction of the joints of the fingers. **B,** Temporomandibular joint radiogram demonstrates destruction of the articular surface of the head of the condyle.

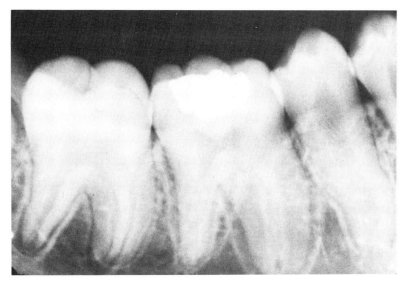

Fig. 16-72. Intraoral radiogram of a patient with scleroderma showing uniform widening of the periodontal space around the roots of the teeth.

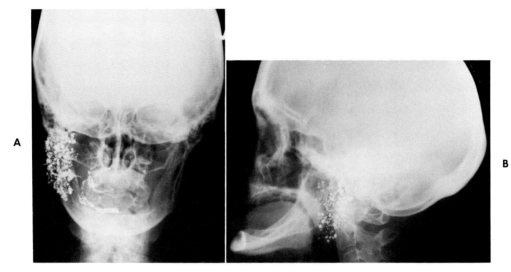

Fig. 16-73. Parotid sialograms of Sjögren's syndrome. **A,** Posteroanterior skull view shows destruction of the glandular structures and the formation of cavity defects seen here as being filled with radiopaque medium. **B,** Lateral skull view made 1 month later shows poor elimination of the nonabsorbable opaque medium.

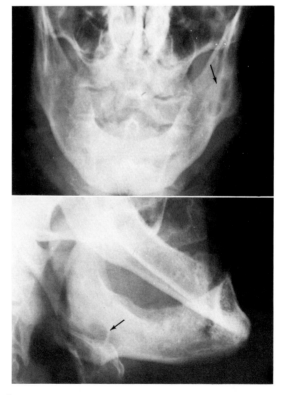

Fig. 16-74. Static bone cavity (idiopathic bone cyst) located at the angle of the mandible. The defect appears like two small cysts adjacent to each other. The lateral jaw and posteroanterior mandibular radiograms show the defect to be within the mandible.

the lingual side of the mandible. The cavities are asymptomatic and are discovered during routine radiographic examination. The radiogram shows a cystlike radiolucency in the mandible that is well defined by a radiopaque border of bone. The cavity is not connected with the mandibular canal. Sialograms are useful in determining if the cavity contains submaxillary gland tissue.

CHAPTER 17

A clinical approach to radiographic interpretation

Traditionally, interpretation has been based on the radiographic appearance of disease entities. Considerably less emphasis has been placed on specific radiographic signs and their meaning in relation to disease processes. The radiographic film should be considered a means or method by which a tentative diagnosis can be made. In combination with clinical tests and observations, and at times with the aid of laboratory data and microscopic analysis, a final diagnosis eventually evolves. Thus an understanding of radiographic signs becomes at least as important as the more didactic and classic approach to radiographic interpretation.

The purpose of this chapter is to note some of the more commonly observed signs and attach significance to them. It must be emphasized that in no instance should a diagnosis be made on the basis of the radiographic film alone. Many disease processes have varying radiographic appearances, depending on the stage of a lesion's development. In spite of this fact, it is possible to correlate in a fairly definitive manner certain radiographic findings with the more usual appearance of types or groups of lesions.

In approaching a radiographic differential diagnosis, one first should consider certain more or less gross factors. This should be followed by a more detailed approach wherein very specific radiographic criteria are noted and evaluated. The ultimate purpose of the two procedures is the same. However, the first step is designed to isolate the disease process in general terms. Is it rapidly destructive or of a chronic nature? Is it neoplastic or infectious? Is it nondestructive? The second step, that of critically evaluating the radiographic film for specific criteria, is used as a means whereby the disease process can be narrowed down to a few possibilities. This information, together with information secured from other sources, is expected to produce a definitive diagnosis.

RADIOGRAPHIC CRITERIA OF A GENERAL NATURE OBSERVED
IN ALTERATIONS OF OSSEOUS TISSUE

Radiographic criteria of a general nature include the following:

1. Is the lesion radiopaque or radiolucent?
2. What kind of a peripheral outline does the lesion have?
3. Has the lesion resulted in a dimensional change?
4. Has the cortical bone at the lower border of the mandible been altered?
5. Has the lesion changed the position and shape of associated tooth roots?
6. Are bone particles retained within the lesion?
7. Has the trabecular pattern of the bone changed? Are nutrient vessels present?
8. Is the lesion a single entity or is it composed of two or more areas in either the same bone or different bones?

Radiolucency versus radiopacity

It is possible to generalize and suggest that radiopacities in osseous tissue are more frequently associated with slowly developing changes that, though causing osseous alterations, can be regarded basically as relatively nondestructive. Conversely, radiolucencies are necessarily destructive in some measure. There are exceptions to this concept, especially when the radiopacity is directly associated with a radiolucent area or areas.

Peripheral outline

After it is observed whether a lesion is radiolucent or radiopaque, the next radiographic characteristic most commonly evaluated is the peripheral outline of the area in question. The lesion, whether it be radiolucent or radiopaque, may have a definite boundary, or its margins may be rough, irregular, or indistinct.

Definite boundary. If the lesion appears self-contained by a definite boundary, it may have the following characteristics:

1. A distinctive opaque lamina or border about a radiolucent area, as seen quite commonly in the "typical" cyst. The shape of the lesion, as seen by its peripheral outline, is significant. A slowly growing, noninvasive lesion develops a spherical shape when no unusual obstruction impedes its growth. Bony septa, cortical plates, teeth, and so forth, tend to distort the spherical shape of such lesions.
2. A definite, relatively smooth, easily identifiable margin between a radiolucent area and the surrounding bone. This can be observed when solid granulation tissue develops in bone.
3. A radiolucent line about a radiopaque area, as seen in the odontomas, particularly the cementoma and the compound composite and complex composite odontomas.
4. A rather easily observed differentiation between an opaque mass and the surrounding bone even though these tissues blend together. This often is observed in the osteoma and in an area of bone sclerosis such as enostosis.

A well-defined boundary suggests a relatively slow rate of growth.

Rough, irregular, or indistinct boundary. Peripheral margins that are rough, irregular, or indistinct suggest tissue growth or a spread of infection beyond the present capacity of the body to wall off or circumscribe. The degree of roughness, irregularity, and indistinctness may provide a clue to the type of destructive lesion. The following examples may be helpful. The squamous cell carcinoma invading bone from the oral soft tissue or metastasizing to bone from elsewhere in the body usually shows no clear-cut delineation between it and the normal bone; the degree of delineation varies inversely with its invasiveness. Somewhat similarly, osteomyelitis, especially in its most fulminating stage, demonstrates only rough, irregular, indistinct borders. However, in the latter instance, there is a tendency for an involucrum, an encircling band of dense bone, to develop around the osteomyelitic area. Fibrotic changes of Paget's disease also demonstrate roughened borders, but delineation of normal from pathologic bone is usually relatively easy. The ameloblastoma produces quite a varied appearance radiographically. In its most common form it is multiloculated and cystlike Its periphery tends to be notched, but because of its relatively slow expansile growth, the periphery is quite easily delineated from the surrounding bone. This is true even though microscopic evidence shows that the neoplastic tissue has encroached into what appears radiographically to be normal bone.

Dimensional changes of surrounding bone

Expansion of bone apparently takes place as a compensatory mechanism resulting from bone resorption in a directly adjacent area. Such resorption results from pressure, chronic infection, or the presence of a slowly growing neoplastic process. Temporary or permanent bone enlargement can also result from severe trauma. The more chronic the resorption process, the greater is the tendency for bone expansion. Expansion of cortical bone in the presence of an ameloblastoma is characteristic as soon as the lesion has reached a size that demands that the bone expand in order to withstand stresses or be fractured. The same phenomenon applies to large cysts. Bone expansion, as a result of periostitis, occurs in chronic infectious processes but not ordinarily in acute, fulminating osteomyelitic conditions. Bone tumors, that is, true neoplastic osteogenic lesions, are inherently expansile, but nonbony tumors that have metastasized to bone expand bone inversely to the rapidity of tumor growth. The squamous cell carcinoma in bone usually demonstrates soft tissue enlargement unaccompanied by osseous expansion. Conversely, slow-growing fibrotic bone changes almost invariably demonstrate enlargement of the part.

Alterations in the cortical bone of the mandible

The cortical bone of the mandible, particularly on its lower border, can give a further clue to the type of process under consideration. A smooth destruction or thinning of the cortical plate over a relatively wide area suggests pressure over an extended period of time. A large cyst could produce this type of evidence; or a similar appearance, possibly with some notching of the periphery, could result from an ameloblastoma or from an osteofibrotic lesion. Areas of breakthrough or tunneling in the cortical bone with intervening segments of relatively normal cortical bone are more indicative of an infectious process such as osteomyelitis. A pitted, punched-out, or totally destroyed cortical plate over a relatively broad area is often a sign of a rapidly invading neoplasm.

Alterations in position and shape of tooth roots

The effect on tooth roots of various types of lesions is basically limited to three characteristics. The roots may be pushed aside, resorbed, or encompassed within the area manifesting bony change. Root displacement is related to chronicity and is most often associated with large cyst formation. Root resorption is infrequent when roots are displaced. Root resorption, which is also related to chronicity, occurs in the presence of more slowly growing neoplasms, such as the ameloblastoma, and in the presence of a chronic infectious process. Rapidly growing neoplasms, such as the squamous cell carcinoma, and fulminating types of infection, such as osteomyelitis tend to include or encircle the tooth root in the destructive process. Root inclusion also occurs in uncomplicated root-end alterations, but here the lesion is self-limiting.

Presence of bone particles

Concepts just expressed concerning the effect of different pathologic processes on changes in root shape or position apply to the inclusion or noninclusion of bone particles within a lesion. Rapidly growing neoplasms and fulminating types of infection tend to encompass bone, including bone particles of various sizes within the growth or area of infection. It is well known that osteomyelitic lesions demonstrate this condition. Rapidly growing neoplasms demonstrate the same phenomenon; however, the included bone spicules are likely to be more numerous and smaller. Conversely, less active neoplasms or infections tend to cause bone resorption at their periphery. Particles of bone are almost never observed within such areas. It must be recognized that some disease processes producing radiolucent lesions also form bone (that is, calcified areas) within themselves, for example, Paget's disease, fibrous dysplasia, and the more osteoid forms of osteoma.

Bone pattern and nutrient vessels

Changes in the size and shape of trabecular spaces and trabeculae in the mandible and maxilla and the existence of nutrient vessels (canals) have at times been considered pathognomonic of a disease process, but no objective evidence has been available to substantiate these claims. On the average, the trabecular spaces in the mandible are larger and more elliptical than those in the maxilla; the elliptical spaces tend to run horizontally. The mandibular spaces are usually larger in areas below the apices of the teeth, and often the trabeculae appear nonexistent because the spaces are very large in proportion to the thickness of the trabeculae. The maxillary trabecular pattern is usually quite fine and without any particular directional arrangement.

As the individual ages, the size of the trabecular spaces, particularly in the mandible, tends to become smaller. (*Note:* This characteristic is open to question; some observers feel that larger spaces predominate in aged persons.) This reduction in the size of spaces is also common when bone is destroyed and is later replaced by new bone. So-called nutrient vessels are found most frequently in the anterior segment of the mandible, although they may appear anywhere in the mandible or maxilla. They are more commonly observed in areas where the trabecular spaces are small and where the bone appears quite dense. Until recently, the significance of such vessels has not been investigated even though experience has suggested that they may tend to be related to advancing age, chronic illness, osteosclerosis, and periodontal disease. The correlation with age has been thought to be possibly related to prior chronic illness.

One of us (A. H. W.) has believed for many years that a correlation may exist between certain radiographic findings and the systemic condition of the individual. This conviction has been based only on experience. Recent research,* limited in scope and in need of further study, now suggests that some of these subjective opinions may have validity. The frequency with which nutrient vessels are seen increases with age except that the frequency decreased in the last age group studied (55 to 65 years of age). Nutrient vessels appear to be more frequently found in blacks than in whites. High blood pressure is known to occur more frequently in blacks. The incidence of nutrient vessels increases with high blood pressure in both blacks and whites. Nutrient vessels tend to be associated more frequently with advanced periodontal disease than with lesser manifestations of the disease. Nonparallelism of trabeculae in the mandibular molar and bicuspid regions and small mandibular trabecular spaces also tend to be associated with more advanced periodontal conditions. It is difficult to know whether the radiographic signs are indicative of certain disease states (and thus can be used to anticipate the likelihood of disease in the future) or whether the radiographic signs are just the sequlae of local or systemic alterations. In any event, the radiographic signs discussed in this section appear, on the basis of initial investigation, to be more than just variations within normal limits.

More dramatic changes in the trabecular pattern do occur that definitely suggest a disease state. The normal pattern may be replaced by a fine, almost weblike network of bone trabeculae, as in fibrous dysplasia. This appearance has been described as being reticulated or as looking like ground glass. The same or a similar appearance can occur in various stages of Paget's disease. Some bone changes may be confined to local areas in the jaws; others may be manifested

---

*See Patel under Suggested readings: Radiographic interpretation.

generally in other areas of the body. When this weblike, reticulated, or ground-glass appearance is associated with a reduction in the opacity of bone generally, particularly in areas that are normally heavily calcified, one must suspect a calcium depletion disease, such as hyperparathyroidism. Enlargement of the part is almost always an accompanying clinical and radiographic finding when fibrous tissue replaces bone. This is not true in calcium depletion diseases.

Accompanying or as sequelae to this ground-glass appearance, reossification and calcification sometimes occur in the altered area, or a deposition of minerals with the fibrous tissue per se can take place. Because this phenomenon can take place in certain areas of the lesion and not in others and/or as a result of varying degrees of remineralization, the radiographic appearance is almost fluffy. Traditionally, these areas are said to have a cotton wool texture. The normal trabecular pattern, particularly of the mandible, can also be altered to show fewer, coarser trabeculae arranged in a horizontal fashion. This gives a so-called stepladder appearance to the trabeculae and is suggestive of a disturbance of the hematopoietic system.

The bone pattern can, of course, vary greatly within the present concepts of normal. How far it can vary without being suggestive of pathologic change is not known. The material discussed in this section should be related to other radiographic, clinical, and laboratory findings and should not be used in a definitive fashion.

Multiple radiolucencies

Multiloculations within a single radiolucency, multiple radiolucencies within one bone (monostotic lesions), and multiple radiolucencies within more than one bone (polyostotic lesions) constitute contributory evidence of value in making a differential radiographic evaluation. Multiloculations in a single radiolucent area suggest the likelihood of a slowly growing neoplasm, but they do not preclude the possibility of an ordinary cyst; the probability of an infectious process is automatically almost eliminated unless the lesion has become secondarily infected. Monostotic lesions are often neoplastic. Polyostotic findings suggest much the same evidence as do the monostotic, but the obvious extent of the alteration into more than one part of the body is significant. It must be remembered that the term *neoplasia* is not necessarily synonymous with malignancy.

SPECIFIC RADIOGRAPHIC CRITERIA OBSERVED IN ALTERATIONS OF OSSEOUS TISSUE

The approach thus far has been of a generalized nature. It now becomes important to consider specific radiographic interpretive criteria. There is some repetition here of prior comments, but this is necessary in order that each individual have the same mental picture of a given radiographic criterion. The following are differential radiographic interpretive criteria. Each criterion is illustrated, and the disease that produced the condition is identified according to a diagnosis established through the combined use of the radiographic film, clinical evidence, microscopic findings, and, where necessary, clinical laboratory tests. Many of the radiograms are the same as those used in Chapter 16 and in other prior chapters. This is done deliberately to enhance learning. It must be remembered that the approach used in this chapter is not traditional; it attempts to place significance on radiographic criteria rather than on what might be termed a *memory* approach.

1. **A well-outlined radiolucent lesion circumscribed by an opaque lamina of bone.** Fig. 17-1 shows an ordinary root end or radicular cyst.

2. **A well-defined radiolucent lesion lacking a limiting bone outline,** such as the opaque lamina seen in Fig. 17-1. The lesion shown in Fig. 17-2, *A*, is an apical granuloma. A more dramatic illustration of this criterion is observed in lesions resulting from eosinophilic granuloma (Fig. 17-2, *B*).

3. **An ill-defined, irregular or ragged radiolucent lesion showing no evidence of calcification.** Fig. 17-3 happens to be of an intraosseous hematoma resulting from trauma, but it could easily be of an acute infection or even a metastatic alteration.

4. **An ill-defined radiolucent lesion showing evidence of calcification within the radiolucency.** This is illustrated by the calcifying cementoma shown in Fig. 17-4.

5. **A radiolucent lesion characterized by a smooth thinning of the cortical bone on its medullary aspect over a relatively large area.** Fig. 17-5 shows a very large dentigerous cyst, but the possibility of an ameloblastoma should not be excluded.

6. **A radiolucent lesion characterized by a rough surface to the thinned cortical bone on its medullary aspect.** In Fig. 17-6 the thinning extends over quite a large area. The lesion is a squamous cell carcinoma. Note that it resembles in some ways the intraosseous hematoma shown in Fig. 17-3.

7. **A radiolucent lesion characterized by a single or an intermittent break through the cortical bone with intervening relatively normal bone.** This tunneling is likely to be caused by an infectious process. Fig. 17-7, *A*, illustrates a case of osteomyelitis. Fig. 17-7, *B*, illustrates a kind of splintering of the cortical bone in one area. The process is similar; this, too, is a case of osteomyelitis.

8. **A radiolucent area showing a diminution in the size of the individual trabeculae with the formation of a reticulated appearance to the bony pattern.** This diminution in trabecular space size is described in some circumstances as having a ground-glass appearance. This radiogram (Fig. 17-8) is of a patient who has Paget's disease. This film also fits the previously stated criterion (4) of an ill-defined radiolucent lesion showing evidence of calcification within the lesion.

9. **A radiolucent area characterized by an enlargement of the trabecular spaces.** In Fig. 17-9, *A*, one observes the maxilla and the mandible of the same individual. This pattern is quite usual. In Fig. 17-9, *B*, one observes some un-

Text continued on p. 437.

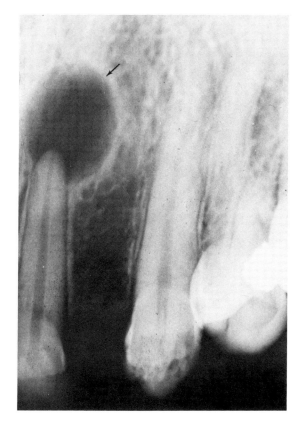

Fig. 17-1

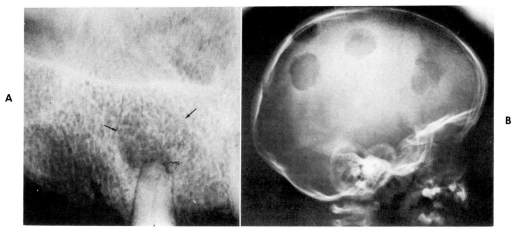

Fig. 17-2

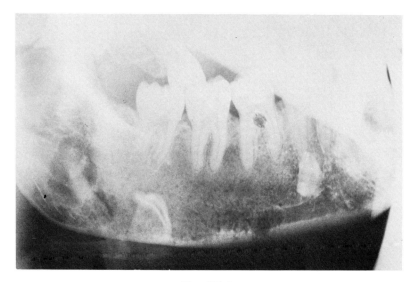

Fig. 17-3

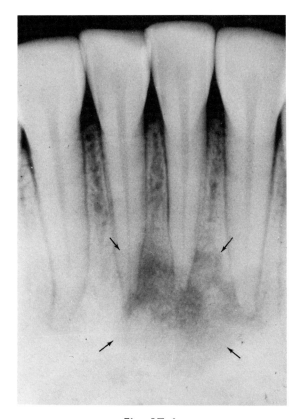

Fig. 17-4

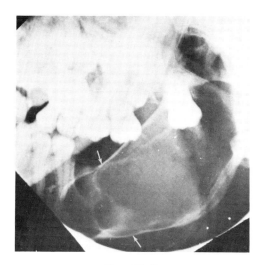

Fig. 17-5

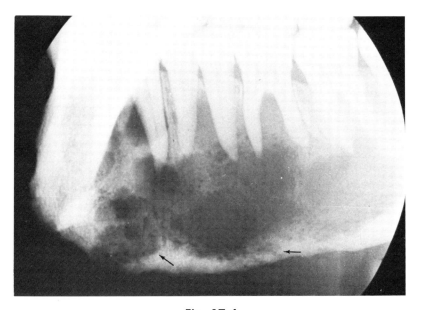

Fig. 17-6

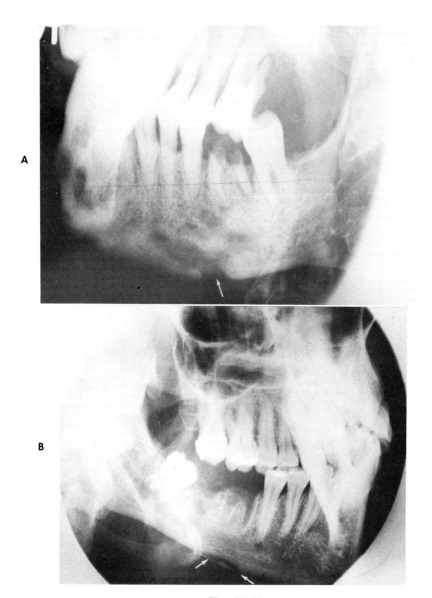

Fig. 17-7

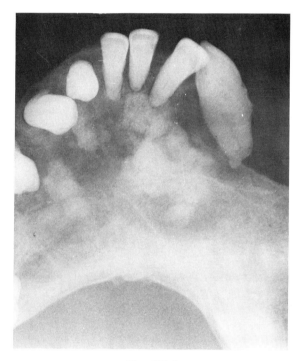

Fig. 17-8

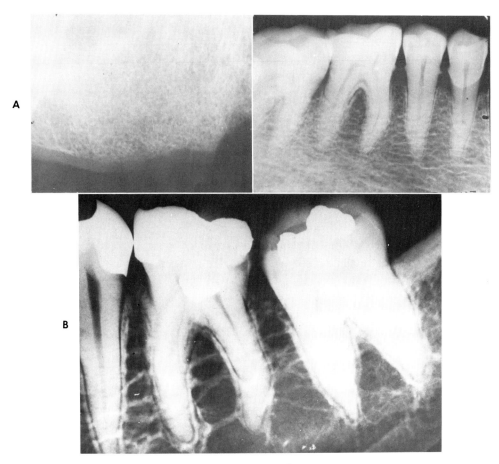

Fig. 17-9

usually large trabecular spaces in the mandible. This patient presented no un-toward symptoms. Note that the heavy, dense trabeculae apparently are sub-stituting for large numbers of finer trabeculae. The possible significance of trabecular pattern variations is discussed further under criterion 32.

10. **Single radiolucent areas as opposed to multiple, separate areas.** This characteristic (Fig. 17-10) is observed almost daily. It is common to most of the lesions observed in the jaws. The lesion is a cyst.

11. **Multiple radiolucent lesions in one bone**—the so-called monostotic le-sion. The case presented (Fig. 17-11) is of an ameloblastoma.

12. **Multiple radiolucent lesions in more than one bone**—the so-called poly-ostotic lesion. Fig. 17-12 illustrates findings in a case of multiple myeloma: the chest, shoulder, and upper arms *(A)*, and the skull *(B)*.

13. **Multiloculated radiolucent areas.** This particular radiogram (Fig. 17-13) is of a large dentigerous cyst; it has many characteristics of an amelo-blastoma.

14. **Honeycombed or soap bubble–like radiolucent areas.** Fig. 17-14 is of an ameloblastoma of a relatively rare type. Note how extensively the jaw has ex-panded. It illustrates well the next criterion.

15. **Expansile radiolucent areas, that is, areas of increased bone dimensions.** In Fig. 17-15 is seen another ameloblastoma, this time in cross section. The lin-gual plate has expanded, but the buccal plate has been partially destroyed.

16. **Porous, spongy, or poorly calcified radiolucent areas, either generalized or locally extensive.** Fig. 17-16 demonstrates fairly well this not very specific criterion. This radiolucency is caused by fibrous dysplasia.

17. **A decrease in the opacity of normally dense bone lamina,** for example, the lamina dura, cortical bone at the lower border of the mandible, the floor and partitions of the maxillary sinus, and so forth. Note that these landmarks are normally quite opaque. In Fig. 17-17 a generalized withdrawal of calcium has occurred. This case of hyperparathyroidism also shows an apparent thinning of the trabecular bone, resulting in a kind of spiderweb appearance.

18. **An inclusion of teeth in a radiolucent area; a complete or partial en-veloping of the tooth in the lesion.** This sign suggests considerable activity of the destructive process. Fig. 17-18 is of a squamous cell carcinoma. The full extent of the lesion is probably not demonstrated on the film.

19. **A resorption of tooth roots by a radiolucent lesion as the pathologic process expands.** Such resorption requires time. The pathologic change must be relatively slow. The resorption shown in Fig. 17-19 was caused by an amelo-blastoma. Root resorption also occurs with chronic apical infection and for a variety of other reasons.

20. **A displacement of teeth to either side of a radiolucent lesion.** This sign is also observed with slowly growing lesions. It is generally associated with processes that are confined within specific borders. The radiogram in Fig. 17-20 illustrates a globulomaxillary cyst.

Text continued on p. 444.

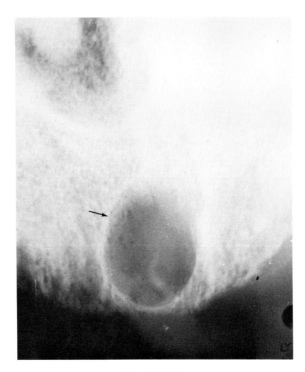

Fig. 17-10

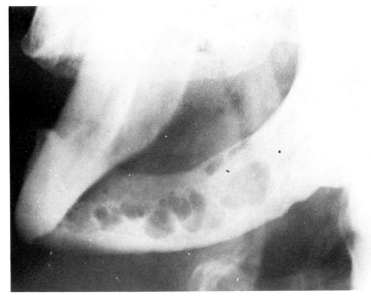

Fig. 17-11. (Courtesy Dr. M. H. Jacobs.)

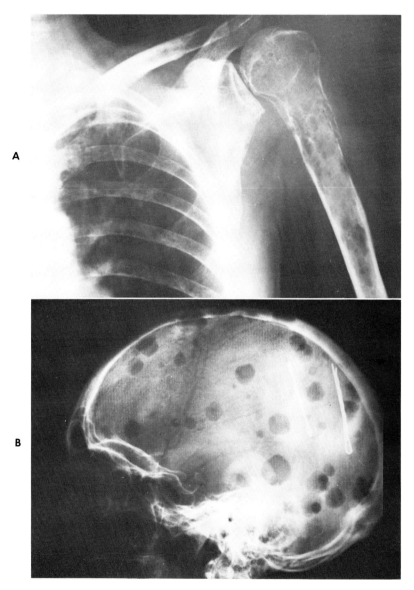

Fig. 17-12

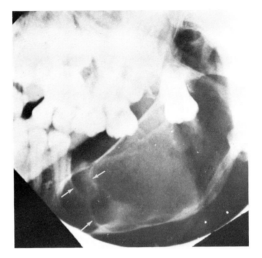

Fig. 17-13

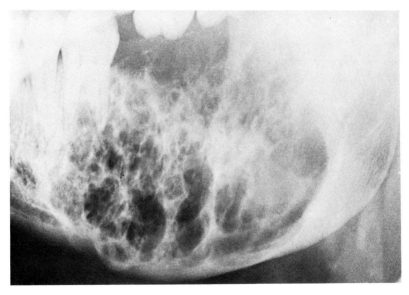

Fig. 17-14

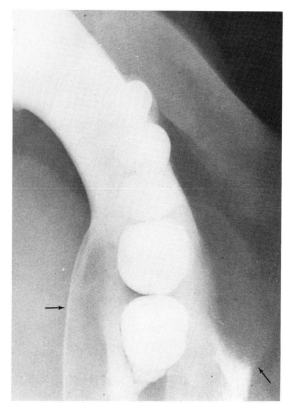

Fig. 17-15

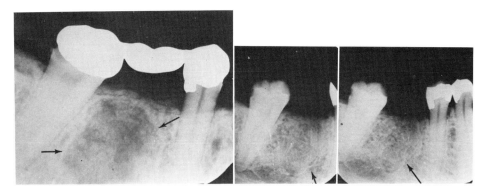

Fig. 17-16

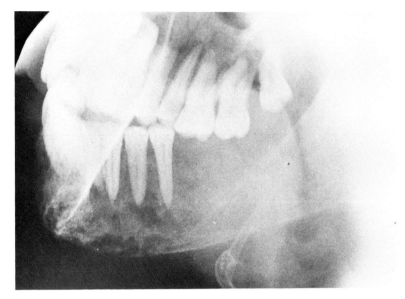

Fig. 17-17. (Courtesy Dr. C. A. McCallum, Jr.)

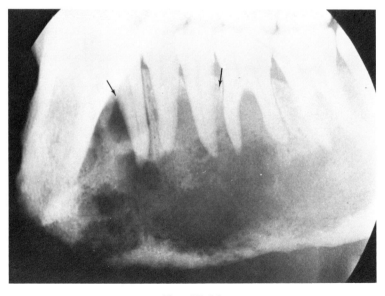

Fig. 17-18

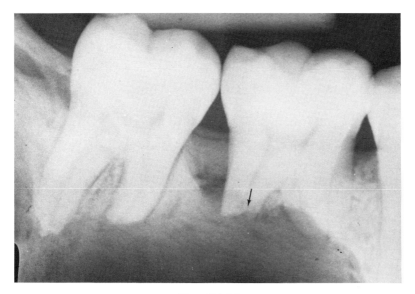

Fig. 17-19

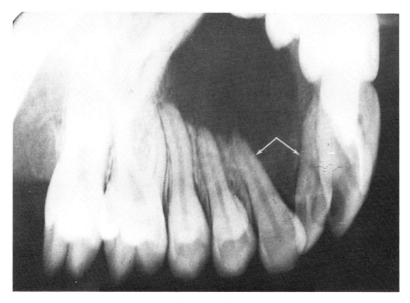

Fig. 17-20

21. **An ill-defined radiolucency showing evidence of entrapment of bone but little or no calcification.** Inclusion of bone, like the inclusion of tooth roots, suggests a rapidly destructive process. Fig. 17-21 is of a fibrosarcoma of the maxilla. Care must be exercised to differentiate between entrapped bone and redevelopment of bone in a radiolucent area.

22. **An essentially radiolucent lesion within and expanding from the surface of the bone in the form of sunray opaque lines.** This sign is said to be a common characteristic of an osteogenic sarcoma. Note that even though the osteogenic sarcoma shown in Fig. 17-22 is of bone, the lesion is still radiolucent in character.

23. **Radiopaque masses within bone having an encapsulating radiolucent border.** In Fig. 17-23 is seen a typical compound composite odontoma. The encapsulation is quite clear, even though it cannot be seen to encircle the opaque mass completely.

24. **Radiopaque masses within bone having a definite union with and no border between it and the surrounding bone.** Fig. 17-24 is of an enostosis—an increase in bone on the medullary aspect of the cortical plate.

25. **Radiopaque masses within bone having interspersed radiolucent areas within the opaque mass, giving a kind of cotton wool appearance.** Fig. 17-25 illustrates a case of Paget's disease. The opaque concretions are common in Paget's disease and are observed when fibrous changes in bone remineralize.

26. **Radiopaque masses within bone having a solid appearance to the opacity, no evidence of interspersed radiolucencies, and a periphery that tends to blend with the bone.** Such characteristics are observed in some types of dentinoma and enameloma (Fig. 17-26), as well as in highly calcified osteomas.

27. **Radiopaque masses within bone having a rough or scalloped periphery to the opaque lesion.** The irregular periphery plus a tendency to be noncircumscribed suggest a possible lack of dormancy. Fig. 17-27 illustrates a case of tuberculous osteitis.

28. **A radiopaque mass on the surface of the bone.** This may be in the form of a gross bone enlargement, as in periostitis (Fig. 17-28, *A*), or it can be observed on the buccal or lingual surfaces in typical cases of torus mandibularis (Fig. 17-28, *B*).

29. **An extraosseous radiopaque mass in the soft tissue associated with the bone surface.** As can be noted in Fig. 17-29, it is important not to confuse opaque masses in the soft tissue with those in bone. A second dimensional view is often essential to avoid this error.

30. **Radiopaque areas of bone sequestration,** in other words, islands of bone surrounded by radiolucent areas of bone destruction. The appearance in Fig. 17-30 is characteristic of osteomyelitis. However, osteomyelitis takes varying forms, depending on its stage of development.

31. **Radiopaque areas of increased bone dimension.** This expansile characteristic has been mentioned several times. The amount of opacity is a function

Text continued on p. 448.

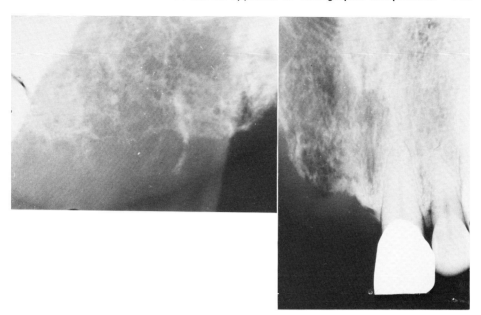

Fig. 17-21

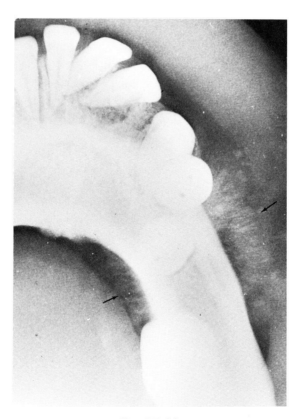

Fig. 17-22

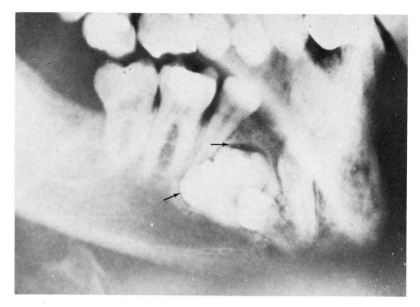

Fig. 17-23. (Courtesy Dr. M. H. Jacobs.)

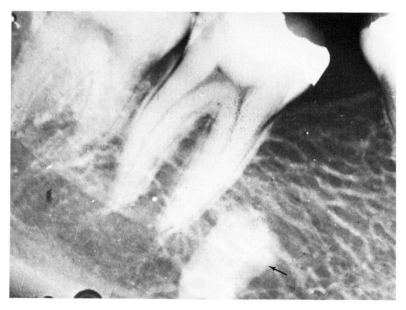

Fig. 17-24

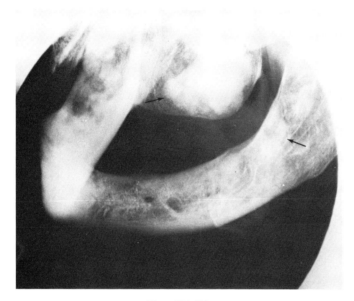

Fig. 17-25

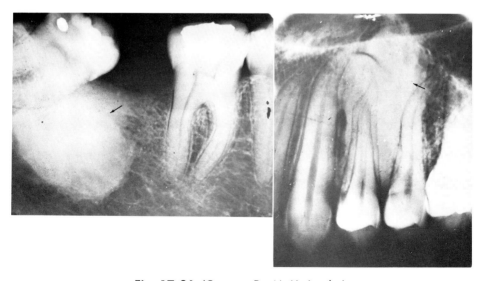

Fig. 17-26. (Courtesy Dr. M. H. Jacobs.)

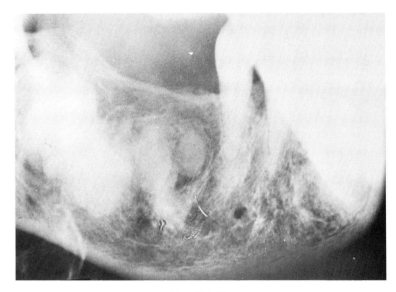

Fig. 17-27

of thickness and degree of mineralization. Fig. 17-31 is of a patient with fibrous dysplasia. The lesion is actually thicker than it is opaque.

32. **Areas showing a change in trabecular pattern characteristics.** Fig. 17-9, *A*, illustrates trabecular pattern characteristics that continue to be considered normal. Fig. 17-9, *B*, shows very large trabecular spaces and correspondingly heavy trabeculae that occurred in an individual showing no discernible symptoms of systemic disease. Fig. 17-32, *A*, illustrates a trabecular pattern that is the antithesis of Fig. 17-9, *B*; no known symptoms of systemic disease were present when this radiogram was made, but the absence of teeth in the area may be significant. This contrast in trabecular patterns is used to emphasize the thinking of the immediate past and, for the most part, current attitudes. Although at great variance, these illustrations are usually considered normal. These traditional attitudes should be reconsidered. Fig. 17-32 illustrates very discernible nutrient vessels in different individuals. Nutrient vessels are often much less discernible; they are observed quite frequently in the mandibular anterior area but only infrequently in the maxilla and in the posterior region of the mandible. Little significance has been placed on such findings in the past; this attitude also should be reconsidered. Fig. 17-33 illustrates variations in trabecular pattern and nutrient vessels between two individuals. The upper radiograms show relatively thin trabeculae and large spaces. The trabeculae tend to be parallel and horizontal. Note lack of bone loss. The lower radiograms show small trabecular spaces and a trabecular pattern that seems to lack organization. Nutrient canals are discernible, especially in the anterior region. Note loss of teeth and of bone supporting the remaining teeth. These two groups of associated characteristics tend to be quite common.

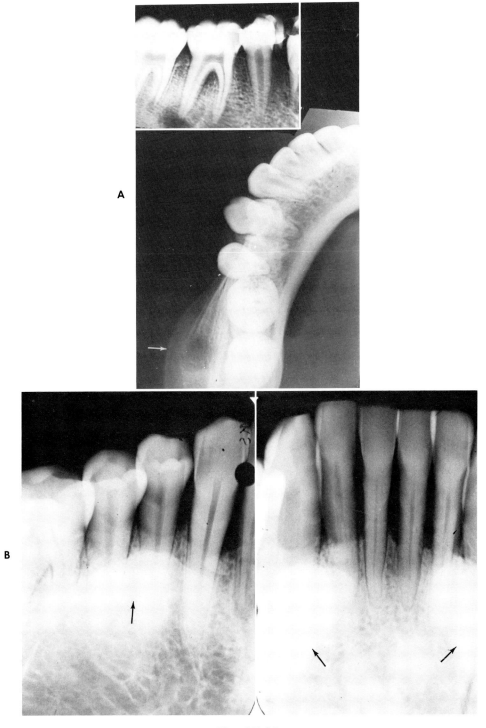

Fig. 17-28

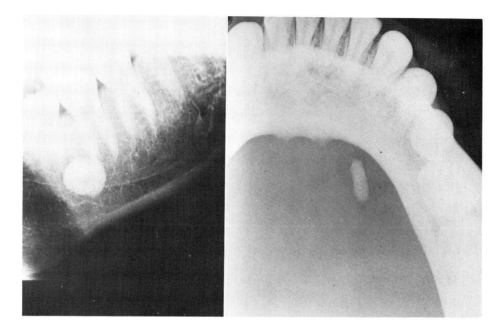

Fig. 17-29

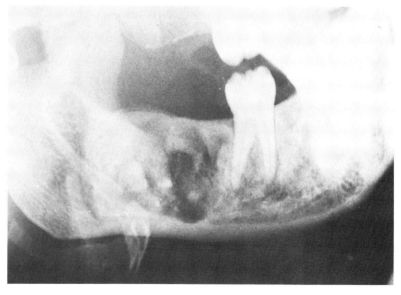

Fig. 17-30

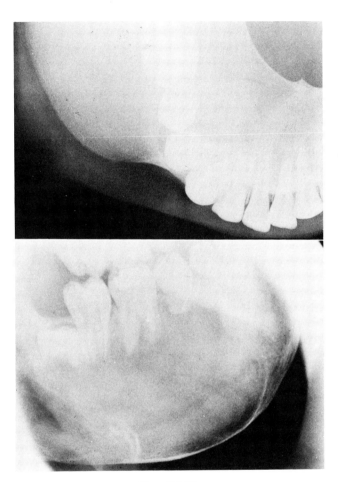

Fig. 17-31

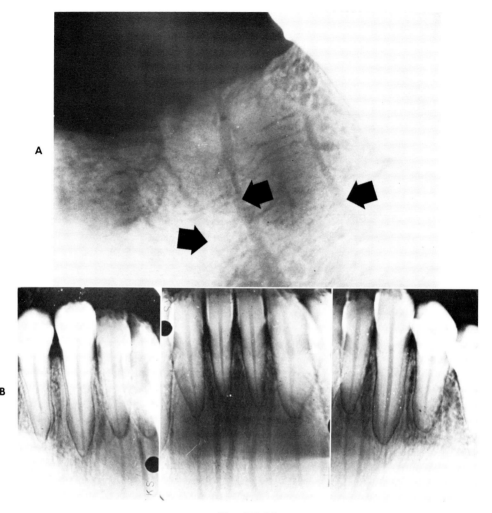

Fig. 17-32

RADIOGRAPHIC DIFFERENTIAL DIAGNOSIS

With these radiographic criteria in mind, it is now possible to proceed to the process of arriving at a radiographic differential diagnosis. Obviously, each area observed radiographically presents more than one radiographic criterion. How can a radiographic *differential diagnosis* best be made? Stress is placed on the term *differential diagnosis* because a definitive diagnosis must await clinical, clinical laboratory, and microscopic findings.

In order to effectively use observed radiographic criteria as a means of separating possible from unlikely diagnoses, one must outline, either on paper or mentally, the various possible radiographic interpretive signs and be cognizant of the diseases that would tend to present each type of criterion. Through the process of eliminating criteria and using only those applicable to a particular

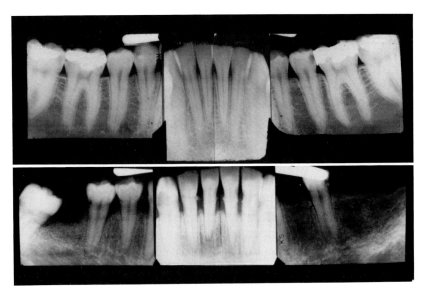

Fig. 17-33

radiogram, one can evolve a list of diseases that could produce radiographic manifestations seen on a questionable film. Although the resulting list of diseases may be long, only a few diseases occur with frequency. The diseases whose names appear on the list constitute the radiographic differential diagnosis. In actual practice, there is a strong likelihood that one of the diseases listed most frequently will be the definitive diagnosis. Diseases whose names are not included in one's thinking are automatically excluded from the differential diagnosis; this is a weakness of the diagnostician.

The method discussed here is not foolproof; it cannot take the place of experience. It does suggest a mechanism for the relatively uninitiated individual to learn to use radiographic information in a manner other than to didactically memorize the names of diseases and correlated radiographic findings. One word of caution is in order. Many of the illustrations presented in this chapter demonstrate dramatic, fully developed signs of disease. It is important to recognize these, but it is equally essential to recognize these signs in their very early stages and to institute procedures that will prevent gross destruction. Differentiation of lesions from each other and from normal conditions is difficult—especially in the early stages. It is the responsibility of the general practitioner to observe the incipient changes and, if necessary, to seek advice. The early use of a biopsy and of clinical laboratory tests can be of considerable value.

CHAPTER 18

Clinical laboratory aids in radiographic interpretation

Throughout the portions of this text devoted to interpretation, stress has been placed on the need for correlating radiographic findings with a clinical examination and, when necessary, with a biopsy report and with the results of clinical laboratory tests. The dental practitioner is well versed in the technics of conducting a clinical examination. Though he is not likely to be qualified to perform histopathologic studies, he has no difficulty understanding biopsy reports. For these reasons, there is no need to stress these aspects of oral diagnosis in this chapter. However, the practitioner is usually not well informed about clinical laboratory tests that can be of assistance in diagnosis. This chapter is designed to emphasize the indications for use and the significance of certain clinical laboratory tests of special value in evaluating radiographic findings.

CLINICAL LABORATORY EXAMINATION

Clinical laboratory studies are ordinarily not included in a clinical dental examination; in a very large proportion of patients such information would be superfluous. However, when the practitioner is forced to deal with complex diagnostic problems, clinical laboratory findings become more important. In most instances the general practitioner will refer such patients to dental specialists or to a medical colleague. Whether or not the patient is referred elsewhere, it is important for the dentist to have a reasonable understanding of the more commonly used clinical laboratory tests and of their normal values.

These facts are especially true if one is to evaluate correctly some of the more obscure radiographic findings. In Chapter 17 mention is made of a differential radiographic diagnosis. This is the final stage insofar as a radiographic evaluation is concerned. A clinical examination frequently contributes little at this point, and the clinician must depend on clinical laboratory tests and histologic examination for a definitive diagnosis. Unlike the clinical examination and the biopsy report, the information returned from the clinical laboratory frequently is confusing to the dental diagnostician unless he makes constant use of such services.

It often has been said that "a little knowledge is a dangerous thing." The scope of laboratory medicine is broad, and extensive clinical experience is needed to accurately interpret results that often are conflicting. It must be emphasized that the material presented in this chapter is not a panacea. It is designed as a ready reference for the dentist; when necessary, further information must be obtained from other sources. Tables 18-1 to 18-5 give normal values for blood and urine. Blood calcium, phosphorus, and alkaline and acid phosphatase, as well as urinary calcium, will be discussed in greater detail; these factors are generally most closely related to alterations in osseous tissue.

Blood calcium

Calcium is absorbed initially from the upper part of the small intestine and is excreted in the urine and feces. It is stored chiefly in bones, from which it can be absorbed for physiologic needs. Blood calcium is found only in the plasma*; it exists in both diffusible and nondiffusible forms. The diffusible portion exists largely in an ionizable form; the nondiffusible calcium is bound to serum protein. Of the total plasma calcium, about 55% is diffusible and 45% is nondiffusible. Measurements are made of the total serum calcium level. Serum protein levels must always be determined when evaluations of blood calcium levels are made because changes in one are in direct proportion to those in the other. Calcium level abnormalities are only significant in the presence of a normal serum protein level.

An increased serum calcium level suggests an intake and absorption of calcium beyond the ability of the body to utilize it or, and far more likely, a condition whereby calcium is being withdrawn from the bones at an abnormal rate. Hypercalcemia occurs in hyperparathyroidism; after excessively high doses of vitamin D and excessive intakes of milk and absorbable alkali; and in the presence of sarcoidosis and bone tumors, for example, multiple myeloma and other neoplastic bone processes including metastatic carcinoma. Hypercalcemia also occurs in patients with Paget's disease, but *only* when the patient is immobilized.

Decreased serum calcium (hypocalcemia) is associated with hypoparathyroidism; vitamin D deficiency; osteomalacia; conditions associated with a poor absorption of calcium and/or vitamin D; certain types of chronic renal failure, such as chronic glomerulonephritis; decreases in serum albumin; and late pregnancy in the absence of sufficient maternal intake of calcium and vitamin D. Osteomalacia implies poor matrix calcification and is ordinarily associated with a low product of $[Ca^{++}] \times [PO_4]$. It can occur with hypocalcemia–normal phosphorus, normal calcium–decreased phosphorus, or increased calcium–decreased phosphorus, but it is most commonly found associated with a normal calcium and a decreased phosphorus.

---

*Blood plasma is the fluid portion of the blood in which the corpuscles are suspended. Plasma is distinguished from serum, which is plasma from which the fibrinogen has been separated through clotting. Plasma contains all the chemical components of whole blood except hemoglobin.

Table 18-1. Normal laboratory values*

Test	Material used and comments	Normal†
Albumin	Serum; see Protein	
Amino acid nitrogen	Serum	3.5-6.0
Amylase	Serum or plasma	80-150 units (Somogyi) (1 unit is 1 mg. of reducing sugar liberated as glucose per 100 ml. of serum)
Ascorbic acid (vitamin C)	Serum or plasma	0.7-2.0
Basal metabolic rate (BMR)		Minus 15% to plus 15%
Bilirubin (van der Bergh)	Serum	Direct: 0-0.2 Total: 0.1-1.0
Bromide	Serum or plasma	Less than 50
Bromsulphalein test (BSP)	Serum; liver function test; method is valueless in patients with obvious jaundice	Less than 10% retained in 30 min. or 5% retained in 45 min.
Calcium, total	Serum; total calcium equals diffusible plus nondiffusible	9.0-11.0 (4.5-5.5 mEq./L.)
Calcium, total	Feces, 24-hr specimen	70%-90% of ingested calcium eliminated in feces
Calcium, total	Urine, 24-hr. specimen	300 mg./day is absolute upper value regardless of intake
Carbon dioxide content	Serum; normal milliequivalent values expressed as bicarbonate	26-28 mEq./L.
Cephalin flocculation	Serum; liver function test	Below 2+ in 48 hr.
Chloride	Serum or plasma	96-105 mEq./L. (as Cl)
Chloride	Spinal fluid	124-130 mEq./L. (as Cl)
Chloride	Urine, 24-hr. specimen	10-12 gm./24 hr. (as NaCl) will equal intake ± a few grams
Cholesterol, esters	Serum of plasma	80-200
Cholesterol, total	Serum of plasma	120-260
Congo red test	Serum or plasma; test for amyloidosis and nephrosis	10%-30% eliminated from blood in 1 hr.
Creatine	Urine, 24-hr. specimen	Adults: 0-200/24 hr. Children: 10-15/24 hr.
Creatinine	Serum	0.6-1.2

*From Shafer, W. G., Hine, M. K., and Levy, B. M.: A textbook of oral pathology, ed. 2, Philadelphia, 1963, W. B. Saunders Co.; with some modifications based on advice received at the University of Alabama in Birmingham Medical Center.
†All values expressed as milligrams per 100 ml. unless otherwise specified.

Table 18-1. Normal laboratory values—cont'd

Test	Material used and comments	Normal†
Creatinine	Urine, 24-hr. specimen	1-1.8 gm./24 hr.
Fatty acids, total	Serum	250-500
Fibrin	Plasma	0.3-0.6 gm./100 ml.
Glucose	Whole blood Serum Postprandial	60-90 70-105 Less than 140 at 2 hr.
Glucose	Spinal fluid	40-60 (roughly ⅔ of blood sugar)
Hydrogen ion concentration (pH)	Arterial blood	7.35-7.40 pH units
Icteric index	Serum	4-6 units
Iodine, protein-bound	Serum	4μg-8μg/100 ml.
Lecithin	Serum or plasma	225-250
Lipase	Serum	0.8-1.5 units (Alper) 0.2-1.5 units (Cherry-Crandall)
Lipids, total	Serum	470-750
Nitrogen, nonprotein	Whole blood	25-35
Nitrogen, urea	Whole blood	9-17
Phenolsulfonphthalein (PSP)	Urine; renal function test	40%-60% 1st hr. 20%-25% 2nd hr.
Phosphatase, acid	Serum	0-2.5 units (King-Armstrong) 0-1.5 phenol units
Phosphatase, alkaline	Serum	Adults: 1.5-4 units (Bodansky) 5-10 units (King-Armstrong) 1-3.5 phenol units Children: 5-14 units (Bodansky) 15-20 units (King-Armstrong) 4-12 phenol units
Phospholipids	Serum	150-350
Phosphorus, inorganic	Serum	Adults: 3-4.5 Children: 4.5-6
Potassium	Serum	3.8-5 mEq./L.
Protein, total Albumin Alpha globulin Beta globulin Gamma globulin Total globulin Albumin-globulin ratio (A/G ratio)	Serum	6-8 gm./100 ml. 3.2-4.1 gm./100 ml. 0.7-1.5 gm./100 ml. 0.7-1.3 gm./100 ml. 0.7-1.3 gm./100 ml. 2.6-3.8 gm./100 ml. 1.5-2.5:1
Protein, total	Spinal fluid	20-40

Continued.

Table 18-1. Normal laboratory values—cont'd

Test	Material used and comments	Normal†
Sodium	Serum	137-147 mEq./L.
Thymol turbidity	Serum; liver function test	0-4 units
Uric acid	Whole blood	2-5 (females) or 6 (males)
Urobilinogen	Feces, 4-day specimen	150-300
Urobilinogen	Urine, 24-hr. specimen	8 or less
Volume, blood	Whole blood and plasma	70-100 ml. blood/kg. 35-50 ml. plasma/kg.

Blood phosphorus

Blood phosphorus is always determined as phosphate but is calculated and reported as elemental phosphorus. Phosphates apparently are absorbed from the upper part of the jejunum; they are excreted by the intestine and kidneys and are resorbed into the blood from the lower part of the small intestine. The amount resorbed varies inversely with the amount of calcium excreted into the intestine. This occurs because calcium and phosphorus in the intestine form an insoluble calcium phosphate that is poorly resorbed. The absorption and utilization of phosphorus are directly related to the amount of vitamin D. Though phosphates are excreted into both the urine and feces, the latter is the more quantitatively important mechanism of phosphate elimination.

Inorganic phosphate blood level is measured in the serum. Physiologic variations occur, particularly in the summer, when an individual is subjected to greater amounts of ultraviolet light. Blood levels also will decrease after high ingestion of large amounts of carbohydrate.

An increase in the serum phosphate level (hyperphosphatemia) occurs in hypoparathyroidism; in hypervitaminosis D; in certain bone diseases, such as multiple myeloma; in the presence of bone tumors; during the healing of fractures; and in renal disease.

Hypophosphatemia occurs in hyperparathyroidism, in osteomalacia caused by vitamin D deficiency or renal tubular disease or defects, in inadequate absorption of phosphorus from the intestine, and to a slight degree in normal pregnancy.

Serum phosphatase

Blood serum contains enzymes that are able to liberate inorganic phosphates by hydrolyzing phosphoric esters of plasma and erythrocytes. The most active phosphatase requires a hydrogen-ion concentration (pH) of 9* for optimum activity and is called alkaline phosphatase. Less active is acid phosphatase, which

---

*A pH of 9 is higher than any body pH. It is available for laboratory procedures.

Table 18-2. Normal red blood cell values (average values and range)*

Age	Red cell count (millions/c.mm. blood)	Hemoglobin (gm./100 ml.)	Hematocrit (vol. packed cells/100 ml.)	Sedimentation rate in 1 hr. (Wintrobe method)	Reticulocytes (% of erythrocytes)
2-10	5.25-4.1 4.6 (values decrease with increasing age; high at birth)	15-10.5 13	42-32 37	3-13 9 (Smith)	Essentially the same as adults
11-15	5.4-4.3 4.6	15.5-11.5 13	45-34 40	—	Essentially the same as adults
12-20	—	—	—	1-20 ♂ 4.7 (Gallagher)	—
Adults	6.2-4.2 4.8 ♀ 5.4 ♂	18-12 14 ♀ 16 ♀	54-38 42 ♀ 47 ♂	0-15 9.6 ♀ 0-6.5 3.7 ♂	0.56-2.72 1.64

*Adapted from Wintrobe, M. M.: Clinical hematology, ed. 6, Philadelphia, 1967, Lea & Febiger.

Table 18-3. Normal white blood cell values*

Total white cell count per c.mm. blood
Infants: 8,000-16,500
4- 7 yr.: 6,000-15,000 (average 10,700)
8-18 yr.: 4,500-13,500 (average 8,300)
Adults: 5,000-10,000 (average 7,000)

Relative (differential) and absolute values for leukocyte counts in normal adults per c.mm. blood†

Type of cell	%	Absolute number		
		Average	Minimum	Maximum
Total leukocytes		7,000	5,000	10,000
Myelocytes	0	0	0	0
Juvenile neutrophils	3-5	300	150	400
Segmented neutrophils	54-62	4,000	3,000	5,800
Eosinophils	1-3	200	50	250
Basophils	0-0.75	25	15	50
Lymphocytes	25-33	2,100	1,500	3,000
Monocytes	3-7	375	285	500

*From Shafer, W. G., Hine, M. K., and Levy, B. M.: A textbook of oral pathology, ed. 2, Philadelphia, 1963, W. B. Saunders Co.
†Data based on Wintrobe, M. M.: Clinical hematology, ed. 5, Philadelphia, 1961, Lea & Febiger.

Table 18-4. Normal blood platelet values and associated phenomena*

Total number of platelets: 150,000-400,000 per c.mm. blood
Bleeding time: under 5 min. (Duke's method)
Clotting time: 1-7 min. (capillary tube method)
              2.5-5 min. (Kruse and Moses method)
              5-10 min. (Lee and White method)
Prothrombin time: 10-20 sec. (Quick method)
Clot retraction time
    Qualitative begins 1-6 hr.; complete at 24 hr.
    Quantitative 80%-90%
Capillary fragility (tourniquet test)
    More than 10 petechiae per 1-in. circle—positive
Heterophil antibodies (sheep cell agglutination)
    Below 1:56 dilution
Incidence of blood groups in normal population
    Group O —40%
            A —45%
            B —12%
          AB— 4%
    Rh positive—85%
    Rh negative—15%

*From Shafer, W. G., Hine, M. K., and Levy, B. M.: A textbook of oral pathology, Philadelphia, 1963, W. B. Saunders Co.

Table 18-5. Normal average values of urine*

Physical characteristics	
Volume, 24-hr. specimen	1,500 ml.
Specific gravity	1.015-1.025
Turbidity	None
Color	Amber
Chemical characteristics	
pH	Slightly acid
Total acidity	25-40 ml. N/10 NaOH to neutralize 100 ml. urine
Water	95% of total urine

*From Shafer, W. G., Hine, M. K., and Levy, B. M.: A textbook of oral pathology, ed. 2, Philadelphia, 1963, W. B. Saunders Co.

acts optimally at a pH of 5. Although both enzymes can function at the normal pH of serum, neither can function at the optimum pH of its counterpart.

Alkaline phosphatase. An increase in alkaline phosphatase is known as hyperphosphatasemia. It occurs in conditions of bone requiring an increased calcium phosphate deposition and is associated with osteoblastic activity. Thus the level elevates in instances of excessive bone production and when destructive processes in bone create a demand for bone repair. Hyperphosphatasemia occurs in hyperparathyroidism (osteitis fibrosa cystica generalisata), Paget's disease (osteitis deformans), osteogenesis imperfecta, severe osteomalacia, osteogenic sarcoma,

Table 18-6. Blood and urine changes under diseased conditions

Disease	Total serum calcium	Total serum phosphorus	Serum alkaline phosphatase	Urinary calcium (Sulkowitch)
Benign tumors	←—————————	All normal values		——————————→
Osteogenic sarcoma	N	N	I	N
Metastatic carcinoma to bone	N-I	N-I	N-I	N-I
Multiple myeloma	N-I	N-I	N-I	I-N
Primary hyperparathyroidism	I	D	N-I	I
Hypoparathyroidism	D	I	N	D
Hyperthyroidism	N-I	N	N-I	N-I
Osteoporosis	N	N	N	N
Osteitis deformans (Paget's disease)	N-I with complete immobilization	N	I	N-I
Fibrous dysplasia	N	N	N	N
Healing fractures	N	I-N	I-N	N
Hypervitaminosis D	I	I	N	I
Osteomalacia*				
Vitamin D deficiency	D-N	D	I	D
Renal insufficiency	D	I	I-N	D
Renal tubular defects	D-N	D	I-N	I
Gastrointestinal malabsorption	D-N	D	I-N	D

*Osteomalacia in most cases is a combined defect of inability to calcify bone matrix and secondary hyperparathyroidism.

metastatic carcinoma to bones resulting in osteoplastic changes, Gaucher's disease, rickets, healing fractures, liver disease (the liver aids in the excretion of this enzyme), advanced hyperthyroidism, and such physiologic conditions as pregnancy, teeth and bone development in childhood, and more than average exposure to ultraviolet light. Hypophosphatasemia occurs in cretinism and renal dwarfism and as a rare congenital inability to produce alkaline phosphatase.

Acid phosphatase. Acid phosphatase change is of significance when it increases, but it is usually a less useful indicator than alkaline phosphatase. It increases in carcinoma of the prostate, particularly when it metastasizes to bone, and in Gaucher's disease. Rarely, there is an elevation in nephritis, Paget's disease, and hyperparathyroidism.

Urine calcium

Calcium is excreted in the urine and the feces. Excretion is equal to intake in the normal person after growth has terminated. A person on an average diet excretes about 200 mg. of calcium daily; an increase in blood calcium ordinarily does not occur until urinary excretion exceeds 500 mg. daily.

An increased urinary calcium, hypercalciuria, occurs in hyperparathyroidism, hypervitaminosis D, neoplastic metastases to bone, hyperthyroidism, multiple myeloma, some renal defects with osteomalacia, and Paget's disease. Hypocalciuria is frequently found in hypoparathyroidism, hypothyroidism, renal insufficiency, and hypovitaminosis D.

Table 18-6 gives an indication of changes in total serum calcium, total serum phosphorus, serum alkaline phosphatase, and urinary calcium under diseased conditions that relate to radiographic interpretation. An *I* indicates an elevated level, a *D* means a depressed level, and an *N* represents normal. Remember that great variability can exist in the results of the few tests listed in Table 18-6. The results are influenced by a multitude of diverse factors that could be involved in a patient's physical condition.

CHAPTER 19

Other radiographic systems of interest

Many technics used in dental research and in other radiographic fields are of importance to dental radiologists. These technics use machines or materials not presently being utilized by the average general dental practitioner. However, they are of potential importance to every dentist and are discussed briefly in this chapter.

CINERADIOGRAPHY

The use of moving x-ray pictures was made practical with the development of the light intensification tube. Prior to this development, very large amounts of radiation were needed to make the fluorescent screen bright enough for a moving picture to be made. This was impractical because of the radiation damage done to the patient. Today, cineradiography uses small amounts of radiation to make a very dim picture on a fluorescent screen. The brightness of the picture on the screen is increased (somewhat in the way a television picture is brightened) by a photomultiplier tube, and a moving picture is made of the brightened image. In the dental field, this technic has been used, among other things, to evaluate temporomandibular joint function and velopharyngeal relationships during speech and swallowing.

Cineradiography as just described implies the use of photographic film. Recently, the utilization of videotapes for use with television has come into existence. These tapes can record the image much as it is recorded on a movie film. Alternatively, a technic can be employed wherein short individual "spot" exposures are made. Each exposure is recorded on television tape and then displayed continuously on a screen until another spot exposure is made. The second exposure ordinarily erases the first set of electronic signals, but it is possible to retain the sequential exposures on the tape if desirable. This technic is used, for example, in heart catheterizations; instead of exposing the patient continuously, the physician makes a series of short exposures as he introduces the catheter and as the catheter tip progresses toward the heart. What the physician sees on the screen are still pictures taken at intervals, rather than a continuous picture, which, by its nature, requires constant patient exposure. Replay of the entire tape can show the movement of the catheter. The application of this type of procedure to the study of some aspects of oral physiology is obvious.

XERORADIOGRAPHY

Xeroradiography utilizes a relatively new principle for recording the radiographic image of an object. A selenium plate is used instead of film. The system is easily understood if one imagines that the plate has the ability to hold an electric charge on its surface without the individual charges moving around.

A uniform electrostatic charge is placed on a layer of photoconductive selenium that has a grounded conductive backing. When the charged plate is used like a film, the x-rays striking it destroy the electric charges at the points where the x-rays are absorbed. This is comparable to the latent image formation in the grains of a film. In order for the image to be seen in the selenium plate, a fine

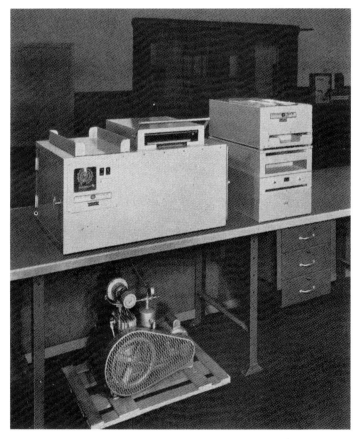

Fig. 19-1. Xeroradiographic unit and an example of a lateral skull projection made by xeroradiography. (Courtesy General Electric Co., Milwaukee, Wis.)

powder is given an electric charge that is opposite the charge on the plate and is sprayed on the surface of the plate. Since opposite electric charges attract each other, the powder clings to the areas where the selenium plate has not been discharged by the x-rays, and the radiographic image is made visible. Basically, the system is the dry processing of an electrostatic image. Permanent records can be made by photographing the image or by transferring the image to a transparent plastic sheet or paper. The selenium plate can be used again by simply wiping off the powder and recharging it. A xeroradiographic unit and an example of the xeroradiographic image are shown in Fig. 19-1. Because the magnetic fields surrounding the electrostatic charges that form the latent image are stronger at the edges of the charged area, the powder that forms the visible image is more attracted to the image edges of the various objects. This edge effect enhances local contrast and resolution. Advantages of xeroradiography are said to be elimination of accidental exposure, superior resolution, visualization of different tissues, ease of viewing, greater exposure latitude, and ease and speed of production.

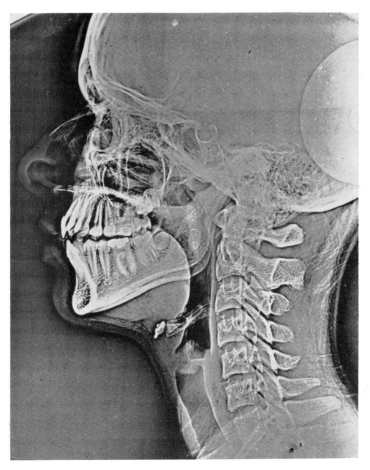

Fig. 19-1, cont'd. For legend see opposite page.

Disadvantages include technical difficulties, fragility of the photoconductor, temporary image retention, and slow imaging speed as compared to films. To date, this equipment has not been developed for general dental and medical use.

LOGETRONOGRAPHY

Logetronography is not a primary radiographic technic but rather a secondary contrast-enhancing method. Essentially, the method accomplishes photographic dodging by an electronic process. The process is one in which the finished radiogram is scanned by a machine that then prints a new picture (simulated) in which the contrast and density of the light areas of the primary radiogram are improved. Similarly, the density and contrast of the dark areas of the primary radiogram are also modified. The reproduced radiogram now shows an image that has the type of contrast most easily visualized by human eyes. A photograph of a lateral skull radiogram and a logetronic print of the same radiogram are shown in Fig. 19-2.

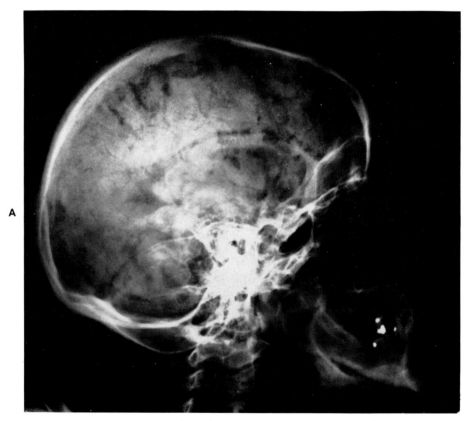

Fig. 19-2. A, Example of a conventional radiogram showing the overly dark nasal area and overly light middle ear area. **B,** Logetronic print made from the radiogram shown in **A,** demonstrating a reduction in film density in the facial areas and an increase in the auditory area. (Courtesy Logetronics, Inc., Alexandria, Va.)

LAND POLAROID PROCESSING

Radiograms can be made with films that consist of an emulsion placed on paper backing. The film is exposed to x-rays by the use of a special casette and screen. The cassette is placed in a Land Polaroid processing machine, in which the film is removed from the cassette and is automatically processed in a manner similar to Polaroid photography. Although conventional double-emulsion x-ray films use less radiation, paperbacked Polaroid film and film processing can be a useful image-recording system. It is most useful when processing speed and inaccessibility of darkroom facilities are important factors.

FLASH RADIOGRAPHY

Radiography using a high-intensity flash of x-rays is obtainable with the use of a new x-ray tube. This tube uses the field-emission electron principle. The technic is comparable to the making of photographs with a flash of light. An intense beam of x-rays can be produced for as short a period as $\frac{1}{10,000,000}$ sec-

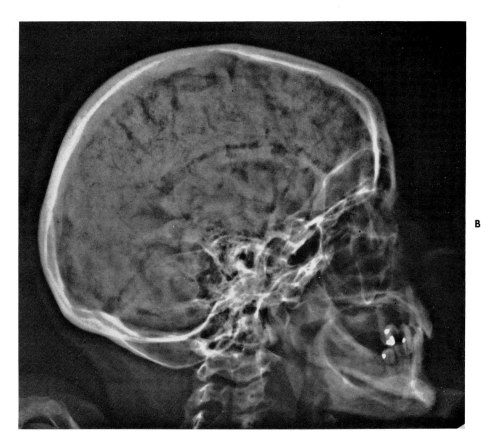

B

Fig. 19-2, cont'd. For legend see opposite page.

ond. The machine is capable of essentially stopping the patient's motion if the radiographic image can be recorded with a single pulse of x-rays. Flash radiography is possible with batteries or conventional power supply, and portable units are being manufactured. The tube is housed in a probelike assembly and is connected to the machine by a flexible cable. Flash radiography promises to make practical many new radiographic technics. A portable flash x-ray unit is shown in Fig. 19-3.

USE OF RADIOISOTOPES

Radioisotopes in dentistry are primarily utilized in the areas of dental research. The use of molecules tagged or labeled with a radioactive element has greatly increased the knowledge of biochemical and physiologic processes.

Autoradiography has been used extensively in studies of clinical importance—for example, the penetration of oral solutions under various filling materials, the penetration of drugs into dentin, and the incorporation of flux in a soldered joint. The penetration of the radioisotope-labeled compound into an object is found by sectioning the object and placing the section against a film surface or embedding the section in a photographic emulsion. When the film is processed, the blackened or exposed areas locate the position of the radioactive element (Fig. 19-4).

Radioisotopes also have been used to make dental radiograms. However, relatively long exposure times are required, and the available radioisotopes have relatively short useful lives. The use of radioisotopes for dental radiography is for the present impractical; however, they do have great potential, especially because of the advances being made in the production of more sensitive films and/or image-recording devices.

MICRORADIOGRAPHY

Microradiography, or radiography of small structures, is useful in dental research but has no apparent clinical application. One system of microradiography utilizes long wavelength x-rays produced in a range of 1 to 5 kVp. Mention of this microradiographic technic is made to emphasize the principle of optimizing contrast through wavelength choice.

Changes occurring in thin sections of teeth (tooth slabs) can be demonstrated through the use of long wavelength x-rays (Fig. 19-5). These changes cannot be demonstrated readily when x-rays in the range of 60 to 90 kVp are used. A comparison of the microradiographic and clinical dental radiographic technics employed in the examination of tooth structure shows that the x-rays used must be selected not only for the density of the object to be examined but also for the thickness of the object.

SUBTRACTION RADIOGRAPHY

Subtraction radiography uses two radiographs to produce a separate image of the difference between the two radiographs. In dentistry, the technic is most

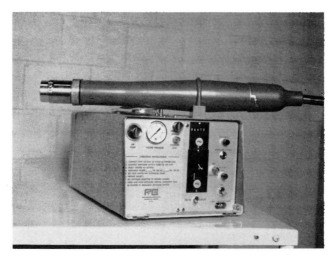

Fig. 19-3. Portable field emission x-ray unit shown with the remote tube head. The unit weighs approximately 45 pounds.

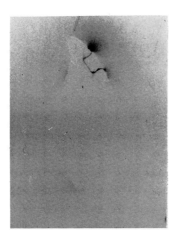

Fig. 19-4. Use of radioisotopes in determining marginal percolation of restorative materials. The illustration is a duplicate of an x-ray film. An outline of the tooth can be seen as well as the black outline of the restorative material. The black outline results from the radioactivity in a solution that infiltrated the space between the tooth substance and the restorative material. After soaking in the radioactive solution, the tooth was sectioned and its cut surface placed in contact with a film for a predetermined time. (Courtesy Dr. R. W. Phillips.)

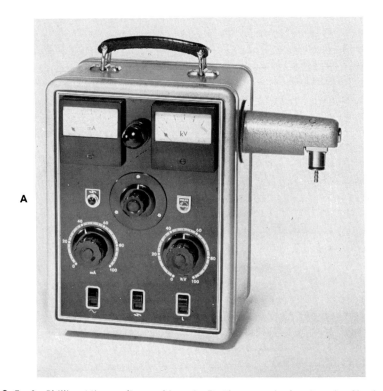

Fig. 19-5. A, Phillips Microradiographic unit. **B,** Photograph showing the film holder, film, section of specimen, metal washer, and locking ring. **C,** Radiogram of an early carious lesion as seen through a microscope. The enamel shows white in the photograph. The initial subsurface demineralization is indicated by the arrow. A very fine grain film is used to record the roentgen image. (**A** and **B,** Courtesy Phillips Electronic Instruments, Mount Vernon, N.Y.; **C,** Courtesy M. B. Quigley.)

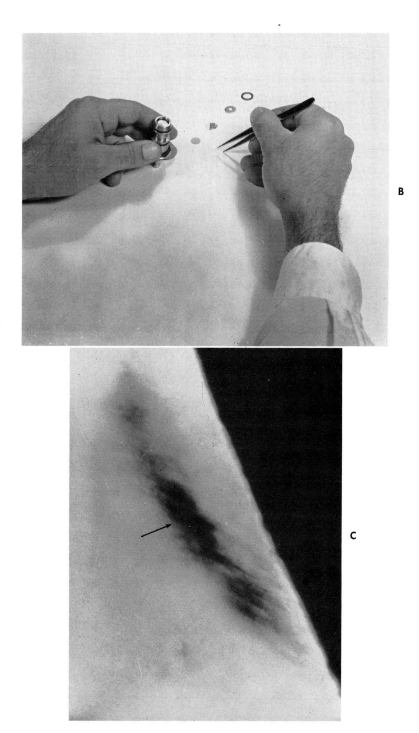

Fig. 19-5, cont'd. For legend see opposite page.

commonly applied in sialography to depict the radiopaque media. The two radiographs are made under similar conditions, one before and one after the injection of the contrast media. Any movement of the object, film, or x-ray machine that produces blurring or magnification differences between the two radiographs will prevent the achievement of total subtraction. An opposite print or negative is made of one radiograph, and this negative is superimposed on the other radiograph. The sandwich of two images results in canceling or blotting out of bone and soft tissue with the opaque media image showing itself more clearly. The subtraction technic will not increase contrast or detail, but it will make the difference between the two radiographs more easily visible.

Color is sometimes added to the films to be superimposed. One light beam is passed through a red filter and the other, through a blue filter. Each colored beam is then passed through a radiograph, and the images are combined. The contrast media can be made to stand out clearly in red. Additional radiographs made during different phases of the contrast media injection can be used to produce spectacular three-colored displays. The technic is only practical with high-contrast radiographs.

Subtraction can also be done with television equipment. Two cameras are used, one for each radiograph. A single camera that stores an image can also be used. One image is electronically converted into a negative image, which is then combined with the other image and displayed as a single image on a monitor. The advantage of two cameras is that each camera can be focused separately; thus small differences in the two radiographs have less deleterious effects on subtraction during superimpositioning or combining of the images. Television subtraction equipment is more complex and expensive than that used by other technics.

THERMOGRAPHY

Diagnostic radiography is most often thought to be accomplished with the use of x-rays. Photons with wavelengths in other regions of the electromagnetic spectrum can also be used to produce photographic or radiographic images of diagnostic importance. The use of photons in the infrared region is one such example. Thermography is the technic of recording an image of the patient's tissues with the infrared radiation emanating from the patient. The technic must not be confused with infrared photography, which is accomplished by irradiating an object with an infrared beam and subsequently photographically recording the reflected infrared image.

Infrared radiations are emitted relative to the temperature of an object. The radiations coming from different parts of the body can be optically collected, converted into proportional electrical signals, and then transformed into a visual picture called a thermogram. Thermograms are pictures of a body's surface temperature. The technic is a nondestructive test and is used in both industry and medicine. Processes characterized by high or low temperatures can be thermographically detected; these include inflammatory conditions, some malignancies, changes in blood supply, and traumatic injuries.

DIAGNOSTIC ULTRASOUND

Ultrasonic examinations use a piezoelectric crystal to generate pulses of low-intensity ultrasonic energy that are sent into the patient's body. The reflected echoes of the individual pulses are detected by the same crystal. Ultrasound is mechanical radiation and needs a medium for propagation. It is characterized by a high frequency above the audible range and cannot be propagated across a vacuum. Although ultrasound is different from electromagnetic energy, it is another method of nondestructive testing of human tissues by a radiating form of energy. The ultrasound pulses are reflected by interfaces where there is a change in tissue density. The greater the density difference, the greater is the reflection of the ultrasound. The time between creation and reception of an ultrasound pulse is related to the depth of the reflecting interface beneath the surface. The ultrasonic transducer can be moved along the surface of the patient and a cross section of the anatomical part mapped out in terms of interfaces. It is thus possible to produce ultrasonic tomograms.

Diagnostic ultrasonic examinations are often done by obstetricians to examine the fetus because no unusual hazard has been found to be associated with this technic; this is in contrast to the genetic and somatic risks inherent in the abdominal x-ray examination of pregnant women. Ultrasound has been used in the examination of teeth and has aided in the detection of surface changes in dental enamel. It has also been applied in the measurement of movements of the pharyngeal wall during speech.

Suggested readings

TECHNICS OF RADIOGRAPHY
Chapters 1-3, 5-10, and 19

Alcox, R. W., and others: Dental radiology—a special area of dental practice, Oral Surg. 32:990, 1971.

American Dental Association Council on Dental Materials and Devices: New American Dental Association Specification No. 26 for dental x-ray equipment, J.A.D.A. 89:386, 1974.

American Dental Association Council on Dental Materials and Devices: Recommendations in radiographic practices, J.A.D.A. 90:171, 1975.

American Dental Association Council on Dental Materials and Devices: Acceptance program for rapid processing devices for dental radiographic film, J.A.D.A. 91:611, 1975.

American Dental Association Council on Dental Materials and Devices: Guide to dental materials and devices, ed. 8, Chicago, The Association.

Ando, S.: Orthopantomography, J. Assoc. Oral Hygiene, Tokyo, October 1971.

Bachman, L.: Pedodontic radiography, Dent. Radiogr. Photogr. 44:51, 1971.

Barber, F. E., and others: Ultrasonic pulse-echo measurements in teeth, Arch. Oral Biol. 14:745, 1969.

Barnes, R. B.: Thermography of the human body, Science 140:870, 1963.

Barnes, R. B., and Gershon-Cohen, J.: Clinical thermography, J.A.M.A. 185:949, 1963.

Barr, J. H., and Garcia, D. A.: X-ray spectra from dental x-ray generators. I. Some general characteristics, Oral Surg. 22:478, 1966.

Baum, G., and others: Observation of internal structures of teeth by ultrasonography, Science 139:495, 1963.

Binford, R. T.: The carpal radiograph—its use in medical and dental diagnostics, Ala. Dent. Rev. 7:18, 1959.

Blackman, S.: Mass dental radiography, Radiography 22:21, 1956.

Blackman, S.: Rotational tomography of the face, Br. J. Radiol. 33:408, 1960.

Blackman, S.: Panagraphy, Oral Surg. 14:1178, 1961.

Blackman, S.: Anatomic structures as visualized on the Panoramix, Oral Surg. 26:321, 1968.

Brown, C. E., Cristen, A. C., and Jerman, A. C.: Dimensions of the focal trough in panoramic radiography, J.A.D.A. 84:843, 1972.

Brynolf, I.: Improved viewing facilities for better roentgenodiagnosis, Oral Surg. 32:808, 1971.

Buchholz, R. E.: X-ray production variability, Oral Surg. 40:282, 1975.

Buchignani, J. S., and Shimkin, P. M.: Subtraction sialography: an improved and simplified technic, Oral Surg. 31:828, 1971.

Chase, G. D., and Rabinowitz, J. L.: Principles of radioisotope methodology, ed. 2, New York, 1962, Burgess Publishing Co.

Chesney, M. O.: The use of high kilovoltage in diagnostic radiography, Radiography 28:46, 1962.

Cooper, H. K.: Application of cinefluorography with image intensification in the fields of plastic surgery, dentistry, and speech, Plast. Reconstructr. Surg. 16:135, 1955.

Crandell, C. E., and Hill, R. P.: Thermography in dentistry: a pilot study, Oral Surg. 21:316, 1966.

Curby, W. A., and Wuehrmann, A. H.: Utilization of constant exposure factors for intraoral roentgenographic studies, J. Dent. Res. 32:790, 1953.

Diagnostic x-ray systems—rules and regulations, Federal Register **37**:16461, 1972.

Donovan, M. H.: Occlusal radiography of the mandibular third molar, Dent. Radiogr. Photogr. **25**:53, 1952.

Ennis, L. M., Berry, H. M., and Phillips, J. E.: Dental roentgenology, ed. 6, Philadelphia, 1967, Lea & Febiger.

Escoe, R., and Escoe, D.: Chairside x-ray processing in broad daylight, N.Y. State Dent. J. **33**:207, 1967.

Files, G. W., editor: Medical radiographic technic, ed. 2, Springfield, Ill., 1959, Charles C Thomas, Publisher.

Fitzgerald, G. M.: Dental roentgenography. I. An investigation in adumbration, or the factors that control geometric unsharpness, J.A.D.A. **34**:1, 1947.

Fuchs, A. W.: Principles of radiographic exposure and processing, ed. 2, Springfield, Ill., 1958, Charles C Thomas, Publisher.

The fundamentals of radiography, ed. 10, Rochester, N.Y., 1960, Eastman Kodak Co.

Garcia, D. A.: X-ray spectra from dental x-ray generators. II. The primary beam, Oral Surg. **23**:610, 1967.

Gershon-Cohen, J., and others: Panography, Am. J. Roentgenol. Radium Ther. Nucl. Med. **101**:988, 1967.

Gibson, H. L.: Infrared photography of patients, Radiol. Clin. Photogr. **21**:72, 1945.

Glasser, O.: Dr. W. C. Roentgen, ed. 2, Springfield, Ill., 1958, Charles C Thomas, Publisher.

Glasser, O., Quimby, E. H., Taylor, L. S., Weatherwax, J. L., and Morgan, R. H.: Physical foundations of radiology, ed. 3, New York, 1961, Paul B. Hoeber, Inc.

Goldman, M., and Darzenta, N.: Endodontic success—Who's reading the radiograph? Oral Surg. **33**:432, 1972.

Goldstein, I. L., Mobley, W. H., and Chellemi, S. J.: The observer process in the visual interpretation of radiographs, J. Dent. Educ. **35**:485, 1971.

Gould, H. R., and others: Xeroradiography of the breast, Am. J. Roentgenol. **84**:220, 1960.

Graber, T. M.: Problems and limitations of cephalometric analysis in orthodontics, J.A.D.A. **53**:439, 1956.

Graber, T. M.: Panoramic radiography, Angle Orthod. **36**:293, 1966.

Greulich, W. W., and Pyle, S. I.: Radiographic atlas of skeletal development of the hand and wrist, ed. 2, Stanford, Calif., 1959, Stanford University Press.

Guzman, C. A.: Principles and function of the Panoramix, Oral Surg. **24**:196, 1967.

Hardy, J. D.: Radiating power of human skin in infrared, Am. J. Physiol. **127**:454, 1939.

Henrikson, C. O.: Speed and contrast of dental films, Acta Radiol. [Diagn.] (Stock.) **1**:66, 1963.

Hudson, D. C., and others: A panoramic dental x-ray machine, U.S. Armed Forces Med. J. **8**:46, 1957.

Hurlburt, C.: Automatic processing of intra-oral films in dental schools, Oral Surg. **40**:423, 1975.

Jacobson, A. F., and Ferguson, J. P.: Evaluation of the S. S. White Panorex x-ray machine, pub. no. (FDA) 72-8020, BRH/DEP 72-6, Washington, D.C., December 1971, U.S. Government Printing Office.

Jacobson, A. F., and Ferguson, J. P.: Evaluation of an S. S. White Panorex x-ray machine, Oral Surg. **36**:426, 1973.

Jacobson, B., and Mackay, R. S.: Radiological contrast enhancing methods, Adv. Biol. Med. Phys. **6**:201, 1958.

Johns, E. H.: The physics of radiology, ed. 2 (revised 2nd printing), Springfield, Ill., 1964, Charles C Thomas, Publisher.

Johnson, W. H.: Oral radiography, London, 1959, William Heinemann, Ltd.

Kelsey, C. A., and others: Ultrasonic measurement of lateral pharyngeal wall displacement, IEEE Trans. Biomed. Eng. **16**:143, 1969.

Kelsey, C. A., and others: Ultrasonic observations of coarticulation in the pharynx, J. Acoust. Soc. Am. **46**:1016, 1969.

Kite, O. W., and others: Radiation and image distortion in the Panorex x-ray unit, Oral Surg. **15**:1201, 1962.

Kornfeld, G.: Latent image distribution by x-ray exposures, J. Opt. Soc. Am. **39**:1020, 1949.

Kossof, G., and Sharpe, C. J.: Examination of the contents of the pulp cavity in teeth, Ultrasonics **4**:77, 1966.

Kraske, L. M., and Mazzarella, M. A.: Evaluation of panoramic x-ray procedures, J. Dent. Res. **39**:693, 1960.

Lawson, R. L., and others: Thermographic assessment of burns and frostbite, Can. Med. Assoc. J. **84**:1129, 1961.

Lees, S.: Specific acoustic impedance of enamel and dentine, Arch. Oral. Biol. **13**:1491, 1968.

Lees, S.: Ultrasonics of hard tissues, Int. Dent. J. 21:403, 1971.

Lees, S., and Barber, F. E.: Looking into teeth with ultrasonics, Science 161:477, 1968.

Lees, S., and Lobene, R. R.: Dental enamel: detection of surface changes by ultrasound, Science 169:1314, 1970.

Lewis, G. R.: Temporomandibular joint radiographic technics, Dent. Radiogr. Photogr. 37:8, 1964.

Lilliequist, B., and Welander, V.: Sialography: new application of the subtraction technic, Acta Radiol. [Diagn.] (Stockh.) 8:228, 1969.

Lund, T. M., and Manson-Hing, L. R.: A study of the focal troughs of three panoramic dental x-ray machines. I. The area of unsharpness, Oral Surg. 39:318, 1975.

Lund, T. M., and Manson-Hing, L. R.: A study of the focal troughs of three panoramic dental x-ray machines. II. Image dimensions, Oral Surg. 39:647, 1975.

Lund, T. M., and Manson-Hing, L. R.: Relations between tooth positions and focal troughs of panoramic machines, Oral Surg. 40:285, 1975.

Manson-Hing, L. R.: Use of dental x-rays in roentgenography of the palato-pharyngeal mechanism, Oral Surg. 13:1085, 1960.

Manson-Hing, L. R.: Kilovolt (peak) and the sensitivity of very fast dental films, Oral Surg. 12: 979, 1959.

Manson-Hing, L. R.: On the evaluation of radiographic techniques, Oral Surg. 27:631, 1969.

Manson-Hing, L. R.: Kilovolt peak and the visibility of lamina dura breaks, Oral Surg. 31:268, 1971.

Manson-Hing, L. R.: Advances in dental pantomography: the GE-3000, Oral Surg. 31:430, 1971.

Manson-Hing, L. R.: William D. Coolidge, Oral Surg. 36:592, 1973.

Manson-Hing, L. R.: Panoramic dental radiography, Springfield, Ill., 1976, Charles C Thomas, Publisher.

Manson-Hing, L. R., and Monnier, P. Y.: Radiographic densitometric evaluation of seven processing solutions, Oral Surg. 39: 493, 1975.

Manson-Hing, L. R., and Turgut, E.: Evaluation of film processing with concentrated solutions, Oral Surg. 36:280, 1973.

McCall, J. O., and Wald, S. S.: Clinical dental roentgenology, ed. 4, Philadelphia, 1957, W. B. Saunders Co.

McLaren, J. W., editor: Modern trends in diagnostic radiology, ed. 3, New York, 1960, Paul B. Hoeber, Inc.

McMaster, R. C.: New developments in xeroradiography, Non-destructive Testing 10:8, 1951.

Merrill, V.: Atlas of roentgenographic positions and standard radiologic procedures, vol. 2, ed. 4, St. Louis, 1975, The C. V. Mosby Co.

Mitchell, G. A. G., and Graham, J. G.: Microradiography, Med. Radiogr. Photogr. 34:1, 1958.

Mitchell, L. D., Jr.: Panoramic roentgenography, J.A.D.A. 66:777, 1963.

Morgan, R. H., and VanAllen, W. W.: The sensitometry of roentgenographic films and screens, Radiology 52:832, 1949.

Nills, T. H., and others: Xeroradiography: the present medical applications, Br. J. Radiol. 28:545, 1955.

Norgaard, F.: Temporomandibular arthrography, Copenhagen, 1947, Einar Munksgaard.

Ollerenshaw, R., and Rose, S.: Sialography— a valuable diagnostic method, Dent. Radiogr. Photogr. 29:37, 1956.

Paatero, Y. V.: A new tomographical method for radiographing curved outer surfaces, Acta radiol. 32:177, 1949.

Paatero, Y. V.: Pantomography and orthopantomography, Oral Surg. 14:947, 1961.

Pappas, G. C.: Panoramic sialography, Dent. Radiogr. Photogr. 43:27, 1970.

Parma, C.: Die Roentgendiagnostik des Kiefergelenkes, Roentgenpraxis 4:633, 1932.

Phillips, J. E.: Principles and function of the Orthopantomograph, Oral Surg. 24:41, 1967.

Preece, J. W.: Roentgen alchemy. I, Oral Surg. 28:680, 1969.

Preece, J. W.: Roentgen alchemy. II, Oral Surg. 28:830, 1969.

Rawls, H. R., and Owen, W. D.: The dental prognosis for xeroradiography, Oral Surg. 33:476, 1972.

Richards, A. G.: New concepts in dental x-ray machines, J.A.D.A. 73:69, 1966.

Roach, J. F., and Hilleboe, H. E.: Xeroradiography, Am. J. Roentgenol. 73:1, 1955.

Rosenberg, H. M.: Laminagraphy: methods and application in oral diagnosis, J.A.D.A. 74:88, 1967.

St. John, E. G., and Craig, D. R.: Logetronography, Am. J. Roentgenol. 88:124, 1957.

Salzmann, J. A., editor: Roentgenographic cephalometrics, Philadelphia, 1961, J. B. Lippincott Co.

Saulnier, V. E., and Barr, J. H.: Compact foreign-made x-ray generators: an evaluation of their acceptability for effective dental radiography. I. A review of the literature, Oral Surg. **38**:810, 1974.

Saulnier, V. E., and Barr, J. H.: Compact foreign-made dental x-ray generators: an evaluation of their acceptability for effective dental radiography. II. Image characteristics and observer performance, Oral Surg. **39**:158, 1975.

Schwarz, G. S.: Subtraction radiography by means of additive color, Radiology **87**: 445, 1966.

Silva, C. A., and Silva, I. A.: Steroscopic roentgenography in dentistry, Oral Surg. **14**:430, 1961.

Spangenberg, H. D., and Pool, M. L.: Experimental evaluation of radioactive nuclides for isotopic radiography, Oral Surg. **16**:159, 1963.

Spangenberg, H. D., and others: Scintillation spectra from dental x-ray machines operated under clinical conditions, J. Dent. Res. **37**:15, 1958.

Stewart, J. L., and Bieser, L. F.: Panoramic roentgenograms compared with conventional intraoral roentgenograms, Oral Surg. **26**:39, 1968.

Tasker, H. S.: Speed and contrast in radiography, Photographic J. **90B**:9, 1950.

Tucker, A. K.: Subtraction in radiology, Radiography **33**:125, 1967.

Turk, M. H., and Katzenell, J.: Panoramic localization, Oral Surg. **29**:212, 1970.

Updegrave, W. J.: Temporomandibular articulation, Dent. Radiogr. Photogr. **26**:41, 1953.

Updegrave, W. J.: Panoramic dental radiography, Dent. Radiogr. Photogr. **36**:75, 1963.

Updegrave, W. J.: The role of panoramic radiography in diagnosis, Oral Surg. **22**:49, 1966.

USPHS Dept. of H.E.W.: Dental X-ray teaching and training replica, pub. no. MORP 68-8, Washington, D.C., 1968, U.S. Government Printing Office.

USPHS Dept. of H.E.W.: Fast film exposure and processing in dental radiography, Washington, D.C., 1970, U.S. Government Printing Office.

Van Aken, J.: Panoramic X-ray equipment, J.A.D.A. **86**:1050, 1973.

Van de Poel, A. C., and others: A comparative study of long-cone and short-cone bitewing radiographs, Oral Surg. **36**:273, 1973.

Waggener, D. T.: Roentgenographic localization of unerupted teeth, Oral Surg. **13**:439, 1960.

Webb, J. H.: The latent image, Physics Today **3**:8, 1950.

Webber, R. L., Benton, P. A., and Ryge, G.: Diagnostic variations in radiographs, Oral Surg. **26**:800, 1968.

Webber, R. L., and Stark, L.: Fitting an image to the eye: a concepted basis for preprocessing radiographs, Oral Surg. **31**: 831, 1971.

Welborn, J. F.: A prosthetic grid for locating foreign bodies and small bone lesions in edentulous jaws, J.A.D.A. **72**:906, 1966.

Williams, S. W.: Occlusal radiography, Dent. Radiogr. Photogr. **27**:50, 1954.

Wilson, J.: Radiography of facial bone injury, Radiography **30**:171, 1959.

Wolfe, J. N.: Xeroradiography of the breast, Radiology **91**:231, 1968.

Wolfe, J. N.: Xeroradiography of bones, joints and soft tissues, Radiology **93**:583, 1969.

Woodcock, R. C., and Properzio, W. S.: Evaluation of a Westinghouse Panoramix x-ray machine, Oral Surg. **32**:650, 1971.

Wuehrmann, A. H.: The long cone technic, P.D.M., pp. 1-30, July 1957.

Wuehrmann, A. H.: Evaluation criteria for intraoral radiographic film quality, J.A.D.A. **89**:345, 1974.

Wuehrmann, A. H., and Curby, W. A.: Radiopacity of oral structures as a basis for selecting optimum kilovoltage for intraoral roentgenograms, J. Dent. Res. **31**:27, 1952.

Yale, S. H., editor: Symposium on oral roentgenology, Dent. Clin. North Am., July 1961.

Zimmer, E. A.: Die Roentgenologie des Kiefergelenkes, Z. Zahnheilk. **12**:51, 1941.

X-RAY HAZARDS AND PROTECTION
Chapter 4

American Dental Association: Radiation hygiene and practice in dentistry. I to V, J.A.D.A. **74**:1032, 1967; **75**:1197, 1967; **76**:115, 363, 602, 1968.

American Dental Association: Radiation hygiene and practice in dentistry: state regulation of dental x-rays, J.A.D.A. **76**:107, 1968.

American Dental Association and Alcox, R. W.: Diagnostic radiation exposures and doses in dentistry, J.A.D.A. **76**:1066, 1968.

Atomic radiation—theory, biological hazards, safety measures, and treatment of injury, Camden, N.J., 1957, R.C.A. Service Co.

Bjärngard, B., and others: Radiation doses in oral radiography, Odontol. Rev. (Malmo) **10**:355, 1959.

Brues, A. M.: Low-level irradiation, pub. 59, Washington, D.C., 1959, American Association for the Advancement of Science.

Budowsky, J., and others: Radiation exposure to the head and abdomen during oral roentgenography, J.A.D.A. **53**:555, 1956.

Bushong, S. C., and others: Panoramic dental radiography for mass screening? Health Phys. **25**:489, 1973.

Chadwick, D. R.: The public health role in controlling radiation, Am. J. Public Health **55**:731, 1965.

Clark, D. E.: Association of irradiation with cancer of the thyroid in children and adolescents, J.A.M.A. **159**:1007, 1955.

Court-Brown, W. M.: Expectation of life and mortality from cancer among British radiologists, Br. Med. J. **2**:181, 1958.

Cronkite, E. P., and Bond, V. P.: Radiation injury in man, Springfield, Ill., 1960, Charles C Thomas, Publisher.

Duffy, B. J., Jr., and Fitzgerald, P. J.: Cancer of the thyroid in children: a report on 28 cases, J. Clin. Endocrinol. **10**:1296, 1950.

Ellinger, F.: Medical radiation biology, Springfield, Ill., 1957, Charles C Thomas, Publisher.

English, J. A.: Radiation biology pertinent to dentistry, J.A.D.A. **70**:1442, 1965.

Federal Radiation Council: Background material for the development of radiation protection standards, Report no. 1, Washington, D.C., 1960, F.R.C. Publications.

Frank, M.: A scheme for teaching radiation protection, Radiography **33**:86, 1967.

Frey, N. W., and Wuehrmann, A. H.: Radiation dosimetry and intraoral radiographic techniques. I. X-ray beam patterns within the head, Oral Surg. **38**:151, 1974.

Frey, N. W., and Wuehrmann, A. H., Radiation dosimetry and intraoral radiographic techniques. II. Internal and external dose measurements, Oral Surg. **38**:639, 1974.

Gentry, J. T., Parkhurst, E., and Bulin, G. V.: An epidemiological study of congenital malformations in New York State, Am. J. Public Health **49**:1, 1959.

Glass, R. L.: Mortality of New England dentists 1921-1960, Environmental Health Series, pub. no. 999-RH-18, Washington, D.C., 1966, U.S. Department of Health, Education and Welfare, Public Health Service.

Goepp, R., and others: The reduction of unnecessary x-ray exposure during intraoral examinations, Oral Surg. **16**:39, 1963.

Greer, D. F.: Determination and analysis of absorbed doses resulting from various intraoral radiographic techniques, Oral Surg. **34**:146, 1972.

Haagensen, C. D.: Occupational neoplastic disease, Am. J. Cancer **15**:641, 1931.

Hearings before the Subcommittee on Research and Development of the Joint Committee on Atomic Energy, Congress of the United States, June 4-8, 1956, May 27-29 and June 3, 1957, June 4-7, 1957, U.S. Government Printing Office, Washington, D.C.

Hodge, P. C.: A radiologist looks at radiation hazards, Radiology **72**:481, 1959.

Jerman, A. C., and others: Absorbed radiation from panoramic plus bitewing exposures vs. full-mouth periapical plus bitewing exposures, J.A.D.A. **86**:420, 1973.

Jung, T.: Gonadal doses resulting from panoramic x-ray examinations of the teeth, Oral Surg. **19**:745, 1965.

Kuba, R. K., and Beck, J. O.: Radiation dosimetry in Panorex roentgenography. I. Use of phantoms in dental research, Oral Surg. **25**:380, 1968.

Kuba, R. K., and Beck, J. O.: Radiation dosimetry in Panorex roentgenography. II. Patterns of radiation distribution, Oral Surg. **25**:386, 1968.

Kuba, R. K., and Beck, J. O.: Radiation dosimetry in Panorex roentgenography. III. Radiation dose measurements, Oral Surg. **25**:393, 1968.

Lea, D. E.: Actions of radiations on living cells, ed. 2, New York, 1956, Macmillan, Inc.

Lee, W., Comparative radiation doses in dental radiography, Oral Surg. **37**:962, 1974.

Lilienfeld, A. M.: Diagnostic and therapeutic x-radiation in an urban population, Public Health Rep. **74**:29, 1959.

Manson-Hing, L. R.: The fundamental biologic effects of x-rays in dentistry, Oral Surg. 12:562, 1959.

Medical Research Council (Great Britain): The hazards to man of nuclear and allied radiations, London, 1956, Her Majesty's Stationery Office.

Menezer, L. F.: The open-ended metal column for the dental x-ray machine, J.A.D.A. 73:1083, 1966.

Merriam, G. R., and Focht, E. F.: A clinical study of radiation cataracts and relationship to dose, Am. J. Roentgenol. 77:759, 1957.

Meyer, I.: Osteoradionecrosis of the jaws, P.D.M., pp. 5-51, November 1958.

Muller, H. J.: Potential hazards of radiation, Excerpta Med. (Amsterdam) 2:223, 1957.

National Academy of Sciences: The biological effect of atomic radiation: a report to the public, Washington, D.C., 1960, National Research Council.

National Academy of Sciences: The effects on populations of exposure to low levels of ionizing radiation, Washington, D.C., 1972, National Research Council.

National Bureau of Standards Handbook 51: Radiological monitoring methods and instruments, Washington, D.C., 1952, U.S. Government Printing Office.

National Bureau of Standards Handbook 57: Photographic dosimetry of x- and gamma rays, Washington, D.C., 1954, U.S. Government Printing Office.

National Bureau of Standards Handbook 59: Permissible dose from external sources of ionizing radiation, Washington, D.C., 1954, U.S. Government Printing Office.

National Bureau of Standards Addendum to Handbook 59: Maximum permissible radiation exposures to man, Washington, D.C., 1957, U.S. Government Printing Office.

National Bureau of Standards Handbook 76: Medical x-ray protection up to three million volts, Washington, D.C., 1961, U.S. Government Printing Office.

National Bureau of Standards Handbook 85: Physical aspects of irradiation (ICRU report of 1962), Washington, D.C., 1964, U.S. Department of Commerce.

National Council on Radiation Protection and Measurements: Dental x-ray protection, NCRP report no. 35, Washington, D.C., 1970, NCRP Publications.

National Council on Radiation Protection and Measurements: Basic radiation protection criteria, NCRP report no. 39, Washington, D.C., 1971, NCRP Publications.

National Council on Radiation Protection and Measurements: Review of the current state of radiation protection philosophy, NCRP report no. 43, Washington, D.C., 1975, NCRP Publications.

Nelson, R. C., and Rupp, T. D.: Phantom depth dose distributions from Panorex dental x-rays, Oral Surg. 32:982, 1971.

Powell, C. C.: The government looks at radiation hazards, Radiology 72:489, 1959.

Report of the Radiation Protection Committee, American Academy of Oral Roentgenology: The effective use of x-radiation in dentistry, Oral Surg. 16:294, 1963.

Report of the United Nations Scientific Committee on the Effects of Atomic Radiation, United Nations Official Records, 13th session, suppl. 17, New York, 1958.

The responsibilities of the medical profession in the use of x-rays and other ionizing radiations, statement by the United Nations Scientific Committee on the Effects of Atomic Radiation, 1957.

Richards, A. G.: Roentgen-ray doses in dental roentgenography, J.A.D.A. 56:351, 1958.

Richards, A. G.: New method for reduction of gonadal irradiation of dental patients, J.A.D.A. 65:15, 1962.

Richards, A. G.: Sources of x-radiation in the dental office, Dent. Radiogr. Photogr. 37:51, 1964.

Richards, A. G.: Radiation barriers, Oral Surg. 25:701, 1968.

Richards, A. G., and Webber, R. L.: Dental x-ray exposure of sites within the head and neck, Oral Surg. 18:752, 1964.

Richards, A. G., and others: X-ray protection in the dental office, J.A.D.A. 56:514, 1958.

Rooney, D. R., and Powell, R. W.: Carcinoma of the thyroid in children after x-ray therapy in early childhood, J.A.M.A. 169:1, 1959.

Scholl, W. J.: A geneticist looks at radiation hazards, Radiology 72:522, 1959.

Seltser, R., and Sartwell, P. E.: Ionizing radiation and longevity of physicians, J.A.M.A. 166:585, 1958.

Somatic radiation dose for the general population: The report of the Ad Hoc Committee on Radiation Protection and Measurements, Science 131:3399, 1960.

Stanford, R. W., and Vance, J.: The quantity of radiation received by the reproductive organs of patients during routine diagnostic x-ray examinations, Br. J. Radiol. **28**:266, 1955.

Thomas, S. F.: Radiation hazards—facts or fancy, Radiology **72**:587, 1959.

Trout, E. D., and others: Conventional building materials as protective barriers in dental roentgenographic installations, Oral Surg. **15**:1211, 1962.

USPHS Dept. of H.E.W.: Population exposure to x-rays U.S.A., 1964, pub. no. 1519, Washington, D.C., 1964, U.S. Government Printing Office.

USPHS Dept. of H.E.W.: Mortality of New England dentists 1921-1960, pub. no. 999-RH-18, Washington, D.C., 1966, U.S. Government Printing Office.

USPHS Dept. of H.E.W.: Guidelines to radiological health, pub. no. 999-RH-33, Washington, D.C., 1968, U.S. Government Printing Office.

USHPS Dept. of H.E.W.: Dental Surpak summary report, pub. no. MORP 68-11, Washington, D.C., 1968, rev. 1969, U.S. Government Printing Office.

USPHS Dept. of H.E.W.: Population dose from x-rays U.S. 1964, pub. no. 2001, Washington, D.C., 1969, U.S. Government Printing Office.

USPHS Dept. of H.E.W.: Regulations, standards, and guides pertaining to medical and dental radiation protection—an annotated bibliography, pub. no. 999-RH-37, Washington, D.C., 1969, U.S. Government Printing Office.

USPHS Dept. of H.E.W.: Regulations for the administration and enforcement of the Radiation Control for Health and Safety Act of 1968, pub. no. BRH/OBD 71-1, Washington, D.C., 1971, U.S. Government Printing Office.

USPHS Dept. of H.E.W.: State radiation control legislation 1970, pub. no. BRH/ORO 71-1, Washington, D.C., 1971, U.S. Government Printing Office.

Van Aken, J., and Van der Linden, L.: The integral absorbed dose in conventional and panoramic complete-mouth examinations, Oral Surg. **22**:603, 1966.

Wallace, B., and Dobzhansky, T.: Radiation, genes, and man, New York, 1959, Henry Holt & Co., Inc.

Warren, S.: Longevity and causes of death from irradiation in physicians, J.A.M.A. **162**:464, 1956.

Webster, E. W.: Hazards of diagnostic radiology: a physicist's point of view, Radiology **72**:793, 1959.

Weissman, D. D., and Feinstein, R. B.: X-ray beam profiles and oral radiography, Oral Surg. **31**:546, 1971.

Weissman, D. D., and Longhurst, G. E.: Comparative absorbed doses in periapical radiography. II. Panorex, Oral Surg. **33**:661, 1972.

Weissman, D. D., and Sobkowski, F. J.: Comparative thermoluminescent dosimetry of intraoral periapical radiography, Oral Surg. **29**:376, 1970.

Wuehrmann, A. H.: Radiation protection and dentistry, St. Louis, 1960, The C. V. Mosby Co.

Wuehrmann, A. H.: Procedure for lining open-end dental x-ray cylinders with lead foil, Oral Surg. **30**:64, 1970.

Yale, S. H., and Goodman, L. S.: Reduction of radiation output of the standard dental x-ray machine utilizing copper for external filtration, J.A.D.A. **54**:354, 1957.

Young, H. H., and Kunkel, M. G.: Diagnosis, treatment and prognosis of roentgen ray injuries to dentists, J.A.D.A. **51**:1, 1955.

RADIOGRAPHIC VISUALIZATION OF NORMAL STRUCTURES
Chapters 13-14

Barber, T. K.: Roentgenographic evaluation of growth and development, J.A.D.A. **67**:329, 1963.

Benkow, H. H.: Interpretive pitfalls in radiodontics, Dent. Radiogr. Photogr. **34**:86, 1961.

Benkow, H. H.: Roentgenological and morphological findings of the mandibular symphysis, Norske Tannlaegeforen. Tid. **71**:13, 1961.

Björk, A.: Facial growth in man, studied with the aid of metallic implants, Acta Odontol. Scand. **13**:9, 1955.

Blackman, S.: Anatomic structures as visualized on the Panoramix, Oral Surg. **26**:321, 1968.

Boyne, P. J., and others: Neutron radiographic examination of soft- and hard-tissue structures of the oral cavity, Oral Surg. **37**:124, 1974.

Brandt, H. F.: The psychology of seeing, New York, 1945, The Philosophical Library.

Brynolf, I.: Improved viewing facilities for better roentgenodiagnosis, Oral Surg. **32**:808, 1971.

Bugyi, B., and Pinter, I.: Neuroradiologie der Schadelnahte, Acta Radiol. [Diagn.] (Stockholm) (n.s.)1:96, 1963.

Chomenko, A. G., and Caulfield, J. J.: Projected artifacts viewed on soft-tissue dental radiographs, Oral Surg. 34:838, 1972.

Christen, A. G., and Segreto, V. A.: Distortion and artifacts encountered in Panorex radiography, J.A.M.A. 77:1096, 1968.

Cohen, M. M.: Pediatric dentistry, ed. 2, St. Louis, 1961, The C. V. Mosby Co.

Degering, C. I., and Buseman, R. H.: A roentgenographic film density study of dental restorative materials, Oral Surg. 15:944, 1962.

Downs, W. B.: Variations in facial relationships: their significance in treatment and prognosis, Am. J. Orthod. 34:812, 1948.

Duke-Elder, W. S.: Textbook of ophthalmology, vol. 1, St. Louis, 1932, The C. V. Mosby Co.

Edge, M. B., and others: Interpretation of the orthopantomogram: complications due to radiographic artifacts, Br. Dent. J. 133: 289, 1972.

Enlow, D. H., and Harris, D. B.: A study of the postnatal growth of the human mandible, Am. J. Orthod. 50:25, 1964.

Etter, L. E.: Atlas of roentgen anatomy of the skull, Springfield, Ill., 1955, Charles C Thomas, Publisher.

Goldman, H. M., and others: Origin of registration of the architectural pattern, the lamina dura, and the alveolar crest in the dental radiograph, Oral Surg. 10:749, 1957.

Gron, A.: Prediction of tooth emergence, J. Dent. Res. 41:573, 1962.

Helmholtz, H. von: Handbuch der physiologischen Optick, ed. 2, Hamburg, 1896, I Voss.

Ingle, D. J.: Principles of research in biology and medicine, Philadelphia, 1958, J. B. Lippincott Co.

Kraus, B. S.: Calcification of human decidious teeth, J.A.D.A. 59:1128, 1959.

LeGrand, Y.: Light, colour, and vision, New York, 1957, John Wiley & Sons, Inc.

Lindblom, G.: Anatomy and function of the temporomandibular joint, Acta Odontol. Scand. 17(suppl. 28):7, 1960.

Manson-Hing, L. R.: Vision and oral roentgenology, Oral Surg. 15:173, 1962.

McCormack, F. W.: A plea for standardized technique for oral radiography, with an illustrated classification of findings and their verified interpretation, J. Dent. Res. 2:467, 1920.

Meschan, I.: An atlas of normal radiographic anatomy, ed. 2, Philadelphia, 1959, W. B. Saunders Co.

Moorrees, C. F., and others: Age variation of formation stages of ten permanent teeth, J. Dent. Res. 42:1490, 1963.

Mourshed, F.: A study of intraoral radiographic errors made by dental students, Oral Surg. 32:812, 1971.

Newell, R. R., and Garneau, R.: The threshold visibility of pulmonary shadows, Radiology 56:409, 1951.

Ohba, T., and Katayama, H.: Comparison of orthopantomography with conventional periapical dental radiography, Oral Surg. 34:542, 1972.

Ohba, T., and Katayama, H.: Panoramic roentgen anatomy of the maxillary sinus, Oral Surg. 39:658, 1975.

Parfitt, G. J.: An investigation of the normal variations in alveolar bone trabeculation, Oral Surg. 15:1453, 1962.

Pineda, F., and Kuttler, Y.: Mesiodistal and buccolingual roentgenographic investigation of 7,275 root canals, Oral Surg. 33:101, 1972.

Reid, J. A.: The "visibility" of x-rays, Oral Surg. 34:330, 1972.

Renshaw, S.: Psychological optics, vols. 1 to 3, Duncan, Okla., 1964, Optometric Extension Program.

Ricketts, R. M.: A foundation for cephalometric communication, Am. J. Orthod. 46: 330, 1960.

Riebel, F. A.: Use of the eyes in x-ray diagnosis, Radiology 70:252, 1958.

Riedel, R. A.: Relation of maxillary structures to cranium in malocclusion and in normal occlusion, Angle Orthod. 22:142, 1952.

Ripa, L. W., and others: The effect of calcium hydroxide and zinc oxide eugenol on dentine in extracted human teeth, Oral Surg. 34:531, 1972.

Shumaker, D. B., and El Hadary, M. S.: Roentgenographic study of eruption, J.A.D.A. 61:535, 1960.

Sicher, H., and DuBrul, E. L.: Oral anatomy, ed. 6, St. Louis, 1975, The C. V. Mosby Co.

Smith, C. J., and Fleming, R. D.: A comprehensive review of normal anatomic landmarks and artifacts as visualized on Panorex radiographs, Oral Surg. 37:391, 1974.

Stafford, G. D., and MacCulloch, W. T.: Radiopaque denture base materials, Br. Dent. J. **131**:22, 1971.

Stafne, E. C., and Hollinshead, W. H.: Roentgenographic observation of the stylohyoid chain, Oral Surg. **15**:1195, 1962.

Steel, G. H.: The relation between dental maturation and physiological maturity, Dent. Pract. **66**:23, 1965.

Storer, R.: A radiographic survey of edentulous mouths, Br. Dent. J. **103**:344, 1957.

Thoma, K.: Principal factors controlling the development of the mandible and maxilla, Am. J. Orthod. **24**:171, 1938.

Updegrave, W. J.: Roentgenographic observations of functioning temporomandibular joints, J.A.D.A. **54**:488, 1957.

Updegrave, W. J.: Normal radiodontic anatomy, Dent. Radiogr. Photogr. **31**:57, 1958.

Van der Linden, L. W., and Van Aken, J.: The origin of localized increased radiopacity in the dentin, Oral Surg. **35**:862, 1973.

Waggener, D. T.: Relationships of third molar roots to the mandibular canal, Oral Surg. **12**:853, 1959.

Walls, G. L.: The filling-in process, Am. J. Optom. **31**:329, 1954.

Weston, H. C.: The relation between illumination and visual performance, London, 1953, Her Majesty's Stationery Office.

Wylie, W. L.: Factors modifying head form in man, Am. J. Orthod. **24**:171, 1938.

Yale, S., and others: An epidemiological assessment of mandibular condyle morphology, Oral Surg. **21**:169, 1966.

RADIOGRAPHIC INTERPRETATION
Chapters 15-18

Bender, I. B.: Roentgenographic significance of the lamina dura in systemic disease, J. Albert Einstein Med. Center **9**:82, 1961.

Berkman, M. D.: Pedodontic radiographic interpretation, Dent. Radiogr. Photogr. **44**:27, 1971.

Bhaskar, S. N.: Periapical lesions—types, incidence and clinical features, Oral Surg. **21**:657, 1966.

Bhaskar, S. N.: Synopsis of oral pathology, ed. 4, St. Louis, 1973, The C. V. Mosby Co.

Bhaskar, S. N.: Roentgenographic interpretation for the dentist, ed. 2, St. Louis, 1975, The C. V. Mosby Co.

Björk, L.: Velopharyngeal function in connected speech, Acta Radiol. [Suppl.] (Stockh.) 202, p. 1, 1961.

Björn, H., and Holmberg, K.: Radiographic determination of periodontal bone destruction in epidemiological research, Odontol. Rev. (Malmo) **17**:232, 1966.

Blackman, S.: Tooth concussion, Dent. Pract. **7**:366, 1957.

Blaney, J. R., and Greco, J. F.: Recognition of early proximal caries, Dent. Radiogr. Photogr. **26**:33, 1953.

Bloom, D.: Mucoceles of the maxillary and sphenoid sinuses, Radiology **85**:1103, 1965.

Boyne, P. J.: Incidence of osteosclerotic areas in the mandible and maxilla, J. Oral Surg. **18**:486, 1960.

Buchholz, R. E.: Radiographic interpretation of proximal carious lesions, Dent. Radiogr. Photogr. **38**:9, 1965.

Cheraskin, E.: Roentgenographic manifestations of osseous changes in the jaws, Oral Surg. **12**:442, 1959.

Cheraskin, E., and Langley, L. L.: Dynamics of oral diagnosis, Chicago, 1956, Year Book Publishers, Inc.

Christen, A. G., and others: Oral health of dentists: analysis of panoramic radiographic survey, J.A.D.A. **75**:1167, 1967.

Clark, J. L., and others: The roentgenographically abnormal temporomandibular joint, Oral Surg. **33**:836, 1972.

Cook, T. J., and Pollock, J.: Sialography: pathologic-radiologic correlation, Oral Surg. **21**:599, 1966.

Curtis, A. B.: Childhood leukemias: osseous changes in the jaws on panoramic radiographs, J.A.D.A. **83**:844, 1971.

DePaola, P., and Alman, J.: Assessment of the reliability of radiographic diagnosis in a clinical caries trial, J. Dent. Res. **51**:1431, 1972.

Duinkerke, A. S., and others: Variations in the interpretation of periapical radiolucencies, Oral Surg. **40**:414, 1975.

Dummett, C. O.: Review of the clinical and roentgenologic manifestations of incipient periodontal disease, Ann. Dent. **4**:47, 1945.

Dunning, J. M., and Ferguson, G. W.: Effect of bite-wing roentgenograms on navy dental examination findings, U.S. Naval Med. Bull. **46**:83, 1946.

Einstein, R. A.: Sialography in the differential diagnosis of parotid masses, Surg. Gynecol. Obstet. **122**:1079, 1966.

Ennis, L. M., Berry, H. M., and Phillips, J. E.: Dental roentgenology, ed. 6, Philadelphia, 1967, Lea & Febiger.

Eselman, J. C.: A roentgenographic investigation of enostosis, Oral Surg. **14**:1331, 1961.

Finley, W., and Finley, S.: Genetic disorders. In Daniel, W. A., Jr., editor: The adolescent patient, St. Louis, 1970, The C. V. Mosby Co.

Finn, S. B.: Clinical pedodontics, ed. 3, Philadelphia, 1967, W. B. Saunders Co.

Galagan, D. J., and Vermillion, J.: Diagnosis of caries by radiographic interpretation, J. Dent. Res. **35**:33, 1956.

Galeone, R. J., and others: Odontodysplasia, Oral Surg. **29**:879, 1970.

Garber, F. N.: Roentgenolucent periapical areas, Oral Surg. **17**:460, 1964.

Goncalves, N., and others: Radiographic evaluation of defects created in mandibular condyles, Oral Surg. **38**:474, 1974.

Gorlin, R. J., and Goldman, H. M.: Thoma's oral pathology, ed. 6, St. Louis, 1970, The C. V. Mosby Co.

Gorlin, R. J., and Pindborg, J. J.: Syndromes of the head and neck, New York, 1964, McGraw Hill Book Co.

Greenfield, G. B., and others: The hand as an indicator of generalized disease, Am. J. Roentgenol. **99**:736, 1967.

Hilbish, T. F., and Bartter, F. C.: Roentgen findings in abnormal deposition of calcium in tissues, Am. J. Roentgenol. **87**:1129, 1962.

Hollender, L., and others: A roentgenographic study of clinically healthy and inflamed periodontal tissues in children, J. Periodont. Res. **1**:146, 1966.

Hutchinson, A. C. W.: Dental and oral x-ray diagnosis, Edinburgh, 1954, E. & S. Livingstone, Ltd.

Jacobson, F. L.: editor: Oral diagnosis and treatment planning, Dent. Clin. North Am. pp. 1-2, March 1963.

Jones, E. H.: Roentgenology in endodontics, Aust. Dent. J. **11**:305, 1966.

Kamen, A., and Schmee, J.: Diagnostic errors and multiple examiners in anticariogenic studies, J. Dent. Res. **53**:1500, 1974.

Keats, T. E.: Cysticercosis: a demonstration of its roentgen manifestations, Mo. Med. **58**:457, 1961.

Klatsky, M.: The incidence of six anomalies of the teeth and jaws, Human Biol. **28**:420, 1956.

Koepp-Baker, H.: Pathomorphology of cleft palate and cleft lip. In Travis, L. E., editor: Handbook of speech pathology, New York, 1957, Appleton-Century-Crofts, Inc.

Laband, P. F., and Leacock, A. G.: Sclerosing osteitis of the jaws, J. Oral Surg. **25**:23, 1967.

Lee, J. L., and Bordenca, C. M.: Self-induced air emphysema of the face and neck, Oral Surg. **36**:603, 1973.

Levy, D. M., and others: Salivary gland calculi, J.A.M.A. **181**:99, 1962.

Lindahl, B.: Transverse intra-alveolar root fractures, Odontol. Rev. (Malmo) **9**:10, 1958.

Lindenberg, W. B., and others: A clinical roentgenographic and histopathologic evaluation of periapical lesions, Oral Surg. **17**:467, 1964.

Lovett, D. W.: Nutrient canals—a roentgenographic study, J.A.D.A. **37**:671, 1948.

Lyon, H. E.: Reliability of panoramic radiography in the diagnosis of maxillary sinus pathosis, Oral Surg. **35**:124, 1973.

McCall, J. O., and Wald, S. S.: Clinical dental roentgenology, ed. 4, Philadelphia, 1957, W. B. Saunders Co.

McGuire, W. B., and Carpenter, C. W.: Multiple fractures of the facial bones, Dent. Radiogr. Photogr. **24**:50, 1951.

Meena, H. E.: Cortical bone atrophy and osteoporosis as a manifestation of aging, Am. J. Roentgenol. **89**:1287, 1963.

Mena, C. A.: Taurodontism, Oral Surg. **32**:812-823, 1971.

Mourshed, F., and Tuckson, C. R.: A study of the radiographic features of the jaws in sickle-cell anemia, Oral Surg. **37**:812, 1974.

Nohrström, P. K., and Anderson, B. D.: A functional cephalometric radiographic investigation of the nasal and oral pharyngeal structures during deglutition in operated cleft palate and noncleft palate persons, Oral Surg. **12**:142, 1959.

Nordin, B. E. C., and Smith, D. A.: Diagnostic procedures in disorders of calcium metabolism, Boston, 1965, Little, Brown & Co.

Ohba, T., and others: Mandibular metastasis of osteogenic sarcoma, Oral Surg. **39**:821, 1975.

Olech, E.: Fracture lines in the mandible, Dent. Radiogr. Photogr. **28**:21, 1955.

Palubinskas, A. J., and Davis, H.: Roentgen features of nasal accessory sinus mucoceles, Radiology **72**:576, 1959.

Patel, J. R., and Wuehrmann, A. H.: A radiographic study of nutrient canals, Oral Surg. **42:**693, 1976.

Pendergrass, E. P., Schaeffer, J. P., and Hodes, P. J.: The head and neck in roentgen diagnosis, ed. 2, Springfield, Ill., 1956, Charles C Thomas, Publisher.

Philip, T.: Some congenital cysts and fistulae of the neck, J. Fac. Radiologists **10:**186, 1959.

Phillips, J. D., and Shawkat, A. H.: A study of the radiographic appearance of osseous defects on panoramic and conventional films, Oral Surg. **36:**745, 1973.

Pinto, R. S., and others: Radiologic features of benign pleomorphic adenoma of the hard palate, Oral Surg. **39:**976, 1975.

Poyton, H. G., and Arora, B. K.: Radiologic evidence of surgical emphysema, Oral Surg. **35:**129, 1973.

Poyton, H. G., Morgan, G. A., and Levine, N.: Median incisor fusion, Oral Surg. **28:** 76, 1969.

Poyton, H. G., and others: Cirsoid aneurysm secondary to an arteriovenous fistula of the facial artery and vein, Oral Surg. **37:**474, 1974.

Prichard, J.: The role of the roentgenogram in the diagnosis and prognosis of periodontal disease, Oral Surg. **14:**182, 1961.

Priebe, W. A., and others: The value of the roentgenographic film in the differential diagnosis of periapical lesions, Oral Surg. **7:**979, 1954.

Prowler, J. R., and Smith, E. W.: Dental bone changes occurring in sickle cell diseases and abnormal hemoglobin traits, Radiology **65:**763, 1955.

Ritchey, B., and Orban, B.: Crests of the interdental alveolar septa, Dent. Radiogr. Photogr. **27:**37, 1954.

Rodahl, K., Nicholson, J. T., and Brown, D. M.: Bone as a tissue, New York, 1960, McGraw-Hill Book Co.

Rose, J. S.: A survey of congenitally missing teeth excluding third molars in 6,000 orthodontic patients, Dent. Pract. **17:**107, 1966.

Rubenfeld, S., and others: Distant metastases from head and neck cancer, Am. J. Roentgenol. **87:**441, 1962.

Rushton, M. A.: Odontodysplasia: "ghost teeth," Br. Dent. J. **119:**109, 1965.

Sabes, W. R., and Bartholdi, W. L.: Congenital partial anodontia of permanent dentition, J. Dent. Child. **29:**211, 1962.

Scandrett, F. R., and others: Radiographic examination of the edentulous patient, Oral Surg. **35:**266, 1973.

Schramek, J. M., and Rappaport, I.: Panoramic x-ray screening for early detection of maxillary sinus malignancy, Arch. Otolaryngol. **90:**347, 1969.

Schramek, J. M., and others: Panoramic radiography in head and neck pathology, Laryngoscope **80:**1797, 1970.

Schwartz, E.: The skull in skeletal dysplasias, Am. J. Roentgenol. **89:**928, 1963.

Schwartz, L.: Disorders of the temporomandibular joint, Philadelphia, 1959, W. B. Saunders Co.

Shafer, W. G., Hine, M. K., and Levy, B. M.: A textbook of oral pathology. ed. 2, Philadelphia, 1963, W. B. Saunders Co.

Shapiro, R.: Metabolic bone disease, Clin. Radiol. **13:**238, 1962.

Sherman, R. S., and Chu, F. C. H.: Carcinomatous invasion of the jaw bones roentgenographically considered, Radiology **65:** 581, 1955.

Shira, R. B.: Roentgenographic interpretation as an aid in oral surgical procedures, J.A.D.A. **65:**449, 1962.

Shore, N. A.: Occlusal equilibration and temporomandibular joint dysfunction, Philadelphia, 1959, J. B. Lippincott Co.

Sibley, C. S., and Zimmerman, E. R.: Odontogenic dysplasia, Oral Surg. **15:**1370, 1962.

Singala, J., and others: Dental involvement in histiocytosis, Oral Surg. **33:**42, 1972.

Spence, A. W.: The diagnostic value of radiology in endocrine disorders, Br. J. Radiol. **21:**341, 1958.

Stafne, E. C.: Oral roentgenogrophic diagnosis, Philadelphia, 1958, W. B. Saunders Co.

Stovin, J. J., and others: Mandibulofacial dysostosis, Radiology **74:**225, 1960.

Suher, T., and others: Localized arrested tooth development, Oral Surg. **6:**1305, 1953.

Sweet, A. P.: Interpretation of lower third molar radiographs, Dent. Radiogr. Photogr. **26:**65, 1953.

Symposium: A medico-dental problem: the temporomandibular joint, Ann. Dent. **15:**89, 1956.

Symposium on bone cysts, Oral Surg. **8:**903, 1955.

Talim, S. T., and others: A roentgenographic evaluation of reimplanted teeth, Oral Surg. **21:**602, 1966.

Thoma, K. H., editor: Cherubism and other intraosseous giant-cell lesions, Oral Surg. **15:** suppl. 2, 1962.

Thoma, K. H., and Robinson, H. B. G.: Oral and dental diagnosis, Philadelphia, 1960, W. B. Saunders Co.

Thomas, J. G.: A study of dens in dente, Oral Surg. **38:**653, 1974.

Tiecke, R. W.: Oral pathology, New York, 1965, McGraw-Hill Book Co.

Tillman, H. H.: Paget's disease of bone, Oral Surg. **15:**1225, 1962.

Uotila, E.: Roentgenologic visualization of the stylohyoid/ligament in patients with rheumatoid arthritis, Odontol. T. **73:**250, 1965.

Weinman, J. P., and Sicher, H.: Bone and bones: fundamentals of bone biology, ed. 2, St. Louis, 1965, The C. V. Mosby Co.

West, R. K.: Differential diagnosis of abnormal dental radiopacities, J.A.D.A. **54:** 271, 1956.

Winter, G. B.: Abscess formation in connection with deciduous molars, Arch. Oral Biol. **7:**373, 1962.

Wintrobe, M. M.: Clinical hematology, ed. 5, Philadelphia, 1961, Lea & Febiger.

Witkop, C. J., Jr., editor: Genetics and dental health, New York, 1962, McGraw-Hill Book Co.

Witkop, C. J.: Manifestations of genetic diseases in the human pulp, Oral Surg. **32:** 278, 1971.

Worth, H. M.: Principles and practice of oral radiologic interpretation, Chicago, 1963, Year Book Medical Publishers, Inc.

Wuehrmann, A. H.: Roentgenographic interpretation of dental caries, P.D.M. pp. 3-46, September 1959.

Zawadski, H.: Maxillary sinus diseases and treatment, New York, 1969, Vantage Press.

Zegarelli, E. V., and Kutscher, A. H.: Fibrous dysplasia of the jaws, Dent. Radiogr. Photogr. **36:**27, 1963.

Zegarelli, E. V., and others: Odontodysplasia, Oral Surg. **16:**187, 1963.

Index